Clinical Aspects of Peroxisome Proliferator-Activated Receptors

Clinical Aspects of Peroxisome Proliferator-Activated Receptors

Edited by Olivia Pitts

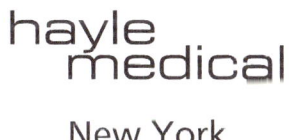

hayle
medical

New York

Hayle Medical,
750 Third Avenue, 9th Floor,
New York, NY 10017, USA

Visit us on the World Wide Web at:
www.haylemedical.com

ISBN: 978-1-63241-863-0

Cataloging-in-Publication Data

Clinical aspects of peroxisome proliferator-activated receptors / edited by Olivia Pitts.
    p. cm.
Includes bibliographical references and index.
ISBN 978-1-63241-863-0
1. Peroxisomes--Receptors. 2. Peroxisomes. 3. Microbodies. I. Pitts, Olivia.
QH603.P47 C55 2020
571.655--dc23

Table of Contents

Preface

Nuclear receptor proteins which function as transcription factors that regulate gene expression are called peroxisome proliferator-activated receptors (PPARs). These have crucial roles in the regulation of cellular metabolism, differentiation and development, as well as in tumorigenesis. There are three types of PPARs that have been identified so far- alpha (α), beta/delta (β/δ) and gamma (γ). There can be disorders of PPARs, which generally lead to a loss in function, insulin resistance, concomitant lipodystrophy and/or acanthosis nigricans. This book provides comprehensive insights into peroxisome proliferator-activated receptors. It aims to shed light on the clinical aspects of peroxisome proliferator-activated receptors and the recent researches in this domain. Coherent flow of topics, student-friendly language and extensive use of examples make this book an invaluable source of knowledge.

The information shared in this book is based on empirical researches made by veterans in this field of study. The elaborative information provided in this book will help the readers further their scope of knowledge leading to advancements in this field.

Finally, I would like to thank my fellow researchers who gave constructive feedback and my family members who supported me at every step of my research.

Editor

Myocardial Expression of PPARγ and Exercise Capacity in Patients after Coronary Artery Bypass Surgery

Izabela Wojtkowska,[1] Tomasz A. Bonda,[2] Jadwiga Wolszakiewicz,[3] Jerzy Osak,[3]
Andrzej Tysarowski,[4] Katarzyna Seliga,[4] Janusz A. Siedlecki,[4] Maria M. Winnicka,[2]
Ryszard Piotrowicz,[3] and Janina Stępińska[1]

[1]Institute of Cardiology, Intensive Cardiac Therapy Clinic, Alpejska St. 42, 04-628 Warsaw, Poland
[2]Department of General and Experimental Pathology, Medical University of Bialystok, Mickiewicza St. 2c, 15-222 Bialystok, Poland
[3]Institute of Cardiology, Department of Cardiac Rehabilitation and Noninvasive Electrocardiology, Alpejska St. 42,
 04-628 Warsaw, Poland
[4]Institute of Oncology, Department of Molecular and Translational Oncology, Wawelska St. 15B, 02-034 Warsaw, Poland

Correspondence should be addressed to Izabela Wojtkowska; izabelawojt@op.pl

Academic Editor: Qinglin Yang

Activation of PPARs may be involved in the development of heart failure (HF). We evaluated the relationship between expression of PPARγ in the myocardium during coronary artery bypass grafting (CABG) and exercise tolerance initially and during follow-up. 6-minute walking test was performed before CABG, after 1, 12, 24 months. Patients were divided into two groups (HF and non-HF) based on left ventricular ejection fraction and plasma proBNP level. After CABG, 67% of patients developed HF. The mean distance 1 month after CABG in HF was 397 ± 85 m versus 420 ± 93 m in non-HF. PPARγ mRNA expression was similar in both HF and non-HF groups. 6MWT distance 1 month after CABG was inversely correlated with PPARγ level only in HF group. Higher PPARγ expression was related to smaller LVEF change between 1 month and 1 year ($R = 0.18$, $p < 0.05$), especially in patients with HF. Higher initial levels of IL-6 in HF patients were correlated with longer distance in 6MWT one month after surgery and lower PPARγ expression. PPARγ expression is not related to LVEF before CABG and higher PPARγ expression in the myocardium of patients who are developing HF following CABG may have some protecting effect.

1. Introduction

Heart failure (HF) is characterized by reduced reserve of the cardiac output. Impaired functional capacity in patients with heart failure is common and results from inability to achieve sufficient oxygen and nutrients delivery and altered washout of metabolites from working muscles.

Decreased stroke volume, altered chronotropic reaction, insufficient increase of myocardial contractility, and altered left ventricular-aortic coupling constitute the major central cardiovascular abnormalities, while decreased capillary density, endothelial dysfunction, and lowered oxygen extraction create the peripheral basic pathomechanisms leading to insufficient oxygenation of skeletal muscles [1, 2]. In addition,

chronic HF is related to dysfunctional metabolism of the skeletal muscles, changes in fibre composition, and progressive muscular atrophy [3, 4]. Overproduction of proinflammatory cytokines like TNF-α or IL-6, which is characteristic for chronic HF, may be responsible for altered muscular structure and function [5, 6]. These cytokines have an influence on normal physiology of the skeletal muscle cells but also affect proper function of endothelium by promoting generation of free oxygen radicals and decreasing availability of nitric oxide that altogether are responsible for insufficient vasorelaxatory function of the blood vessels [7]. The unfavorable effects of chronic inflammation in heart failure may be opposed by different endogenous mechanisms. One of these mechanisms may be related to the function of peroxisome proliferator-activated receptor gamma (PPARγ), which gained attention in recent decade mainly because of its metabolism-improving activities. Thiazolidinediones, the pharmacological activators of PPARγ, are used in patients with diabetes to decrease insulin resistance and improve glycemic control. Some positive effects of this therapy were also noted in relation to the cardiovascular system. Thiazolidinediones improved function of the endothelium, enhanced fatty acid oxidation in the cardiac muscle, decreased myocardial fibrosis, and diminished the risk of myocardial infarction and stroke [8]. Numerous experimental studies using rodents showed protective activity of PPARγ agonists on cardiac function [9–12]. However the significance of PPARγ activation is not univocal, as pioglitazone failed to provide any protective effect on the myocardium after ischemia-reperfusion in pigs [13] and rosiglitazone failed to prevent cardiac remodeling and caused increased mortality after acute infarction in rats [14]. Moreover, a meta-analysis of clinical studies showed increased risk for developing heart failure in patients with diabetes treated with PPARγ agonist pioglitazone [15]. The mechanisms leading to development of heart failure in patients treated with pioglitazone remain vague. These data were further blurred by improvement of aerobic capacity and skeletal muscle energy metabolism in patients with metabolic syndrome treated with pioglitazone [16].

In the present study we aimed to evaluate the relationship between expression of PPARγ in the myocardium, plasma levels of IL-6, and exercise tolerance in patients with ischemic heart disease undergoing coronary artery bypass grafting (CABG) before the operation and during the follow-up.

2. Methods

Patients with angiographically confirmed multivessel coronary artery disease, qualified to the CABG, were recruited to the study. Only subjects with normal blood levels of NT-proBNP and preserved cardiac function in resting echocardiographic examination and without clinical manifestations of heart failure or diabetes mellitus were included.

The clinical examination, biochemical tests, resting echocardiography, and six-minute walk test (6MWT) were performed before CABG and at 3-time points during the follow-up: one, twelve, and twenty-four months after the operation.

6MWT is a submaximal exercise test for evaluation of physical functional capacity measured in walked distance. The methodology of the examination was in agreement with the published guidelines [17]. Briefly, before the test patients were informed about the procedure and were allowed to rest in a sitting position for 10 minutes. Then they were asked to walk as fast and long as possible on a 50-meter walkway. Patients were allowed to stop and rest or reduce their walking speed if they felt fatigue. The dyspnea was estimated using the Borg scale. Samples of the left ventricular myocardium were harvested during the CABG procedure, and tissue fragments were placed in the "RNA later" solution (Qiagen) immediately after surgery and stored until RNA isolation. Expression of PPARγ mRNA was determined in these

samples by means of quantitative real-time PCR using TaqMan probes as previously described [18].

Blood samples were drawn initially and during each follow-up step. Serum concentrations of IL6 were measured using solid phase sandwich enzyme-linked immunosorbent assay kits (HS600B, R&D Systems) according to the manufacturer's guidelines.

Patients were examined during the follow-up and the measures of heart failure development were sought. During follow-up all patients were divided into two groups: with heart failure (HF) and without heart failure (non-HF). The criteria for the diagnosis of heart failure were left ventricular ejection fraction (LVEF) < 40% or NT-proBNP > 400 pg/mL. Presence of any of the abovementioned values during the follow-up was considered a marker of heart failure.

2.1. Ethics Statement. The procedures followed in the study were conducted ethically according to the principles of the World Medical Association Declaration of Helsinki and ethical standards in sport and exercise science research. All procedures were approved by the Ethics Committee of the Regional Medical Chamber in Warsaw [IK NP-0021/13/998/2007]. Informed consent was obtained from all participants.

2.2. Statistics. Data are presented as mean ± SD for quantitative variables or percent of study group for qualitative variables. Specific parameters of both groups (group with and without heart failure at baseline) and change in parameter values during follow-up were compared using chi square test and ANOVA with post hoc analysis. Correlations between variables were tested using Pearson's method. A value of $p < 0.05$ was considered statistically significant. Analysis was performed using Statistica 9.0PL.

3. Results

157 patients were qualified to the study. All patients did not have heart failure before CABG. After 1 month of CABG, 67% of patients developed heart failure. During 2-year follow-up the number of patients has been reduced in 1 year to 124 and in 2 years to 86 because of the loss of connection. In the HF group one patient died because of myocardial infarction in 1 year after CABG. The baseline characteristics of the study group were presented in the previous paper [18]. One month after CABG 106 patients (67%) were diagnosed with heart failure based on NT-proBNP exceeding 400 pg/mL or LVEF < 40%. Mean NT-proBNP concentration in this group was 675.2 ± 134.7 pg/mL and increased NT-proBNP was the most frequent indicator of HF. Only 13 subjects out of 106 had LVEF < 40%. The initial distance in 6MWT was 439 ± 73 m (408 ± 61 m in HF group and 458 ± 59 m in non-HF group). Patients developing HF during the follow-up had insignificantly lower exercise capacity 1 month after CABG than patients without HF. The mean 6MWT distance in HF group was 397 ± 85 m versus 420 ± 93 m in patients without HF. The distance improved significantly during the follow-up only in patients without HF ($p = 0.002$) and 24 months after CABG it was significantly longer than in HF group (410 ± 134 m in HF group versus 522 ± 82 m in non-HF

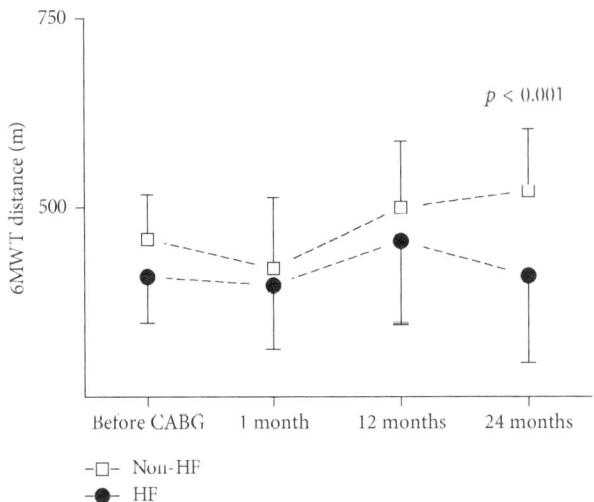

FIGURE 1: Changes of distance in 6-minute waking test in patients with (HF) and without heart failure (non-HF) during the follow-up. The improvement of the distance 24 months after CABG was observed only in non-HF group, and the distance was significantly longer as compared to the HF patients.

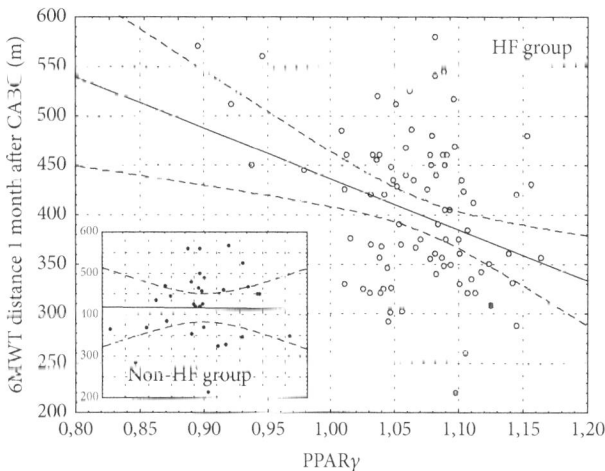

FIGURE 2: 6MWT distance 1 month after CABG was negatively correlated with PPARγ only in patients with HF during follow-up ($R = -0.24$; $p < 0.05$).

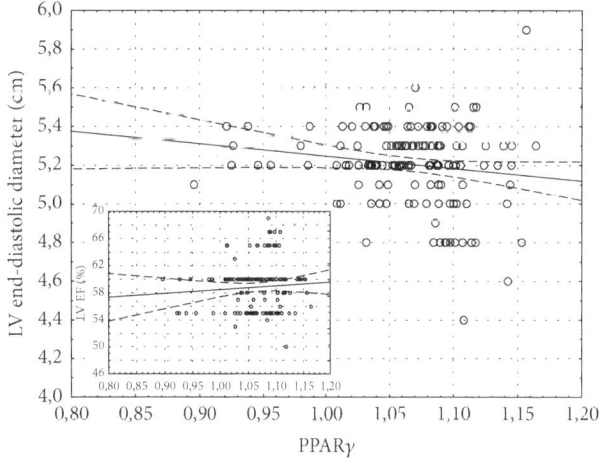

FIGURE 3: There were no significant correlations between PPARγ and either left ventricular end-diastolic dimension ($R = -0.11$, p = NS, the main graph) or left ventricular ejection fraction (LVEF; $R = 0.05$, p = NS, small graph) after CABG.

group, $p < 0.001$, Figure 1). Rate of perceived exertion scale was 6–12 for majority of patients. The parameters of 6MWT in both HF and non-HF groups are presented in Table 1. PPARγ gene expression in left ventricular myocardium taken during CABG was at the same level in patients included in HF and non-HF group during follow-up (1.069 ± 0.049 and 1.069 ± 0.034, resp.). However the distance of 6MWT one month after CABG was inversely correlated with myocardial PPARγ level ($R = -0.24$, $p < 0.05$) only in patients developing HF during the follow-up and was not present in those without HF (Figure 2). Although the expression of PPARγ gene in the myocardium was not correlated with left ventricular ejection fraction (LVEF) before or after CABG (Figure 3), higher PPARγ level was related to smaller attenuation of LVEF between 1-month and 1-year observations ($R = 0.18$, $p < 0.05$). The relation described was more pronounced in those patients, who developed HF during the follow-up ($R = 0.25$, $p < 0.01$) and was not significant in patients without HF (Figure 4). The concentration of IL-6 was highest before CABG (7.2 ± 5.5 pg/mL) and was significantly declining during the follow-up to reach level of 2.4 ± 2.1 pg/mL after one year and remained at that level ($p < 0.0001$ for the trend). Before CABG there was negative correlation between concentration of IL-6 in plasma and PPARγ expression ($R = -0.31$, $p < 0.05$, Figure 5) and positive correlation between IL-6 and NT-proBNP ($R = 0.35$, $p < 0.001$). In patients who developed heart failure higher initial levels of IL-6 were correlated with longer distance in 6MWT one month after surgery ($R = 0.47$, $p < 0.001$).

4. Discussion

The six-minute walk test (6MWT) is a submaximal exercise test for evaluating physical functional capacity. Fiorina et al. suggest that 6MWT is feasible and well tolerated in adult and older patients shortly after uncomplicated cardiac surgery and provides reference values for distance walked after cardiac surgery [19]. In our observations patients diagnosed with heart failure after CABG had a shorter distance in 6MWT, than patients without heart failure. In the HF group there was no significant improvement of the distance in 6MWT, while in patients without HF the distance increased significantly. Differences in exercise capacity can be attributed to the altered cardiac function; however there were no correlations between distance in 6MWT and LVEF or LV diastolic dimension. It should be emphasized that the abovementioned two parameters are related to the systolic function of the heart and poorly related to its diastolic performance.

Literature describing potential links between myocardial PPARγ expression and cardiac function or exercise capacity after CABG is very scant. In addition existing experimental

TABLE 1: Temporal changes of parameters related to six-minute walk test (6MWT) in patients with heart failure (HF) and without heart failure (non-HF).

	HF						Non-HF				
	Before CABG n = 157	Before CABG n = 106	1 month n = 106	After CABG 1 year n = 91	2 years n = 54	p	Before CABG n = 33	1 month n = 33	After CABG 1 year n = 33	2 years n = 32	p
6MWT distance (±SD) [m]	439 (±73)	408 (±61)	397 (±85)	456 (±110)	410 (±134)	NS	458 (±59)	420 (±93)	499 (±87)	522 (±82)	0.002
Rate of perceived exertion scale (Borg)											
6–12	90%	75%		80%	75%	NS	80%		85%	90%	NS
12–16	10%	20%		15%	20%		20%		15%	10%	
17–20	0%	5%		5%	5%		0%		0%	0%	
Respiratory rate/min.											
<14	90%	75%		80%	75%	NS	80%		85%	90%	NS
<20	10%	20%		15%	20%		20%		15%	10%	
<25	0%	5%		5%	5%		0%		0%	0%	
HR/min.											
<100	90%	75%		80%	75%	NS	80%		85%	90%	NS
<120	10%	20%		15%	20%		20%		15%	10%	
<160	0%	5%		5%	5%		0%		0%	0%	

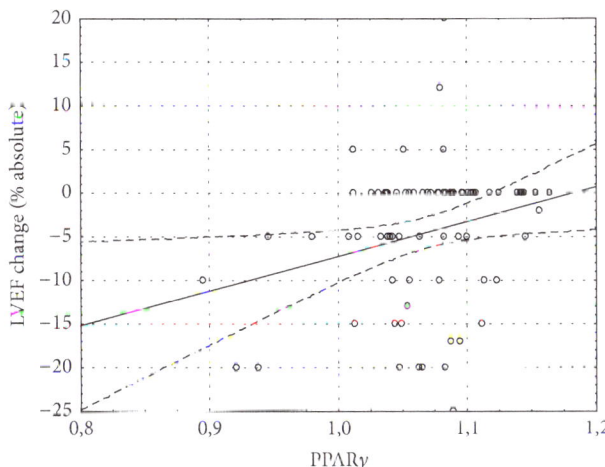

FIGURE 4: LVEF change between 1- and 12-month follow-up was significantly correlated with myocardial PPARγ in patients, in whom heart failure was diagnosed ($R = 0.25$, $p < 0.05$).

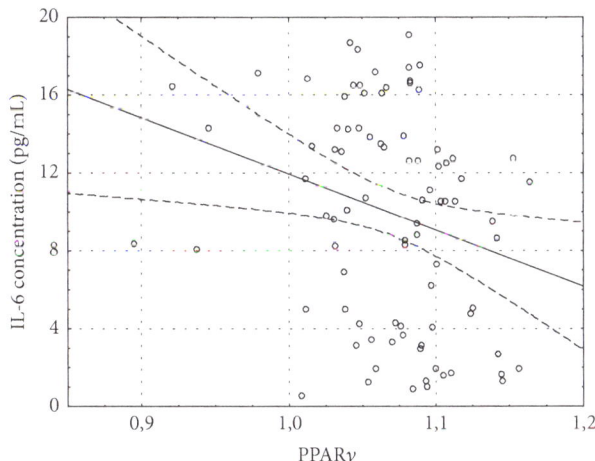

FIGURE 5: Significant negative correlation between serum IL6 level before CABG and expression of PPARγ ($R = -0.31$, $p < 0.05$) was observed only in patients in whom later in the follow-up heart failure was diagnosed.

data present contrasting results about the influence of PPARγ on cardiac function. On one hand, overexpression of PPARγ in transgenic mice was reported to evoke accumulation of lipids and glycogen and distortion of mitochondrial architecture leading to dilated cardiomyopathy [20]. On the other hand, activation of PPARγ with its agonist reduced lipotoxicity and improved cardiac function [21]. Expression of PPARs and their coactivators is diminished in cardiomyopathy and heart failure [22]. Cernecka et al. reported downregulation of PPARγ in the myocardium of anthracycline-induced cardiomyopathy in rodents, and treatment with an angiotensin converting enzyme inhibitor restored normal level of PPARγ but was not sufficient to restore normal cardiac function [23].

Our data showed no clear relation between PPARγ expression at the time of CABG and left ventricular size or ejection fraction at any time point. The level of PPARγ

in the myocardium was not able to predict development of heart failure after CABG, as was shown in our previous work [18]. However, in the group of patients, in whom heart failure develops during the follow-up, higher myocardial PPARγ level seems to preserve the systolic function of the left ventricle. On the other hand, also only in patients developing HF, PPARγ expression was inversely correlated with exercise capacity during the follow-up. It should be emphasized that left ventricular systolic function, if not significantly depressed, is not related to the exercise tolerance, but abnormalities of its diastolic function are independently associated with exercise capacity [24]. In our study however, NT-proBNP, which can be considered a marker of increased myocardial strain during systole and during diastole, was not related to PPARγ in the myocardium at all. Possible protective effect of PPARγ on the cardiac function may be related to suppression of the excessive inflammatory process and inhibition of apoptosis [25, 26]. Persistent inflammation, with chronically elevated concentrations of proinflammatory cytokines like TNF-α, ET-1, and IL-6, plays a pathogenic role in heart failure [27, 28]. In patients with heart failure, inflammation has been associated with worse functional capacity [29, 30] and concomitant cytokines and angiotensin II overproduction was shown to promote skeletal muscle atrophy in animals' models [31] that resemble changes seen in chronic heart failure. Without heart failure however, IL-6 seems to exert protective role on the skeletal muscles, stimulates hypertrophy and myogenesis, and regulates the energy metabolism [31]. We found negative correlation between myocardial PPARγ expression and IL-6 level only before CABG, when none of patients had features of heart failure. A subgroup of patients who developed HF and had higher initial levels of IL-6 had also better exercise capacity at one-month follow-up, which may reflect the protective role of IL-6 on skeletal muscle physiology, which is more important for skeletal muscle function and exercise capacity than weak PPARγ-related phenomena affecting cardiac muscle.

5. Conclusions

Higher levels of PPARγ in myocardium of patients who developed HF after CABG were correlated with smaller attenuation of LVEF, reduced plasma level of IL-6, and worsening of exercise tolerance.

These results indicate that PPARγ expression in the myocardium was not related to left ventricular systolic function before CABG. However higher levels of PPARγ gene transcript in the myocardium of patients who develop heart failure following CABG may have some protecting effect on cardiac contractility, which seem not to be directly related to exercise capacity.

Additional Points

Study Limitations. Significant number of patients was lost during follow-up: 12% 1 month after CABG, 18% after one year, and 36% after two years. The significance of the PPARγ expression may not be directly translated into its activity and biological role. The correlations presented in the work do not imply the causality and may be accidental; however it is not possible to evaluate them in the clinical observational study.

Conflicts of Interest

The authors declare that they have no conflicts of interest.

Acknowledgments

The study was supported by the Polish Ministry of Science and Higher Education, Warsaw, Poland (Research Grant N N 402 177934).

References

[1] B. P. Dhakal, R. Malhotra, R. M. Murphy et al., "Mechanisms of exercise intolerance in heart failure with preserved ejection fraction: the role of abnormal peripheral oxygen extraction," *Circulation: Heart Failure*, vol. 8, no. 2, pp. 286–294, 2015.

[2] R. Arena, J. Myers, and M. Guazzi, "The clinical importance of cardiopulmonary exercise testing and aerobic training in patients with heart failure," *Revista Brasileira de Fisioterapia*, vol. 12, no. 2, pp. 75–87, 2008.

[3] D. Harrington, S. D. Anker, T. P. Chua et al., "Skeletal muscle function and its relation to exercise tolerance in chronic heart failure," *Journal of the American College of Cardiology*, vol. 30, no. 7, pp. 1758–1764, 1997.

[4] H. Drexler, U. Riede, T. Münzel, H. König, E. Funke, and H. Just, "Alterations of skeletal muscle in chronic heart failure," *Circulation*, vol. 85, no. 5, pp. 1751–1759, 1992.

[5] S. D. Anker, P. P. Ponikowski, A. L. Clark et al., "Cytokines and neurohormones relating to body composition alterations in the wasting syndrome of chronic heart failure," *European Heart Journal*, vol. 20, no. 9, pp. 683–693, 1999.

[6] T. Tsujinaka, C. Ebisui, J. Fujita et al., "Muscle undergoes atrophy in association with increase of lysosomal cathepsin activity in interleukin-6 transgenic mouse," *Biochemical and Biophysical Research Communications*, vol. 207, no. 1, pp. 168–174, 1995.

[7] V. M. Conraads, E. M. Van Craenenbroeck, C. De Maeyer, A. M. Van Berendoncks, P. J. Beckers, and C. J. Vrints, "Unraveling new mechanisms of exercise intolerance in chronic heart failure. Role of exercise training," *Heart Failure Reviews*, vol. 18, no. 1, pp. 65–77, 2013.

[8] W. S. Lee and J. Kim, "Peroxisome proliferator-activated receptors and the heart: lessons from the past and future directions," *PPAR Research*, vol. 2015, Article ID 271983, 18 pages, 2015.

[9] D. Kamimura, K. Uchino, T. Ishigami, M. E. Hall, and S. Umemura, "Activation of Peroxisome Proliferator-activated Receptor γ Prevents Development of Heart Failure With Preserved Ejection Fraction; Inhibition of Wnt-β-catenin Signaling as a Possible Mechanism," *Journal of Cardiovascular Pharmacology*, vol. 68, no. 2, pp. 155–161, 2016.

[10] T. Shiomi, H. Tsutsui, S. Hayashidani et al., "Pioglitazone, a peroxisome proliferator-activated receptor-γ agonist, attenuates left ventricular remodeling and failure after experimental myocardial infarction," *Circulation*, vol. 106, no. 24, pp. 3126–3132, 2002.

[11] H. Ito, A. Nakano, M. Kinoshita, and A. Matsumori, "Pioglitazone, a peroxisome proliferator-activated receptor-γ agonist, attenuates myocardial ischemia/reperfusion injury in a rat model," *Laboratory Investigation*, vol. 83, no. 12, pp. 1715–1721, 2003.

[12] T. Honda, K. Kaikita, K. Tsujita et al., "Pioglitazone, a peroxisome proliferator-activated receptor-gamma agonist, attenuates myocardial ischemia-reperfusion injury in mice with metabolic disorders," *Journal of Molecular and Cellular Cardiology*, vol. 44, no. 5, pp. 915–926, 2008.

[13] Y. Xu, M. Gen, L. Lu et al., "PPAR-gamma activation fails to provide myocardial protection in ischemia and reperfusion in pigs," *American Journal of Physiology. Heart and Circulatory Physiology*, vol. 288, no. 3, pp. H1314–H1323, 2005.

[14] C. A. Lygate, K. Hulbert, M. Monfared, M. A. Cole, K. Clarke, and S. Neubauer, "The PPARγ-activator rosiglitazone does not alter remodeling but increases mortality in rats post-myocardial infarction," *Cardiovascular Research*, vol. 58, no. 3, pp. 632–637, 2003.

[15] H.-W. Liao, J. L. Saver, Y.-L. Wu, T.-H. Chen, M. Lee, and B. Ovbiagele, "Pioglitazone and cardiovascular outcomes in patients with insulin resistance, pre-diabetes and type 2 diabetes: A systematic review and meta-analysis," *BMJ Open*, vol. 7, no. 1, Article ID e013927, 2017.

[16] T. Yokota, S. Kinugawa, K. Hirabayashi et al., "Pioglitazone improves aerobic capacity and skeletal muscle energy metabolism in patients with metabolic syndrome," *Journal of Cardiac Failure*, vol. 22, no. 9, p. S205, 2016.

[17] ATS Committee on Proficiency Standards for Clinical Pulmonary Function Laboratories, "ATS statement: guidelines for the six-minute walk test," *American Journal of Respiratory and Critical Care Medicine*, vol. 166, no. 1, pp. 111–117, 2002.

[18] I. Wojtkowska, A. Tysarowski, K. Seliga et al., "PPAR gamma expression levels during development of heart failure in patients with coronary artery disease after coronary artery bypass-grafting," *PPAR Research*, Article ID 242790, 242790 pages, 2014.

[19] C. Fiorina, E. Vizzardi, R. Lorusso et al., "The 6-min walking test early after cardiac surgery. Reference values and the effects of rehabilitation programme," *European Journal of Cardiothoracic Surgery*, vol. 32, no. 5, pp. 724–729, 2007.

[20] N. H. Son, T. S. Park, H. Yamashita et al., "Cardiomyocyte expression of PPARgamma leads to cardiac dysfunction in mice," *Journal of Clinical Investigtion*, vol. 11, no. 10, pp. 2791–2801, 2007.

[21] R. K. Vikramadithyan, K. Hirata, H. Yagyu et al., "Peroxisome proliferator-activated receptor agonists modulate heart function in transgenic mice with lipotoxic cardiomyopathy," *Journal of Pharmacology and Experimental Therapeutics*, vol. 313, no. 2, pp. 586–593, 2005.

[22] M. A. Burke, S. Chang, H. Wakimoto et al., "Molecular profiling of dilated cardiomyopathy that progresses to heart failure," *JCI Insight*, vol. 1, no. 6, 2016.

[23] H. Cernecka, G. Doka, J. Srankova et al., "Ramipril restores PPARβ/δ and PPARγ expressions and reduces cardiac NADPH oxidase but fails to restore cardiac function and accompanied myosin heavy chain ratio shift in severe anthracycline-induced cardiomyopathy in rat," *European Journal of Pharmacology*, vol. 791, pp. 244–253, 2016.

[24] J. Grewal, R. B. McCully, G. Kane, C. Lam, and P. A. Pellikka, "Left ventricular function and exercise capacity," *JAMA*, vol. 301, no. 3, pp. 286-94, 2009.

[25] Y. Ye, Z. Hu, Y. Lin, C. Zhang, and J. R. Perez-Polo, "Downregulation of microRNA-29 by antisense inhibitors and a PPAR-γ agonist protects against myocardial ischaemia–reperfusion injury," *Cardiovascular Research*, vol. 87, no. 3, pp. 535–544, 2010.

[26] A. Cabrero, J. C. Laguna, and M. Vázquez, "Peroxisome proliferator activated receptors and the control of inflammation.," *Curr Drug Targets Inflamm Allergy*, vol. 1, no. 3, pp. 243–248, 2002.

[27] L. Gullestad, T. Ueland, L. E. Vinge, A. Finsen, A. Yndestad, and P. Aukrust, "Inflammatory cytokines in heart failure: mediators and markers," *Cardiology*, vol. 122, no. 1, pp. 23–35, 2012.

[28] A. Deswal, N. J. Petersen, A. M. Feldman, J. B. Young, B. G. White, and D. L. Mann, "Cytokines and cytokine receptors in advanced heart failure: an analysis of the cytokine database from the Vesnarinone Trial (VEST)," *Circulation*, vol. 103, no. 16, pp. 2055–2059, 2001.

[29] J. Thierer, A. Acosta, N. Vainstein et al., "Relation of left ventricular ejection fraction and functional capacity with metabolism and inflammation in chronic heart failure with reduced ejection fraction (from the MIMICA Study)," *American Journal of Cardiology*, vol. 105, no. 7, pp. 977–983, 2010.

[30] M. M. Fernandes-Silva, G. V. Guimarães, V. O. Rigaud et al., "Inflammatory biomarkers and effect of exercise on functional capacity in patients with heart failure: insights from a randomized clinical trial," *European Journal of Preventive Cardiology*, vol. 24, no. 8, pp. 808–817, 2017.

[31] P. Muñoz-Cánoves, C. Scheele, B. K. Pedersen, and A. L. Serrano, "Interleukin-6 myokine signaling in skeletal muscle: a double-edged sword?" *The FEBS Journal*, vol. 280, no. 17, pp. 4131–4148, 2013.

A Reduction in ADAM17 Expression is Involved in the Protective Effect of the PPAR-α Activator Fenofibrate on Pressure Overload-Induced Cardiac Hypertrophy

Si-Yu Zeng ⓘ,[1] **Hui-Qin Lu ⓘ,**[1] **Qiu-Jiang Yan ⓘ,**[2] **and Jian Zou ⓘ**[3]

[1]*Department of Drug Clinical Trials, Guangdong Second Provincial General Hospital, Guangzhou 510317, China*
[2]*Department of Cardiac & Thoracic Surgery, The Third Affiliated Hospital of Guangzhou Medical University, Guangzhou 510000, China*
[3]*Department of Pharmacy, The People's Hospital of Pengzhou, Chengdu 611900, China*

Correspondence should be addressed to Si-Yu Zeng; cosmo81@qq.com and Jian Zou; 70336641@qq.com

Academic Editor: Brian N. Finck

The peroxisome proliferator-activated receptor-α (PPAR-α) agonist fenofibrate ameliorates cardiac hypertrophy; however, its mechanism of action has not been completely determined. Our previous study indicated that a disintegrin and metalloproteinase-17 (ADAM17) is required for angiotensin II-induced cardiac hypertrophy. This study aimed to determine whether ADAM17 is involved in the protective action of fenofibrate against cardiac hypertrophy. Abdominal artery constriction- (AAC-) induced hypertensive rats were used to observe the effects of fenofibrate on cardiac hypertrophy and ADAM17 expression. Primary cardiomyocytes were pretreated with fenofibrate (10 μM) for 1 hour before being stimulated with angiotensin II (100 nM) for another 24 hours. Fenofibrate reduced the ratios of left ventricular weight to body weight (LVW/BW) and heart weight to body weight (HW/BW), left ventricular anterior wall thickness (LVAW), left ventricular posterior wall thickness (LVPW), and ADAM17 mRNA and protein levels in left ventricle in AAC-induced hypertensive rats. Similarly, *in vitro* experiments showed that fenofibrate significantly attenuated angiotensin II-induced cardiac hypertrophy and diminished ADAM17 mRNA and protein levels in primary cardiomyocytes stimulated with angiotensin II. In summary, a reduction in ADAM17 expression is associated with the protective action of PPAR-α agonists against pressure overload-induced cardiac hypertrophy.

1. Introduction

Hypertension, a critical cardiovascular disease, is responsible for many disabilities and deaths worldwide. It is characterized by sustained pressure overload and concurrent development of pathological cardiac hypertrophy, which plays a critical role in the onset and development of chronic heart failure, the end stage of the cardiovascular event chain [1, 2]. The five-year-survival rate has been reported to be very low in symptomatic patients with chronic heart failure [3, 4]. Thus, improving pathological cardiac hypertrophy may prevent the progression from hypertension to chronic heart failure.

Pressure overload and cardiac hypertrophy share common inducers (e.g., endothelin and angiotensin II) that activate downstream matrix metalloproteinases (MMPs, such as MMP2 and MMP7) and a disintegrin and metalloproteinases (ADAMs, such as ADAM12 and ADAM17) via activating Gq protein-coupled receptors [2, 5–7]. Among these metalloproteinases, MMP2, MMP7, ADAM12, and ADAM17 are the most well studied in the context of the cardiovascular system. Previous studies have verified that ADAM17 lies on upstream of ADAM12 and MMP2 in the network of the metalloproteinase signaling pathway [2, 8], indicating that ADAM17 could be a key member of the metalloproteinases family. ADAM17 has essential functions in cell-cell interactions, signaling, and proteolysis of key cytokines, cytokine receptors, and other targets [9, 10]. Systemic ADAM17 knockdown was shown to ameliorate cardiac hypertrophy in angiotensin II-induced hypertensive mice and spontaneously hypertensive rats [7, 8]. Therefore,

ADAM17 is a crucial factor that mediates pressure overload-induced cardiac hypertrophy.

PPAR-α is present in high levels in tissues with high energy demands that depend on the oxidation of mitochondrial fatty acids as a primary energy source, including the heart and liver [11]. Recently, PPAR-α activators have been evaluated as therapeutic agents to modulate cardiac hypertrophy alone or in conjunction with other agents [12–16]. However, it remains unclear whether ADAM17 participates in the protective effect of fenofibrate against cardiac hypertrophy.

In this research, we found that PPAR-α activation by fenofibrate ameliorated pressure overload-induced cardiac hypertrophy and reduced ADAM17 expression in left ventricular tissue in AAC-induced hypertensive rats. In cultured primary cardiomyocytes, PPAR-α activation inhibited angiotensin II-induced cardiac hypertrophy and decreased ADAM17 protein and mRNA levels. Our previous results showed that ADAM17 siRNA markedly attenuated angiotensin II-induced cardiac hypertrophy in primary cardiomyocytes [17]. Therefore, these lines of indirect evidence indicate that a decrease in ADAM17 expression is involved in the protective effect of fenofibrate on pressure overload-induced cardiac hypertrophy.

2. Materials and Methods

2.1. Animals. Animal protocols were performed according to the guidelines principles for the Care and Use of Laboratory Animals issued by National Institutes of Health of the United States. Further, the animal experiments were approved by the Medical Ethics Committees of Guangdong Second Provincial General Hospital. A total of 46 male Sprague-Dawley rats (about 200-250 g) were purchased from the Experimental Animals Center of Sun Yat-Sen University.

2.2. AAC-Induced Cardiac Hypertensive Model. After rats were anesthetized via intraperitoneal injection of 3% sodium pentobarbital (40mg /kg), midline celiotomy was performed to expose the abdominal artery just above the kidney artery. Aortic banding was carried out according to the method described by Irukayama-Tomobe Y [15]. AAC was performed in 36 rats, which were divided into the AAC rats group (vehicle, oral gavage), AAC+Fenofibrate (60mg/kg, oral gavage) group, and AAC+ Fenofibrate (120mg/kg, oral gavage) group. The 60 mg/kg and 120 mg/kg doses of fenofibrate in rats are two times and four times, respectively, as much as the equivalent dose in humans. Likewise, these same procedures were carried out in rats of the Sham group except for the binding of the abdominal artery. There were 10 rats in each group. Sustained AAC for 4 weeks caused no deaths in the rats even though there was about 15% mortality within 24 hours in rats subjected to AAC.

2.3. Echocardiography and Hemodynamic Measurements. Ultrasonic electrocardiograph images were obtained with a Vevo 2100 high-resolution *in vivo* microimaging system (Visual Sonics, Canada) after rats were anesthetized through inhalation of 2% enflurane as described previously; left ventricular anterior and posterior wall thickness (LVAW and LVPW) were measured and analysed [17, 18]. Next, aortic systolic pressure (AoSP), left ventricular systolic pressure (LVSP), and maximal rate of left ventricular pressure increase (dp/dtmax) and decrease (dp/dtmin) were measured using a BL-420S system (Chengdu Tai-Meng Technology Co., Ltd., China). Finally, heart mass index and left ventricular mass index were calculated separately.

2.4. Cell Culture. Primary cultures of ventricular cardiomyocytes were obtained from 2-day-old Sprague- Dawley rats as previously described [19].

2.5. Cellular Surface Area. After staining with tetramethyl-rhodamine- (TRITC-) labelled phalloidin, cardiomyocytes were used to evaluate cell surface area by automatically analysing the mean cell area of 40 visual fields using Cellomics/High Content Screening (Thermo Scientific, America) as previously described [17].

2.6. Real Time Quantitative PCR. RNA extraction and real time quantitative PCR were carried out as described previously [17]. For real time quantitative PCR, specific primers against ADAM17, BNP, and ANP were used and the GADPH gene was used as an inner control. The following premiers were used: ADAM17: 5′-GTGAGCAGTTTC-TCGAACGC-3′ (forward primer) and 5′-AGCTTCTCA-AGTCGCAGGTG-3′ (reverse primer); BNP: 5′-ATGCAG-AAGCTGCTGGAGCTGATA-3′ (forward primer) and 5′-TTG TAGGGCCTTGGTCCTTTGAGA-3′ (reverse primer); ANP: 5′-GGAAGTCAACCCGTCTCA-3′ (forward primer) and 5′-AGCCCTCAGTTTGCTTTT-3′ (reverse primer); GADPH: 5′-ATCAA GAAGGTGGTGAAGCA-3′ (forward primer), 5′-AAGGTGGAAGAATGGGAGTTG-3′ (reverse primer).

2.7. Western Blotting. Protocols for western blotting were based on a previously reported method [17]. Antibodies included antibody against ADAM17 (Abcam, America), antibody against tubulin (Santa Cruz, America), and goat anti-rabbit lgGHRP (Affinity, America).

2.8. Statistical Analysis. Data are expressed as the mean ± SD. Results were analysed using an unpaired t-test between two groups and one-way ANOVA among at least three groups. Results were considered to be statistically significant when $p < 0.05$.

3. Results

3.1. Fenofibrate Protected against Pressure Overload-Induced Cardiac Hypertrophy. As shown in Table 1, there were significant increases in aortic systolic pressure [AoSP, 180.6 ±13.7 mm Hg versus 124.3±8.6 mm Hg] and left ventricular systolic pressure [LVSP, 184.4±11.4 mm Hg versus 134.3±9.8 mm Hg] in the AAC group compared with those in the Sham group, indicating the successful construction of an AAC-induced hypertensive model. Cardiac hypertrophy was commonly assessed by ventricular mass and ventricular wall thickness,

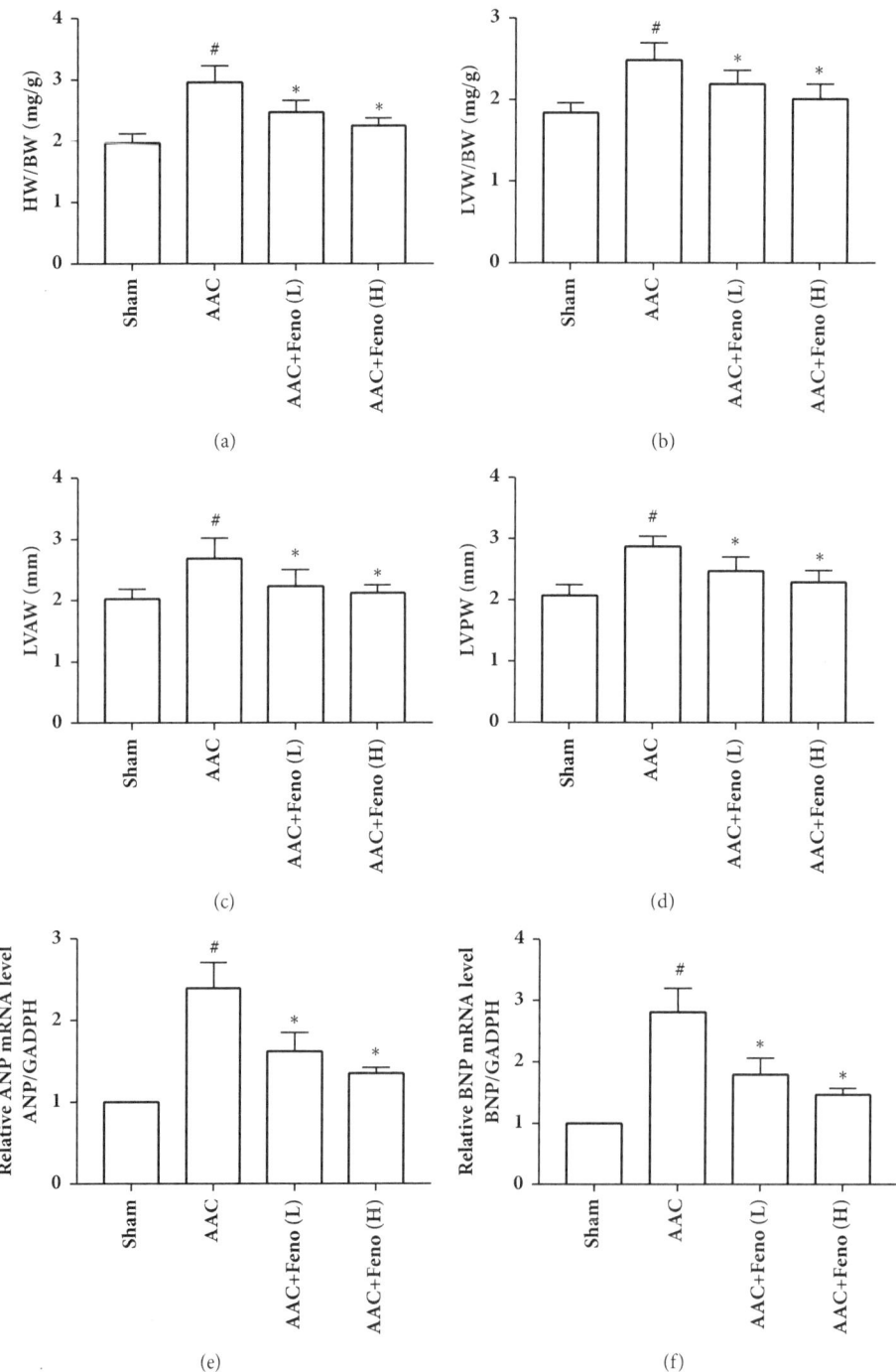

FIGURE 1: Fenofibrate inhibited pressure-overload-induced cardiac hypertrophy in abdominal artery constriction- (AAC-) induced hypertensive rats. (a) HW/BW; (b) LVW/BW; (c) LVAW; (d) LVPW; (e) ANP mRNA level; (f) BNP mRNA level. Feno represents fenofibrate; HW/BW represents ratio between heart weight and body weight; LVW/BW represent ratio between left ventricular weight and body weight; LVAW represents left ventricular anterior wall thickness; LVPW represents left ventricular posterior wall thickness; $^{\#}$p<0.05 versus Sham group; *p<0.05 versus AAC group, n=6 per group.

indicated by HW/BW, LVW/BW, LVAW, and LVPW [20]. After treatment with a low or high dose of fenofibrate for 28 days, rats subjected to AAC showed weakened hypertrophy in the left ventricle supported by decreased HW/BW, LVW/BW, LVAW, LVPW, and mRNA levels of hypertrophic genes (ANP and BNP), although treatment with fenofibrate caused no

significant change in LVSP (Figure 1 and Table 1). Thus, fenofibrate can inhibit pressure overload-induced cardiac hypertrophy.

3.2. Fenofibrate Reduced ADAM17 Expression in Left Ventricular Tissue from AAC-Induced Hypertensive Rats.

As shown

TABLE 1: The effect of fenofibrate on hemodynamic data in rats with abdominal artery constriction.

	Sham	AAC	AAC+Feno (L)	AAC+Feno (H)
AoSP (mmHg)	124.3±8.6	180.6±13.7[#]	178.6±14.1	176.1±10.4
LVSP (mmHg)	134.3± 9.8	184.4±11.4[#]	180.8±10.9	178.5±10.7
HR (bpm)	348.8±18.2	358.6±16.1	354.0±15.2	350.8±12.8
+dp/dt$_{max}$ (mmHg/sec.)	4.98±0.28	3.37±0.61[#]	4.53±0.45[*]	4.79±0.29[*]
-dp/dt$_{max}$ (mmHg/sec.)	4.84±0.35	3.08±0.37[#]	4.27±0.41[*]	4.56±0.28[*]

AoSP, aortic systolic pressure; LVSP, left ventricular systolic pressure; HR, heart rate; dp/dt$_{max}$, maximal rate of left ventricular pressure increase; dp/dt$_{min}$, maximal rate of left ventricular pressure decrease. n=6 for each group, values are mean ± SD. [#]p<0.05 versus sham group, *p<0.05 versus AAC group. Feno represents fenofibrate, n=6 for each group.

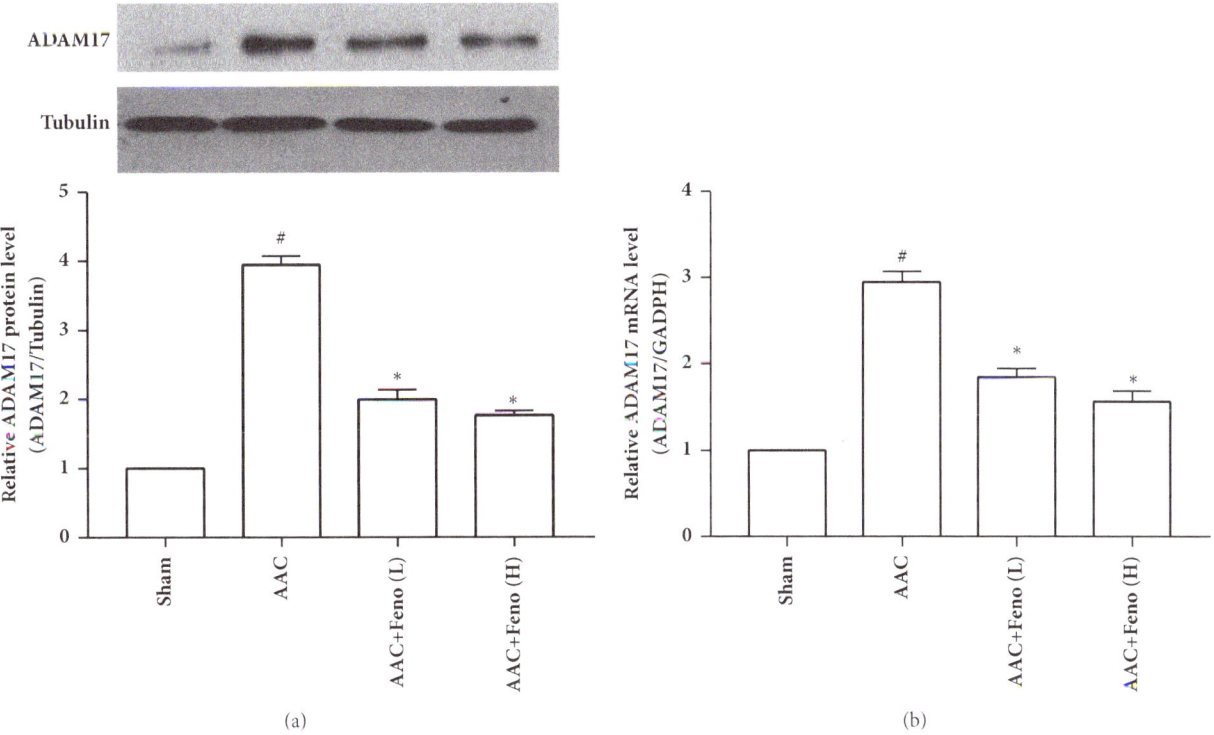

(a)   (b)

FIGURE 2: Fenofibrate reduced the expression of a disintegrin and metalloproteinase-17 (ADAM17) in left ventricular tissue from abdominal artery constriction- (AAC-) induced hypertensive rats. (a) ADAM17 protein level (n=4 independent experiments); (b) ADAM17 mRNA level (n=3 independent experiments). Feno represents fenofibrate; [#]p<0.05 versus Sham group; *p<0.05 versus AAC group.

in Figures 2(a) and 2(b), ADAM17 protein and mRNA levels were significantly upregulated in the AAC group compared with those in the Sham group, whereas the low or high dose of fenofibrate significantly reduced ADAM17 protein and mRNA levels in left ventricular tissue from AAC-induced hypertensive rats. These findings showed that fenofibrate decreased ADAM17 expression in left ventricular tissue from AAC-induced hypertensive rats.

3.3. Fenofibrate Inhibited Angiotensin II-Induced Cardiac Hypertrophy in Cultured Primary Cardiomyocytes.

Cardiac hypertrophy involves the reexpression of foetal genes, including β-myosin heavy chain (β-MHC), ANP, and BNP, and these foetal genes were commonly used as cell markers to diagnose cardiac hypertrophy [21]. Furthermore, cell surface area is also used to evaluate cardiac hypertrophy in cultured cardiac cells [22]. As shown in Figure 3, cell surface area and

mRNA levels of hypertrophic markers (ANP and BNP) were markedly elevated in cardiomyocytes treated with 100nM angiotensin II for 24 hours compared with those in the control group, whereas treatment with fenofibrate reduced cell surface area and mRNA levels of ANP and BNP. These findings indicated that fenofibrate can alleviate angiotensin II-induced cardiac hypertrophy.

3.4. ADAM17 Mediated the Protective Action of Fenofibrate against Angiotensin II-Induced Cardiac Hypertrophy.

In vitro experiments showed that pretreatment with fenofibrate (10 μM) inhibited angiotensin II-induced upregulation of ADAM17 expression (Figure 4). Our previous results revealed that ADAM17 siRNA could attenuate cardiac hypertrophy, as indicated by its effects on cell surface area and mRNA levels of hypertrophic genes (ANP and BNP) in primary cardiomyocytes stimulated with 100nM angiotensin II for

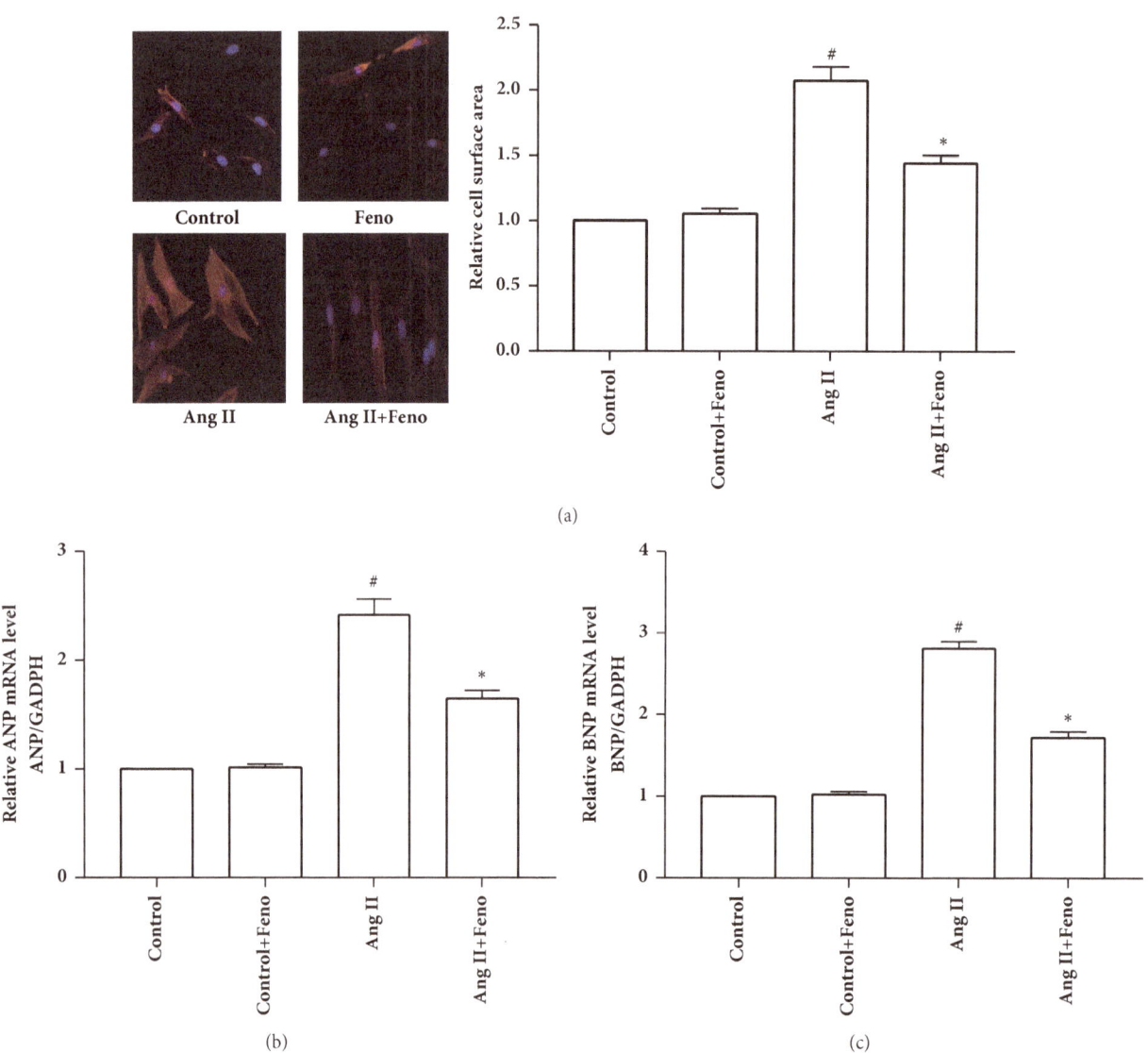

FIGURE 3: Fenofibrate attenuated angiotensin II-induced cardiac hypertrophy in cultured primary cardiomyocytes. After pretreated with fenofibrate (10 μM) for 1 hour, cardiomyocytes were then stimulated with 100 nM angiotensin II for 24 hours. (a) Cell surface area; (b) ANP mRNA level; (c) BNP mRNA level. Ang II represents angiotensin II; Feno represents fenofibrate; [#]$p < 0.05$ versus control group; *$p < 0.05$ versus Ang II group. n=3 independent experiments.

24 hours [17]. Together, these lines of indirect evidence showed that inhibition of ADAM17 modulated the protective action of fenofibrate against angiotensin II-induced cardiac hypertrophy.

4. Discussion

PPAR-α is a critical mediator of cardiac hypertrophy. An approximately 4-fold increase in PPAR-α expression in PPAR-α transgenic (Tg) mice compared with that in nontransgenic (NTg) littermates does not cause significant cardiac hypertrophy in PPAR-α Tg mice [23]. There was, however, a report of the induction of significant ventricular hypertrophy in normal mice in PPAR-α TG mice that express a higher PPAR-α levels compared with those of NTg littermates [24]. Nevertheless, Rana S et al. [25]

reported that PPAR-α overexpression during pathological cardiac hypertrophy ameliorated cardiac hypertrophy and improved heart function. PPAR-α expression is downregulated in the failing human hearts [26] but increased in the hearts of diabetic mice induced by streptozotocin and patients with dilated cardiomyopathy [24, 27]. Moreover, the absence of PPAR-α results in a more pronounced hypertrophic growth response and cardiac dysfunction associated with the enhanced expression of inflammatory markers and extracellular matrix remodelling [28]. These findings suggest that a certain amount of PPAR-α expression and activity is required for maintaining heart morphology and function, but excessive or lower expression and activity levels of PPAR-α promote cardiac hypertrophy and heart dysfunction under physiological conditions, whereas PPAR-α overexpression

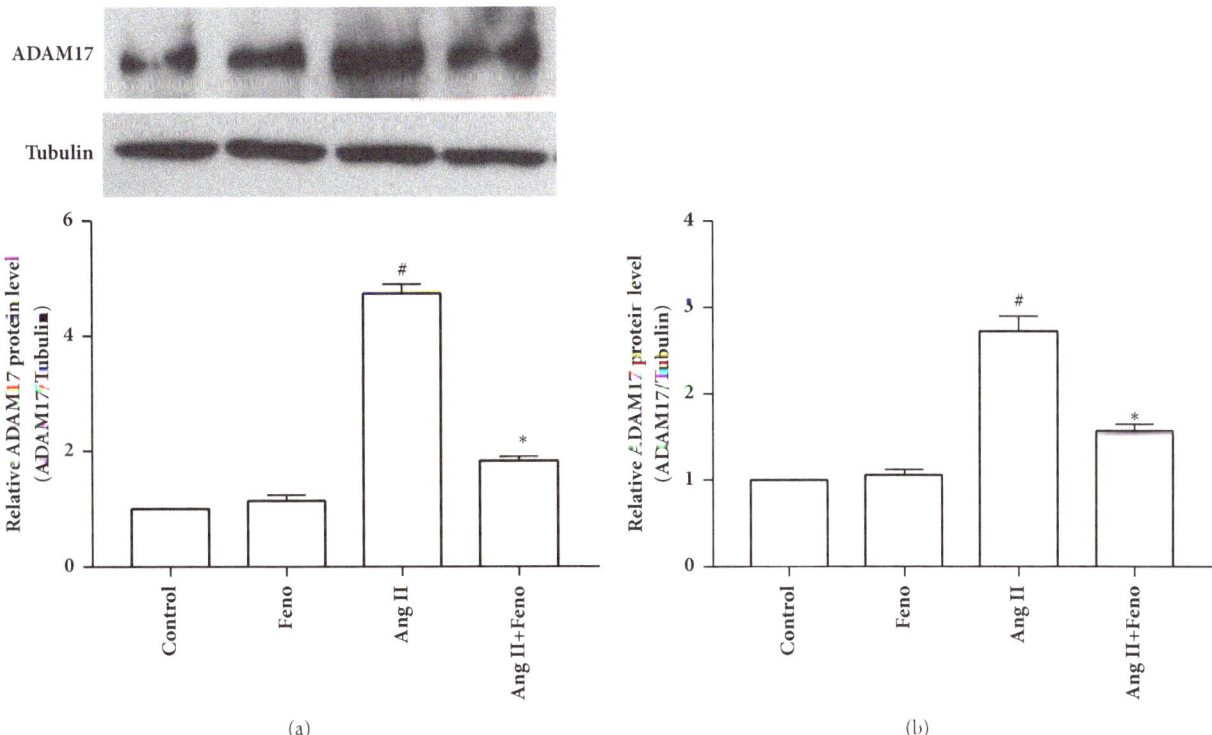

FIGURE 4: Fenofibrate reduced the expression of a disintegrin and metalloproteinase-17 (ADAM17) in primary cardiomyocytes stimulated with 100 nM angiotensin II for 24 hours. After pretreated with fenofibrate (10 μM) for 1 hour, cardiomyocytes were then stimulated with 100 nM angiotensin II for 24 hours. (a) ADAM17 protein level (n=4 independent experiments); (b) ADAM17 mRNA level (n=3 independent experiments). Ang II represents angiotensin II; Feno represents fenofibrate; #p<0.05 versus control group; *p<0.05 versus Ang II group.

attenuates cardiac hypertrophy under pathological conditions.

The modest activation of PPAR-α with its agonist fenofibrate represents a potentially pharmacological intervention against pressure overload-induced cardiac hypertrophy. The PPAR-α agonist fenofibrate is commonly applied to treat hyperglyceridaemia, hypercholesterolemia, and mixed dyslipidaemia [29, 30]. It has been reported that fenofibrate suppresses cardiac hypertrophy, fibrosis, and inflammation in pressure overloaded rats [12–16, 31, 32], in agreement with our results that fenofibrate inhibited pressure overload-induced cardiac hypertrophy in rats subjected to AAC.

The mechanisms by which fenofibrate inhibits pressure overload-induced cardiac hypertrophy are very complicated. Fenofibrate attenuates pressure overload-induced cardiac hypertrophy partly by inhibiting the binding of p65-NFκB to NFATc4, the c-Jun NH2-terminal kinase pathway, ERK activation, and MMP2 activity, as well as increasing high mobility group box 1 (HMGB1) levels in nuclei [12, 15, 33, 34]. However, additional details are needed to improve our understanding about how PPAR-α agonist fenofibrate suppresses cardiac hypertrophy.

Activated ADAM17 promotes the shedding of substrates, including proinflammatory factors [such as tumour necrosis factor α (TNF-α)] and growth factors [such as epidermal growth factor (EGF) and heparin-binding EGF-like growth factor (HB-EGF)] [10], thus triggering a cascade of mitogen-activated protein kinase to advance cardiac hypertrophy

via the transcriptional activation of immediate-early genes and foetal genes referred to as hypertrophic genes [8]. Our previous results also showed that ADAM17 siRNA inhibited angiotensin II-induced cardiac hypertrophy in primary cardiomyocytes. Temporal systemic ADAM17 deletion suppresses the increase in systolic blood pressure and levels of fasting glucose and lipid in mice fed with a high-fat diet, indicating that ADAM17 might participate in the balance between fatty acid uptake and utilization in the heart [35]. Fatty acid uptake/utilization mismatch in the heart leads to lipid accumulation that is related to initial cardiac hypertrophy [36]; however, it needs to elucidate whether ADAM17 mediates cardiac hypertrophy through lipids accumulation in the heart. In the present study, our findings indicated that fenofibrate alleviated cardiac hypertrophy and reduced ADAM17 expression in hypertrophic cardiomyocytes in vivo and in vitro experiments. Collectively, decreased ADAM17 expression is associated with the protective effect of the PPAR-α activator fenofibrate on pressure overload-induced cardiac hypertrophy.

5. Conclusion

In conclusion, our indirect evidence indicates that a decrease in ADAM17 expression is related to the beneficial role of PPAR-α activation in pressure overload-induced cardiac hypertrophy. These results may aid in improving our understanding about how fenofibrate inhibits cardiac hypertrophy, thereby providing additional evidence for preventing from cardiac hypertrophy with fenofibrate. However, further research is needed to elucidate whether and how ADAM17 mediates the protective effects of fenofibrate on cardiac hypertrophy in hypertensive rats overexpressing ADAM17 gene in combination with fenofibrate treatment.

Conflicts of Interest

The authors have no conflicts of interest to disclose.

Acknowledgments

This work was supported by The Science and Technology Planning Project of Guangdong Province (Grant no. 2016A020226005); The Natural Science Foundation of Guangdong Province (no. 2015A030310076); and The Nature Scientific Foundation of Guangdong Second Provincial General Hospital (Grant no. YQ2015-008). The authors thank Ms. Menzhen Zhang for her technical assistance with echocardiography measurement.

Supplementary Materials

Figure S1: additional western blot protein bands. A: ADAM17 protein level in the left ventricle in abdominal artery constriction- (AAC-) induced hypertensive rats. B: ADAM17 protein level in cardiomyocytes stimulated with angiotensin II for 24 hours. *(Supplementary Materials)*

References

[1] S. M. Hamza and J. R. B. Dyck, "Systemic and renal oxidative stress in the pathogenesis of hypertension: modulation of long-term control of arterial blood pressure by resveratrol," *Frontiers in Physiology*, vol. 5, article 292, 2014.

[2] J. Odenbach, X. Wang, S. Cooper et al., "MMP-2 mediates angiotensin ii-induced hypertension under the transcriptional control of MMP-7 and TACE," *Hypertension*, vol. 57, no. 1, pp. 123–130, 2011.

[3] D. Lloyd-Jones, R. Adams, M. Carnethon et al., "Heart disease and stroke statistics—2009 update. A report from the American heart association statistics committee and stroke statistics subcommittee," *Circulation*, vol. 119, no. 3, pp. 480–486, 2009.

[4] Chinese Society of Cardiology of Chinese Medical Association, "Guidelines for the diagnosis and management of chronic heart failure," *Chinese Journal of Cardiology*, vol. 35, no. 12, pp. 1076–1095, 2007.

[5] M. Asakura, M. Kitakaze, S. Takashima et al., "Cardiac hypertrophy is inhibited by antagonism of ADAM12 processing of HB-EGF: Metalloproteinase inhibitors as a new therapy," *Nature Medicine*, vol. 8, no. 1, pp. 35–40, 2002.

[6] L. Hao, M. Du, A. Lopez-Campistrous, and C. Fernandez-Patron, "Agonist-induced activation of matrix metalloproteinase-7 promotes vasoconstriction through the epidermal growth factor-receptor pathway," *Circulation Research*, vol. 94, no. 1, pp. 68–76, 2004.

[7] T. Takayanagi, S. J. Forrester, T. Kawai et al., "Vascular ADAM17 as a novel therapeutic target in mediating cardiovascular hypertrophy and perivascular fibrosis induced by angiotensin II," *Hypertension*, vol. 68, no. 4, pp. 949–955, 2016.

[8] X. Wang, T. Oka, F. L. Chow et al., "Tumor necrosis factor-α-converting enzyme is a key regulator of agonist-induced cardiac hypertrophy and fibrosis," *Hypertension*, vol. 54, no. 3, pp. 575–582, 2009.

[9] D. F. Seals and S. A. Courtneidge, "The ADAMs family of metalloproteases: multidomain proteins with multiple functions," *Genes & Development*, vol. 17, no. 1, pp. 7–30, 2003.

[10] U. Sahin, G. Weskamp, K. Kelly et al., "Distinct roles for ADAM10 and ADAM17 in ectodomain shedding of six EGFR ligands," *The Journal of Cell Biology*, vol. 164, no. 5, pp. 769–779, 2004.

[11] S. H. Han, M. J. Quon, and K. K. Koh, "Beneficial vascular and metabolic effects of peroxisome proliferator-activated receptor-alpha activators," *Hypertension*, vol. 46, no. 5, pp. 1086–1092, 2005.

[12] J. Zou, K. Le, S. Xu et al., "Fenofibrate ameliorates cardiac hypertrophy by activation of peroxisome proliferator-activated receptor-alpha partly via preventing p65-NFkappaB binding to NFATc4," *Molecular and Cellular Endocrinology*, vol. 370, no. 1-2, pp. 103–112, 2013.

[13] M. Iglarz, R. M. Touyz, E. C. Viel et al., "Peroxisome proliferator-activated receptor-α and receptor-γ activators prevent cardiac fibrosis in mineralocorticoid-dependent hypertension," *Hypertension*, vol. 42, no. 4, pp. 737–743, 2003.

[14] Q. N. Diep, K. Benkirane, F. Amiri, J. S. Cohn, D. Endemann, and E. L. Schiffrin, "PPARα activator fenofibrate inhibits myocardial inflammation and fibrosis in angiotensin II-infused rats," *Journal of Molecular and Cellular Cardiology*, vol. 36, no. 2, pp. 295–304, 2004.

[15] Y. Irukayama-Tomobe, T. Miyauchi, and S. Sakai, "Endothelin-1-induced cardiac hypertrophy is inhibited by activation of peroxisome proliferator-activated receptor-alpha partly via blockade of c-Jun NH2-terminal kinase pathway," *Circulation*, vol. 109, no. 7, pp. 904–910, 2004.

[16] N. K. LeBrasseur, T.-A. S. Duhaney, D. S. De Silva et al., "Effects of fenofibrate on cardiac remodeling in aldosterone-induced hypertension," *Hypertension*, vol. 50, no. 3, pp. 489–496, 2007.

[17] S.-Y. Zeng, X. Chen, S.-R. Chen et al., "Upregulation of Nox4 promotes angiotensin II-induced epidermal growth factor receptoractivation and subsequent cardiac hypertrophy by increasing ADAM17 expression," *Canadian Journal of Cardiology*, vol. 29, no. 10, pp. 1310–1319, 2013.

[18] X. Chen, S. Zeng, J. Zou et al., "Rapamycin attenuated cardiac hypertrophy induced by isoproterenol and maintained energy homeostasis via inhibiting NF-κB activation," *Mediators of Inflammation*, vol. 2014, Article ID 868753, 15 pages, 2014.

[19] J. Fu, J. Gao, R. Pi, and P. Liu, "An optimized protocol for culture of cardiomyocyte from neonatal rat," *Cytotechnology*, vol. 49, no. 2-3, pp. 109–116, 2005.

[20] J. N. Cohn, R. Ferrari, and N. Sharpe, "Cardiac remodeling—concepts and clinical implications: a consensus paper from an International Forum on Cardiac Remodeling," *Journal of the American College of Cardiology*, vol. 35, no. 3, pp. 569–582, 2000.

[21] P. S. Azevedo, B. F. Polegato, M. F. Minicucci, S. A. R. Paiva, and L. A. M. Zornoff, "Cardiac remodeling: concepts, clinical impact, pathophysiological mechanisms and pharmacologic treatment," *Arquivos Brasileiros de Cardiologia*, vol. 106, no. 1,

pp. 62–69, 2016.

[22] J. Endo, M. Sano, J. Fujita et al., "Bone marrow-derived cells are involved in the pathogenesis of cardiac hypertrophy in response to pressure overload," *Circulation*, vol. 116, no. 10, pp. 1176–1184, 2007.

[23] C. N. Karam, C. M. Warren, M. Henze, N. H. Banke, E. D. Lewandowski, and R. J. Solaro, "Peroxisome proliferator-activated receptor-α expression induces alterations in cardiac myofilaments in a pressure-overload model of hypertrophy," *American Journal of Physiology—Heart and Circulatory Physiology*, vol. 312, no. 4, pp. H681–H690, 2017.

[24] B. N. Finck, J. J. Lehman, T. C. Leone et al., "The cardiac phenotype induced by PPARα overexpression mimics that caused by diabetes mellitus," *The Journal of Clinical Investigation*, vol. 109, no. 1, pp. 121–130, 2002.

[25] S. Rana, R. Datta, R. D. Chaudhuri, E. Chatterjee, M. Chawla-Sarkar, and S. Sarkar, "Nanotized PPARα overexpression targeted to hypertrophied myocardium improves cardiac function by attenuating the p53-GSK3β mediated mitochondrial death pathway," *Antioxidants & Redox Signaling*, 2018.

[26] J. Karbowska, Z. Kochan, and R. T. Smoleński, "Peroxisome proliferator-activated receptor alpha is downregulated in the failing human heart," *Cellular & Molecular Biology Letters*, vol. 8, no. 1, pp. 49–53, 2003.

[27] M. Schupp, U. Kintscher, J. Fielitz et al., "Cardiac PPARα expression in patients with dilated cardiomyopathy," *European Journal of Heart Failure*, vol. 8, no. 3, pp. 290–294, 2006.

[28] P. J. H. Smeets, B. E. J. Teunissen, P. H. M. Willemsen et al., "Cardiac hypertrophy is enhanced in PPARα-/- mice in response to chronic pressure overload," *Cardiovascular Research*, vol. 78, no. 1, pp. 79–89, 2008.

[29] C. Hottelart, N. El Esper, F. Rose, J.-M. Achard, and A. Fournier, "Fenofibrate increases creatininemia by increasing metabolic production of creatinine," *Nephron*, vol. 92, no. 3, pp. 536–541, 2002.

[30] P. Balakumar, M. K. Arora, and M. Singh, "Emerging role of PPAR ligands in the management of diabetic nephropathy," *Pharmacological Research*, vol. 60, no. 3, pp. 170–173, 2009.

[31] T. Ogata, T. Miyauchi, S. Sakai, Y. Irukayama-Tomobe, K. Goto, and I. Yamaguchi, "Stimulation of peroxisome-proliferator-activated receptor alpha (PPAR alpha) attenuates cardiac fibrosis and endothelin-1 production in pressure-overloaded rat hearts," *Clinical Science*, vol. 103, supplement 48, pp. 284S–288S, 2002.

[32] L. Castiglioni, A. Pignieri, M. Fiaschè et al., "Fenofibrate attenuates cardiac and renal alterations in young salt-loaded spontaneously hypertensive stroke-prone rats through mitochondrial protection," *Journal of Hypertension*, vol. 36, no. 5, pp. 1129–1146, 2018.

[33] T.-A. S. Duhaney, L. Cui, M. K. Rude et al., "Peroxisome proliferator-activated receptor α-independent actions of fenofibrate exacerbates left ventricular dilation and fibrosis in chronic pressure overload," *Hypertension*, vol. 49, no. 5, pp. 1084–1094, 2007.

[34] Z. Jia, R. Xue, G. Liu et al., "HMGB1 is involved in the protective effect of the PPARα agonist fenofibrate against cardiac hypertrophy," *PPAR Research*, vol. 2014, Article ID 541394, 9 pages, 2014.

[35] H. Kaneko, T. Anzai, K. Horiuchi et al., "Tumor necrosis factor-α converting enzyme inactivation ameliorates high-fat diet-induced insulin resistance and altered energy homeostasis," *Circulation Journal*, vol. 75, no. 10, pp. 2482–2490, 2011.

[36] H.-C. Chiu, A. Kovacs, D. A. Ford et al., "A novel mouse model of lipotoxic cardiomyopathy," *The Journal of Clinical Investigation*, vol. 107, no. 7, pp. 813–822, 2001.

Nutrigenomic Functions of PPARs in Obesogenic Environments

Soonkyu Chung,[1] Young Jun Kim,[2] Soo Jin Yang,[3] Yunkyoung Lee,[4] and Myoungsook Lee[5]

[1]Department of Nutrition and Health Sciences, University of Nebraska-Lincoln, Lincoln, NE, USA
[2]Department of Food & Biotechnology, Korea University, Sejong, Republic of Korea
[3]Department of Food and Nutrition, Seoul Women's University, Seoul, Republic of Korea
[4]Department of Food Science and Nutrition, Jeju National University, Jeju, Republic of Korea
[5]Department of Food and Nutrition and Research Institute of Obesity Science, Sungshin Women's University, Seoul, Republic of Korea

Correspondence should be addressed to Myoungsook Lee; mlee@sungshin.ac.kr

Academic Editor: John P. Vanden Heuvel

Peroxisome proliferator-activated receptors (PPARs) are ligand-activated transcription factors that mediate the effects of several nutrients or drugs through transcriptional regulation of their target genes in obesogenic environments. This review consists of three parts. First, we summarize current knowledge regarding the role of PPARs in governing the development of white and brown/beige adipocytes from uncommitted progenitor cells. Next, we discuss the interactions of dietary bioactive molecules, such as fatty acids and phytochemicals, with PPARs for the modulation of PPAR-dependent transcriptional activities and metabolic consequences. Lastly, the effects of PPAR polymorphism on obesity and metabolic outcomes are discussed. In this review, we aim to highlight the critical role of PPARs in the modulation of adiposity and subsequent metabolic adaptation in response to dietary challenges and genetic modifications. Understanding the changes in obesogenic environments as a consequence of PPARs/nutrient interactions may help expand the field of individualized nutrition to prevent obesity and obesity-associated metabolic comorbidities.

1. Introduction

In the past few decades, the prevalence of chronic diseases has been shown to be linked to nutrition deficiencies and overnutrition. Nutritional genomics/nutrigenomics, a unique approach for investigation of the genome-wide effects of nutrients at the molecular level, has contributed to the development of nutritional science and applications in medicinal and pharmacological research. Peroxisome proliferator-activated receptors (PPARs) are ligand-activated transcription factors (TFs) that mediate the effects of several nutrients or drugs through transcriptional regulation of their target genes. PPAR isotypes of the NR1 family, such as PPARα (nuclear receptor; NR1C1), PPARβ/δ (NR1C2), and PPARγ (NR1C3), can be distinguished based on their different biological roles and are the most relevant subtypes in the field of nutrition research. PPARs exert their biologically distinct functions in an isotype- and tissue-specific manner; however, the molecular details of tissue-dependent PPAR function remain unclear. PPARs are also able to repress transcription by interacting with other TFs and/or coactivators, thereby interfering with other signaling pathways to control physiology. Understanding the changes in the obesogenic environment as a consequence of PPAR/nutrient interactions may help expand the field of individualized nutrition to prevent obesity and its associated metabolic comorbidities.

In this review, we summarized current knowledge regarding (1) the role of PPARs in governing the development of white and brown/beige adipocytes from uncommitted progenitor cells, (2) interactions between dietary bioactive molecules and PPARs for the modulation of PPAR-dependent transcriptional activity and metabolic consequences, and (3) the effects of PPAR polymorphisms on obesity and metabolic outcomes.

2. Transcriptional Regulation of PPARs in White, Brown, and Beige Adipose Tissue

2.1. Functions of PPARs in White Adipose Tissue

2.1.1. Regulation of Adipogenesis.

The process of adipogenesis is divided into two distinct stages: determination and terminal differentiation. Each stage is governed by the orchestrated regulation of TFs. TFs involved in the stage of adipocyte determination include CCAAT/enhancer-binding protein β and δ (C/EBPβ and C/EBPδ), glucocorticoid receptor (GR), signal transducer and activator of transcription 5A (STAT5A), and cAMP-response element-binding protein (CREB) [22, 23]. These TFs induce the transcriptional activation of target genes responsible for the second stage of adipogenesis. Regulators of early-stage adipogenesis, that is, C/EBPβ and C/EBPδ, directly induce the expression of C/EBPα and PPARγ, which transcriptionally activate their own expression and the expression of other adipogenesis-related genes, for example, PPARγ coactivator 1 alpha (PGC-1α) and fatty acid synthase (FAS) [24–26].

PPARγ is known for its role in the regulation of adipogenic and lipogenic pathways [4, 27, 28]. Initial studies examining the role of PPARγ in adipogenesis showed that PPARγ-knockout mice had little adipose tissue [29]. PPARγ cooperatively acts with early adipogenic TFs, such as C/EBPs [30]. C/EBPβ and C/EBPδ induce PPARγ expression, and C/EBPα and PPARγ commutatively induce the expression of each other by facilitating chromatin binding [4, 31]. Some studies have suggested that the involvement of PPARs in adipogenesis is limited to the effects of PPARγ during later stages of adipogenesis and terminal differentiation of adipocytes. However, evidence has shown that PPARγ also plays a role in the early stages of adipogenesis. A subset of adipocyte progenitors is present within the WAT perivascular region in which PPARγ is expressed, suggesting that this protein may have a role in adipocyte self-renewal [32, 33]. The involvement of PPARγ in adipogenesis is more evident at the later stages of adipogenesis in mature adipocytes. Because the ablation of PPARγ is lethal, cell-specific knockout of PPARγ has been utilized in mature mouse adipocytes by applying the tamoxifen-dependent Cre-ER (T2) recombination system. A few days after ablation of the PPARγ gene, mature adipocytes and brown adipocytes died, and a subset of PPARγ-positive cells appeared [34], suggesting the involvement of PPARγ in maintaining mature adipocytes.

2.1.2. PPARs and Adipokines.

PPARγ controls the expression of adipokines, including adiponectin, leptin, fibroblast growth factor 1 (FGF1), FGF21, resistin, and tumor necrosis factor-α (TNF-α). Adiponectin is a main adipokine that stimulates insulin sensitization by increasing glucose uptake and decreasing gluconeogenesis. Between the two adiponectin receptors (AdipoR1 and AdipoR2), AdipoR2 activates hepatic PPARα [35]. Hepatic PPARα activation by AdipoR2 decreases lipid accumulation and lipid peroxidation, contributing to improvements in hepatic steatosis and nonalcoholic steatohepatitis [35]. Adipose PPARα and PPARγ activation increases adipocyte uptake of glucose and free fatty acids and enhances insulin sensitivity by inducing the expression of AdipoR1 and AdipoR2 [36]. In contrast to adiponectin, PPARγ indirectly suppresses adipose leptin expression by inhibiting the binding of C/EBP to the leptin promoter region [37].

FGF1 is known to be selectively induced in adipose tissues by consumption of a high-fat diet through PPARγ, which acts on adipose tissue remodeling [38]. The phenotypes of FGF1-knockout mice depend on the conditions. FGF1-knockout mice do not show abnormal phenotypes under normal physiological conditions; however, the mice show disruption of fat expansion and subsequent development of diabetes in an obesogenic environment from high-fat feeding. FGF21 is expressed in the adipose tissue and liver and exerts tissue-specific effects. In adipose tissues, FGF21 increases energy expenditure and prevents weight gain in diet-induced obese and ob/ob mice [39]. Moreover, FGF21 also sensitizes cells to the effects of insulin by increasing adipose PPARγ activity [40]. The PPARγ agonist rosiglitazone induces FGF21 in the epididymal WAT of C57Bl/6 mice, and adipose FGF21 stimulates PPARγ, affecting adipogenesis and insulin sensitization. In the livers of these mice, FGF21 is induced by the PPARα agonist GW7647, and hepatic FGF21 acts as a hormone, regulating carbohydrate and lipid metabolism [40]. FGF21-knockout mice exhibited lipodystrophy with little adipose tissue owing to the low expression levels of PPARγ and its target genes.

Resistin is another adipokine that is upregulated in patients with type 2 diabetes and inflammation-related diseases [41]. Transcriptional regulation of resistin is governed by cooperative regulation of PPARγ and C/EBP in murine adipocytes, but not in human adipocytes. Additionally, PPARγ reduces the expression of proinflammatory cytokines in adipose tissue by acting on nuclear factor-kappa B (NF-κB) signaling. PPARγ inhibits NF-κB activity and induces its degradation by direct binding to NF-κB [42], leading to downregulation of the proinflammatory cytokines TNF-α, interleukin-6 (IL-6), and plasminogen activator inhibitor-1. As a transrepressive effect of PPARγ and NF-κB, NF-κB also inhibits PPARγ transcriptional activity by acting on histone deacetylase 3 [43].

2.1.3. Regulation of PPARs in Subcutaneous and Visceral WAT.

Three subtypes of PPAR, that is, PPARα, PPARβ/δ, and PPARγ, have tissue-specific regulatory functions. The tissue-specificity of each PPAR isoform is due to differences in the tissue-specific expression and specific target genes of each PPAR isoform. The tissue distribution, target genes, and main functions of PPAR subtypes are summarized in Table 1. Among the three PPAR subtypes, PPARγ is highly expressed in adipose tissues and stimulates glucose uptake and adipokine secretion [1]. Through its interactions with adipokines, PPARγ is involved in adipogenesis, lipid metabolism, glucose homeostasis, adipose remodeling, and WAT browning in WAT [2]. PPARγ agonists have been used as oral hypoglycemic agents by sensitizing cells to insulin action; however, the application of these agents is often limited because of their effects on increasing body fat content [3]. The PPARγ agonist thiazolidinedione (TZD) selectively

TABLE 1: Tissue distribution, target genes, and main functions of PPAR subtypes.

PPAR isoform	PPARα	PPARβ/δ	PPARγ
Tissue distribution	Liver, heart, BAT	Many tissues (mainly in skeletal muscle, liver, heart)	PPARγ1: many tissues PPARγ2: WAT and BAT
Target genes	ACAA2, ACAD, CPT1A, CPT2, ETFA, ETFDH, HADHA, HADHB, SLC25A20, SLC22A5, TXNIP, apoA-1	ACOX1, CPT1, LCAD, UCP1, VLCAD, CPT1	ACBP, ACS, aP2, CD36, C/EBPα, GLUT4, LPL, GyK, IRS-1, IRS-2, PEPCK, PI3K, STAT1, STAT5A, STAT5B
Physiological functions	Fatty acid oxidation, amino acid catabolism, oxidative phosphorylation, lipoprotein synthesis [1, 2]	Fatty acid oxidation, oxidative phosphorylation, muscle type determination [3]	Adipogenesis, lipid metabolism, glucose homeostasis [2, 4]

ACAA2, acetyl-CoA acyltransferase 2; ACAD, acyl-coenzyme A dehydrogenase; ACBP, acyl-CoA-binding protein; ACOX1, acyl-coenzyme A oxidase 1; ACS, acyl-CoA synthetase; aP2, fatty acid binding protein 2; BAT, brown adipose tissue, C/EBPα, CCAAT/enhancer-binding protein α; CD36, cluster of differentiation 36; CPT, carnitine palmitoyl transferase; ETFA, electron transfer flavoprotein alpha subunit; ETFDH, electron transfer flavoprotein dehydrogenase; GLUT4, glucose transporter 4; GyK, glycerol kinase; HADHA, hydroxyacyl-CoA dehydrogenase, alpha subunit; IRS, insulin receptor substrate; LCAD, long-chain acyl-CoA dehydrogenase; LPL, lipoprotein lipase; PEPCK, phosphoenolpyruvate carboxykinase; PI3K, phosphoinositide 3-kinase; SLC25A20, solute carrier family 25 member 20; STAT, signal transducer and activator of transcription; TXNIP, thioredoxin-interacting protein; UCP1, uncoupling protein 1; VLCAD, very long-chain acyl-CoA dehydrogenase.

induces the differentiation of immature preadipocytes in subcutaneous fat. Newly differentiated adipocytes are small and exhibit increased insulin sensitivity without altering the total weight of the WAT [44]. Interestingly, the opposite is true of visceral fat pads; TZD treatment decreases the numbers of large adipocytes in visceral fat by increasing apoptosis in large and relatively insulin-resistant visceral adipocytes [45]. Fat deposition in subcutaneous adipose tissue is relatively beneficial compared with increased visceral fat contents in terms of the risk of metabolic syndrome and cardiovascular diseases (CVDs). Lipoprotein lipase (LPL) has been suggested to be involved in PPARγ-dependent fat redistribution from visceral to subcutaneous tissues in PPARγ agonist-treated experimental models. The mass and catalytic activities of LPL are increased in subcutaneous fat, but not in visceral fat depots, accompanied by alterations in factors involved in the regulation of LPL activity, fatty acid transport, and lipogenesis [46, 47]. Nonetheless, in addition to increased subcutaneous fat, other side effects, including adverse cardiac outcomes, have been reported in patients receiving rosiglitazone, resulting in withdrawal of rosiglitazone from the market. Novel approaches have been applied for the use of PPARγ agonist as antidiabetic drugs, including development of new types of PPARγ agonists, dual PPARα and PPARγ agonists, and combination with agents that can suppress adipocyte differentiation and fat accumulation. In particular, dual PPARα and PPARγ agonists have been accepted to be promising for the treatment of type 2 diabetes with dyslipidemia. Administration of lobeglitazone and saroglitazar was effective in lowering HbA1c and in improving glucose control and lipid profiles in subjects of type 2 diabetes [48–51]. It does not mean that these dual PPARα and PPARγ agonists have no side effects. For example, weight gain was still observed in lobeglitazone-treated diabetic subjects [50]. Collectively, existing evidence suggests that the usage of dual PPARα and PPARγ agonists was relatively well tolerated and acceptable considering the balance between efficacy and side effects.

2.2. Regulation of PPARs in BAT

2.2.1. Cellular Origin of Brown and Beige Adipocytes.
At least two metabolically distinct brown adipocytes are found in humans: "classical brown" and "beige" adipocytes [52–54]. Classical brown adipocytes possess molecular attributes similar to interscapular BAT (iBAT) of rodents based on constitutive uncoupling protein-1 (UCP1) expression, homogeneous multilocular morphology, and a myogenic origin (Myf5$^+$) [55, 56]. Conversely, beige adipocytes are differentiated from nonmyogenic lineage progenitors (Myf5$^-$) and possess low levels of UCP1 expression under unstimulated conditions. Although there is still some controversy regarding the cellular identity, anatomical location, and recruitment versus transdifferentiation of beige adipocytes [57, 58], the metabolic relevance of beige adipocytes in terms of energy expenditure [52, 59] has well been established in response to environmental stimuli, such as low temperature [60, 61], and to physical activity [62]. Because BAT activity is negatively associated with adiposity, insulin resistance (IR), and aging, therapeutics targeting BAT recruitment and activity have attracted attention as a potential novel treatment strategy. PPARγ regulates the general differentiation program and metabolic function of brown adipocytes as well as white adipocytes. Given the metabolic relevance of BAT in metabolism, we will summarize the role of the PPARs in regulating brown and beige fat development in this section. We also propose that reduced PPARγ activity may explain the compromised BAT activities in obesity and metabolic syndrome.

2.2.2. Transcriptional Regulation of PPARγ in Brown and Beige Adipocytes.
PPARγ is the single most important TF that governs white adipocyte differentiation. However, PPARγ alone is insufficient to drive the entire brown adipogenic transcriptional program, and its transcriptional partner, PR domain-containing protein 16 (PRDM16), is also required. Nonetheless, PPARγ activity is essential for the development of both classical brown and beige adipocytes. Using a brown preadipocyte cell line, researchers have shown that PPARγ

binding to the PPAR response element of UCP1 is required for the transcriptional activity of UCP1 [63]. Inhibition of PPARγ activity using a dominant-negative mutant promotes the whitening of interscapular brown fat [64]. In addition, genome-wide binding analyses have demonstrated that PPARγ binds to many other genes unique to brown adipocytes, suggesting that PPARγ binding to PPRE response elements in brown target genes confers lineage specificity during brown fat differentiation [65, 66]. In addition to promoting classical brown adipocyte differentiation, PPARγ has also been implicated in white-to-beige conversion. Lack of functional PPARγ activity leads to defective beige fat recruitment, suggesting that beige fat development is dependent on PPARγ function [64]. Conversely, synthetic PPARγ ligands, particularly those in the TZD class, are potent regulators of mitochondrial biogenesis and cause significant increases in brown-specific phenotypes in white adipocytes, including UCP1 upregulation and uncoupled respiration [67–73]. In later studies, Ohno et al. showed that the white-to-beige conversion by PPARγ agonism could be explained by stabilization of PRDM16 protein, the master transcriptional regulator of brown adipocytes [74]. Interestingly, energy expenditure is not increased in TZD-treated animals. This could be due to the observation that TZD-mediated systemic lipogenesis overshadows the improved mitochondrial function and suppresses β3-adrenergic receptor- (ADRB3-) mediated activation in vivo [75–77]. Another important mechanism through which PPARγ agonism enhances BAT activity involves the activation of SIRT1, a Sir2 homolog and NAD-dependent deacetylase [78]. Moreover, activation of SIRT1 and deacetylation of PPARγ by resveratrol increase the recruitment of PRDM16, resulting in implementation of the transcriptional cascade for brown signature genes [74]. In addition to PPARγ, PPARα plays a role in brown adipocyte formation. Because PPARα is a primary regulator of mitochondrial β-oxidation, it is not surprising that PPARα expression levels are higher in brown adipocytes than in white adipocytes. Although PPARα expression is often regarded as a downstream brown marker gene, other studies have demonstrated that PPARα functions simultaneously with PPARγ to increase the brown-specific expression of PRDM16, PGC1α, and UCP1 [79, 80]. PPARβ/δ is ubiquitous, showing highest expression in the gut, but is now thought to be important in exercise-induced white-to-beige conversion and thermogenesis [81]. In conclusion, the plasticity of adipocytes in response to different environmental stimuli is likely regulated by the dynamic associations among TFs (e.g., PPARs and PRDM16) and their coregulators (e.g., PGC1α and SIRT1). These interactions between environmental and transcriptional regulators determine the lineage commitment of adipogenic progenitor cells, that is, white, brown, and beige adipocytes, and the metabolic fate of existing adipocytes, that is, browning or its reversal, whitening.

2.2.3. Compromised Activities of PPARs in Obese and Metabolically Unhealthy BAT. Chronic activation of ADRB3 is a key signaling event enhancing BAT activity and/or mass. In healthy humans, at least three distinct metabolic responses occur concurrently in response to ADRB3 signaling: (1)

an increase in BAT activity in preexisting classical brown adipocytes, (2) metabolic switch of some, if not all, existing white adipocytes to beige adipocytes in subcutaneous fat, and (3) new beige adipocyte formation from adipogenic progenitor cells [82, 83]. Emerging evidence has revealed that these metabolic adaptations of BAT are preceded by cellular remodeling of WAT via type 2 innate immune responses, that is, IL-4 and IL-13 secretion [84, 85], M2 macrophage polarization [86], and local catecholamine production from macrophages and eosinophils [86, 87]. Unfortunately, BAT activity in humans is inversely correlated with body fat mass [88, 89], age, and blood glucose levels [90, 91]. Compromised BAT activation in conditions of obesity and metabolic vulnerability is associated with impairment of immunological remodeling in WAT upon ADRB3 activation. Given the critical role of PPARs in BAT regulation, the molecular mechanisms through which these defective immune responses affect the transcriptional regulation of PPARs/PRDM16 and the recruitment of these proteins to brown-specific target genes need to be defined. One of the most plausible and reasonable mechanisms for defective BAT activation in obesity involves the inverse regulation of NF-κB and PPARγ transactivation [92–95]. Toll-like receptor 4- (TLR4-) mediated NF-κB activation in obesity severely impairs cold-induced type 2 immune responses [85], downregulates PPARγ and PPARα expression, and markedly reduces beige fat development [96]. Similarly, Goto et al. showed that IL-1β, which causes systemic IR, strongly reduces PPARγ expression and blocks BAT development upon cold exposure [97]. Hence, pharmaceutical or nutritional strategies to restore PPAR activities by NF-κB suppression should be revisited as a new approach to reinstate type 2 immune responses and PPAR/PRDM16 recruitment for beige fat development.

3. Effects of Nutrition on the Modulation of PPARs

3.1. Fatty Acids (FAs) and Their Derivatives. Food components that act as ligands for PPARs can show multiple effects, including antidiabetic, antiadipogenic, and anti-inflammatory effects [98–100]. A wide range of PPAR agonists have been identified; synthetic PPAR agonists, such as fibrates and TZD, as well as natural PPAR ligands, such as dietary FAs and their derivatives, have been shown to bind to and activate PPARs [101–103]. Indeed, fibrates and TZD are already used to treat hyperlipidemia and diabetes mellitus, respectively. Ligand-activated PPARs play a critical role in regulating metabolic activities associated with lipid metabolism, glucose metabolism, and the inflammatory state [99]. As shown in various ligand-binding assays, PPARs generally prefer to bind to polyunsaturated FAs, whereas saturated FAs are poor PPAR ligands. Thus, the activity of PPARs can be modulated by FAs derived from the diet; however, the capacity of FAs to activate PPAR-dependent gene transcription varies according to the type of FA [101, 104]. A variety of FAs and their derivatives as PPAR ligands are shown in Table 2.

TABLE 2: FAs and their derivatives as PPARs ligands.

Receptor	PPARα	PPARβ/δ	PPARγ
Ligands	Saturated FAs (weaker)	Unsaturated FAs	Unsaturated FAs (LA, LNA, CLA, DHA, EPA)
	Unsaturated FAs (LA, LNA, PUFAs, including AA, EPA, phytanic acid)	Saturated FAs (much weaker) Prostacyclin	15-d-PGJ2 15-HETE
	Leukotriene B4	4-HNE	9-HODE
	8-HETE	4-HDDE	13-HODE
	8,9-Epoxyeicosatrienoic acids		
	11,12-Epoxyeicosatrienoic acids		
	OEA		
	PEA		

AA, arachidonic acid; CLA, conjugated linoleic acid; DHA, docosahexaenoic acid; EPA, eicosapentaenoic acid; 15-d-PGJ2, 15-deoxy-Δ12,14 prostaglandin J2; LA, linoleic acid; LNA, α-linolenic acid; OEA, oleoylethanolamide; PEA, palmitoylethanolamide; 4-HDDE, 4-hydroxydodeca-(2E,6Z)-dienal; 4-HNE, 4-hydroxy-2-nonenal; 15-HETE, 15(S)-hydroxyeicosatetraenoic acid; HODE, hydroxyoctadecadienoic acid.

FAs are ubiquitous biological molecules that act as metabolic fuels and essential components of cellular functions [101]. Although FAs are essential biological components, elevated levels of circulating FAs are closely related to most common metabolic disorders, such as CVD, hyperlipidemia, obesity, and IR [105]. Not all fats are created equal; high consumption of foods enriched in saturated FAs has been shown to be associated with the development of common diseases, such as coronary artery disease, obesity, diabetes, and cancer, whereas consumption of a diet high in polyunsaturated FAs (PUFAs), such as fish oil, appears to have protective effects against atherosclerosis and heart disease [106, 107]. As FA sensors, PPARs should also be considered when evaluating the distinctly different physiological effects of different FAs owing to small structural variations in FAs and their derivatives [99, 108].

PUFAs are classified as n-3 and n-6 FAs that have opposing effects in the modulation of receptor signaling and gene expression; n-6 (i.e., arachidonic acid [AA])-derived eicosanoids are mostly proactive, whereas n-3 (i.e., eicosapentaenoic acid [EPA])-derived eicosanoids are inhibitory [109]. After the essential FAs linoleic acid (LA, n-6) and α-linolenic acid (LNA, n-3) are consumed, they are further metabolized by various desaturases and elongases to generate long-chain FAs including AA, EPA, and docosahexaenoic acid (DHA; n-3) [110]. AA, EPA, and DHA are then further metabolized by cyclooxygenases, lipoxygenases, and/or epoxygenases to various FA-derived eicosanoids, some of which are listed in Table 2 as PPAR ligands [111]. FAs bind directly to PPARα at physiologically relevant levels and induce transcriptional activation. In fact, unsaturated FAs and PUFAs bind to PPARα in the μM range, which can be achieved by dietary intake [108]. With regard to activation potency, the n-3 FAs EPA and DHA are more potent as in vivo activators of PPARα than n-6 FAs [112–114]. Moreover, various eicosanoids can activate PPARα with a stronger affinity than their PUFA precursors [103, 115, 116]. Recent findings have shown that acylethanolamides (AEs), such as anandamide (AEA), palmitoylethanolamide (PEA), and oleoylethanolamide (OEA), which are biosynthesized in

the gastrointestinal tract, also act as PPARα activators [117]. PPARα activation by OEA results in appetite suppression and lipolysis, whereas activation of PPARα by PEA results in anti-inflammatory effects [118]. Known PPARβ/δ ligands are similar to those for PPARα with much lower levels of activation [108]. PPARγ ligands include unsaturated FAs, such as LA, LNA, CLA, DHA, and EPA, as well as FA derivatives in the physiologically relevant range [119]. Additionally, PPARγ agonists can have systemic anti-inflammatory effects [100]. For example, the prevention of high-fat or high-energy diet-induced adipose tissue inflammation and remodeling by long-chain n-3 PUFAs is reported to involve PPARγ activation [120, 121]. Collectively, various FAs and their derivatives are natural ligands for PPARs, with a fair amount of overlap among the three PPAR subtypes, and these molecules act as metabolic regulators by controlling the PPAR activity. Although many studies have helped to elucidate the role of PPARs in FA-mediated activation, more research is needed to determine the tissue distribution of PPAR subtypes in humans and evaluate the concentration and availability of FAs and their derivatives in human tissues.

3.2. Conjugated Linoleic Acids (CLAs). CLAs are FAs that are mainly found in foods derived from ruminant animals [122]. CLAs are geometrical and positional isomers (cis- or trans-double bond positioning at 7, 9; 8, 10; 9, 11; 10, 12; or 11, 13) of the parent molecule LA (cis-9, cis-12-18:2, n-6). The cis-9, trans-11 (9Z, 11E-octadecenoic acid, C18:2) isomer, also known as rumenic acid, is generated through biohydrogenation of dietary LAs by ruminant microflora and is the most abundant natural CLA isomer (over 75–80% of total CLAs). Due to their multiple health benefits, CLAs are currently being used as dietary supplements for altering body composition in humans and livestock [123, 124]; however, little is known regarding the mechanisms of these beneficial properties of CLAs.

CLA isomers are ligands for PPARα, PPARβ/δ, and PPARγ [125, 126], exhibiting differences in health benefits and PPAR activation [124, 127]. For example, 9Z, 11E-CLA is a potent PPARα ligand in the low nM range and exerts potent anticancer effects [125, 128]. In contrast, 10E, 12Z-CLA causes adipocyte delipidation, IR, and inflammation by acting as a PPARγ antagonist [129]. In addition, a mixture of CLA isomers as well as 9Z, 11Z-CLA and 9Z, 11E-CLA isomers can significantly activate PPARβ/δ in preadipocytes [108]. Thus, there are important cellular mechanisms that are able to differentiate subtle structural changes in various CLA isomers to allow tissue- and species-specific responses [130, 131]. Taken together, these findings support that CLA affects the production of eicosanoids either directly or indirectly, enhances PPARγ activation, attenuates the NF-κB pathway, and directly decreases proinflammatory cytokines to have beneficial effects on inflammation, ultimately influencing metabolic syndrome-related conditions, including obesity, IR, and atherosclerosis [132]. Thus, CLAs can directly exert anti-inflammatory effects by regulating the expression of inflammatory mediators, potentially through NF-κB-dependent and/or PPARγ-dependent pathways [133, 134].

3.3. Flavonoids. Flavonoids are a class of polyphenolic compounds that are secondary plant products [135]. The structure of flavonoids is based on C6-C3-C6, which involves two aromatic rings (A and B) linked to a heterocyclic ring (C) containing one oxygen and three carbons. Flavonoids are classified as flavanols, flavones, flavonols, flavanones, isoflavones, and anthocyanidins according to structural differences in the C ring. Many studies have reported the functionalities of flavonoids. One of the main functionalities of flavonoids is their antioxidant effects, for example, metal chelating activity [136], reactive oxygen species (ROS) scavenging [137, 138], antioxidant enzyme activation [139], and α-tocopherol reduction [140], which collectively result in inhibition of ROS-mediated cellular aging [141], inhibition of mutations [142], anticancer effects [143], inhibition of LDL oxidation and CVDs [144–146], and reduction of ischemic damage [147]. Moreover, many studies have examined the antiobesity effects of flavonoids with regard to energy expenditure and lipid metabolism [148–151]. However, additional studies are needed because the antiobesity effects of flavonoids are still unclear. Thus, in this review, we discuss the effects of flavonoids on PPARγ-mediated obesity based on the role of PPARγ as a master regulator of adipogenesis. Abundant evidence has shown that PPARγ influences the adipogenic transcriptional cascade as a master regulator of adipogenesis [26, 152]. PPARγ is also involved in glucose and cholesterol metabolism. Regulation of PPARγ activation is a primary focus in studies of the control of obesity and type 2 diabetes. TZD, a synthetic ligand for PPARγ activation, is used in the treatment of type 2 diabetes. However, because TZD has major side effects, such as edema, weight gain, and heart failure, many researchers have attempted to identify natural PPARγ activators [153–155]; indeed, identification of effective therapeutic modulators of PPARγ without side effects or with reduced side effects has become a major research focus. Many studies have investigated the therapeutic effects of natural substances owing to the potential or practical negative effects of synthetic medications. Natural substances originating from plants and fruits are traditionally used for the treatment of various diseases. Additionally, the value of natural substances as sources for new drug discovery is increasing because natural substances can be used as a therapeutic strategy to avoid side effects of synthetic drugs [156]. Taken together, these findings highlight the role of natural substances in PPARγ-mediated mechanisms. In this review, we discuss recent reports of the effects of flavonoids on PPAR activity based on an antiobesity perspective.

Recent findings have suggested that dietary flavonoids inhibit adipogenesis during differentiation of preadipocytes and prevent obesity by downregulation of PPARγ expression. Catechin significantly suppresses body fat accumulation and downregulates PPARγ in visceral WAT [5]. Quercetin also downregulates PPARγ in WAT but does not alter the amount of body fat [18]. Notably, most evidence has been reported from *in vitro* studies rather than *in vivo* studies. Several flavonoids, including hesperetin [12], isoflavones [13], licochalcone A [15], luteolin [16], quercetin [19], and tangeritin [21], have been shown to have inhibitory effects on adipogenesis during differentiation of preadipocytes into adipocytes, accompanied by downregulation of PPARγ. Activation of PPARγ induces upregulation of various downstream target genes involved in lipogenesis and FA synthesis. Although it in unclear whether the inhibition of adipocyte differentiation occurs directly through PPARγ activity, it is feasible that flavonoids may effectively inhibit the transcriptional activity of PPARγ by inhibiting adipocyte differentiation via downregulation of PPARγ [13].

Recently, numerous natural substances have been reported to potentially modulate PPARγ activity as a source of PPARγ ligands; the natural compounds involved in mediating these effects have been identified as flavonoids, lignans, and stilbenes [157]. In particular, the role of flavonoids in the regulation of PPARγ activity has been extensively studied owing to the agonist potential of these molecules. Moreover, several studies have reported and highlighted the role of flavonoids as latent PPARγ agonists against GW9662 or T0070907 (PPARγ antagonists) [6–8]. The agonistic effects of flavonoids on PPARγ-mediated obesity, however, vary according to the chemical characteristics of the flavonoids. Some flavonoids selectively modulate PPARγ activity and suppress adipogenesis or obesity [5, 12, 13, 15, 16, 18, 19, 21]. In contrast, other flavonoids promote adipogenesis by activation of PPARγ [6–11, 14, 17, 20], as shown in Table 3. Inhibition of the transcriptional activation of PPARγ by flavonoids is closely related to suppression of adipogenesis [13, 158]. Accordingly, PPARγ activity can be altered through various pathways, including posttranslational modification, ligand type, or ligand-binding domain. For example, inhibition of PPARγ phosphorylation at serine 273 by PPARγ ligands leads to antiobesity effects with fewer side effects because serine 273 phosphorylation prevents the transcription of antiobesity genes [156, 159]. Although flavonoids are known to show agonistic effects toward PPARγ, the detailed molecular mechanisms of their antiobesity effects have not been fully elucidated. Taken together, these findings support the importance of identifying novel flavonoids that modulate PPARγ activity through posttranslational modification, for example, through phosphorylation, in order to improve

Table 3: Summary of recent publications on the effects of flavonoids: adipogenesis and PPARγ activity.

Flavonoid	Model	Effect	PPARγ activity	Ref.
Catechin	Adipocyte differentiation in human bone marrow mesenchymal stem cells High-fat diet- (HFD-) induced obese SD rats	Adipogenesis ↑ Fat ↓	Activity ↑ Not measured	[5, 6]
Daidzein	3T3-L1 preadipocyte differentiation High-fat high-sucrose diet-induced obese C57BL/6J mice	Adipogenesis ↑ Adipocyte area ↓	Activity ↑ Not measured	[7]
Equol	3T3-L1 preadipocyte differentiation	Adipogenesis ↑	Activity ↑	[8]
EGCG	AML-I human preadipocyte differentiation	Adipogenesis ↑	Not measured	[9]
Fisetin	3T3-L1 preadipocyte differentiation	Adipogenesis ↑	Activity ↑	[10]
Flavanone	3T3-L1 preadipocyte differentiation	Adipogenesis ↑	Activity ↑	[11]
Hesperetin glucuronides	3T3-L1 preadipocyte differentiation	Adipogenesis ↓	Not changed	[12]
Isoflavonoids	3T3-L1 preadipocyte differentiation	Adipogenesis ↓	Activity ↓	[13]
Kaempferol	3T3-L1 preadipocyte differentiation	Adipogenesis ↓	Activity ↑	[14]
Licochalcone A	3T3-L1 preadipocyte differentiation HFD-induced obese ICR mice	Adipogenesis ↓ Body weight ↓ Plasma lipid ↓	Not measured Not measured	[15]
Luteolin	3T3-L1 preadipocyte differentiation	Adipogenesis ↓	Not changed	[16]
Pentamethylquercetin	3T3-L1 preadipocyte differentiation	Adipogenesis ↑	Not measured	[17]
Quercetin	HFD-induced obese Wistar rats	Plasma TG ↓	Not changed	[18]
Quercetin-3-O-(6″-Feruloyl)-β-D-galactopyranoside	3T3-L1 preadipocyte differentiation	Adipogenesis ↓	Not changed	[19]
Sakuranetin	3T3-L1 preadipocyte differentiation	Adipogenesis ↑	Not changed	[20]
Tangeritin	3T3-L1 preadipocyte differentiation	Adipogenesis ↓	Not measured	[21]

TG, triglyceride; HFD, high-fat diet.

our understanding of the interactions of flavonoids with PPARγ; such studies are expected to enhance the therapeutic potential of flavonoids. Furthermore, additional studies of the PPAR-dependent effects of flavonoids on tissue-specific events, for example, in the WAT and BAT, are needed. Based on the importance of the tissue-specific roles of PPAR, as demonstrated in this review, future studies may focus on tissue-specific PPAR regulation by flavonoids.

4. Nutrigenetics and PPARγ Polymorphisms

4.1. PPARγ Gene and Polymorphism. PPARα is located on chromosome 22q13.3 and spans 93.15 kb. Single nucleotide polymorphisms (SNPs) in PPARα, that is, L162V, V227A, and intron 7G>C, are associated with metabolic features, such as dyslipidemia, CVD, and type II diabetes [160]. In this review, we have focused on PPARγ SNPs associated with the obesogenic environment because of the limited availability of information regarding the clinical/biological effects of genetic variants in PPARα and PPARβ/δ.

The PPARγ gene, which encodes a TF belonging to the same family of NRs as steroid hormone receptors, is a master regulator of the relationships between nutrients (such as FAs), prostanoids, insulin-sensitizing agents, susceptibility to obesity, control of peptides released from adipocytes, and insulin sensitivity [161]. In macrophages, PPARγ has been shown to regulate the suppression of inflammatory cytokine production and improvement of insulin sensitivity [162].

Alternative promoter regions within the PPARγ gene allow the formation of three PPARγ subtypes: PPARγ1, PPARγ2, and PPARγ3. Although PPARγ1 mRNA has been identified in many tissues, including the heart, liver, skeletal muscle, and adipose tissue, PPARγ2 mRNA is abundantly expressed in adipose tissue, whereas PPARγ3 mRNA is expressed in macrophages, epithelial tissue, and adipose tissue [163]. The PPARγ gene extends over 100 kb and includes nine exons, which give rise to three different PPARγ transcripts with differential promoter usage and differential splicing (PPARγ1, PPARγ2, and PPARγ3). The PPARγ1 and PPARγ2 expressed during the differentiation of 3T3-L1 into adipocytes are derived from two alternative transcripts which share six identical C-terminal exons. Although PPARγ is well known for its role in adipogenesis, it also plays a crucial role in maintaining normal physiology, including insulin sensitization.

This role of PPAR is consistent with many human genetic studies of various single amino acid mutations, such as Pro12Ala, Pro115Gln, Cys114Arg, Cys131Tyr, Cys162Trp, Val290Met, Pro388Leu, Arg425Cyc, C1431T, and Pro467Leu, which are located in several domains [164]. Of these identified mutations in the PPARγ gene, a common polymorphism occurs in the PPARγ2-specific exon B. The Pro12Ala polymorphism rs1801282 (C34G) and the silent C1431T mutation (His449His, CAC478CAT) are frequently observed in PPARγ2. Many mutations in the PPARγ gene are associated with obesity and diabetes-related phenotypes [165]. For example, the Pro115Gln mutation is associated with obesity but not IR, and the mutations Val290Met and Pro467Leu are related to severe IR but not obesity [164]. The CCA-to-GCA missense mutation in codon 12 of exon B of the *PPARγ* gene encodes an NH2-terminal residue that defines the adipocyte-specific *PPARγ2* isoform [166]. Obesity is a multifactorial disorder involving the regulation of food intake and energy expenditure, and ethnicity-dependent-genetic factors play significant pathogenic roles. *PPARγ* genes independently or dependently regulate the transcription of target genes involved in obesity-related processes, such as adipogenesis, IR, angiogenesis, and inflammation, in a tissue-dependent manner. Therefore, *PPARγ2* gene polymorphisms influence obesity in a complex manner, likely involving ethnicity-dependent variations in obesity-related phenotypes.

4.2. The Common Pro115Ala Polymorphism in PPARγ and Obesity. The Pro12Ala polymorphism in PPARγ2 was first identified in 1997, and a point mutation found in the B exon of the NH2-terminal of PPARγ at position 12 (rs1801282) was shown to cause a moderate decrease in the transcription activity and adipogenic potential of this protein [162]. The rare allele frequencies are high in Caucasians (12%) and relatively low in Asians (4% of Japanese and 1% of Chinese) and African Americans (3%) [167]. The Ala allele generated by the Pro12Ala polymorphism is associated with obesity and confers a 25% reduction in the risk of type II diabetes, IR, and CVD in Caucasians [167]. However, although PPARγ is associated with IR and type II diabetes, the 12Ala allele does not reduce the risk of diabetes in South Asians, Chinese, and Malaysians [168, 169]. The 12Pro-161T haplotype is associated with lower body mass index (BMI) and lower fasting serum triglycerides (TGs) in Koreans but not in Iranians [170, 171]. In a meta-analysis of BMI subgroups, the Ala allele was shown to be associated with an increase in 0.96 units for BMIs of 35 or more, and this association was observed in individuals with BMIs of 27 to less than 35 or with BMIs of 35 or more when the meta-analysis was restricted to Caucasians [172]; this pattern was not found in Asians. Further analysis suggested that this discrepancy may be explained by differences in body weight distributions and lifestyles of these ethnic groups [173]. In Italian population, carriers of the *PPARγ2* Ala allele were found to have higher BMIs and fat-mass levels than carriers of the wild-type allele, although a metabolically healthy profile was associated with the *PPARγ2* Ala allele due to the more favorable distribution of adipose tissue. Researchers also found that there was a genetic interaction between Pro12Ala and ACE I/D with regard to BMI and fat mass [174]. According to a gene-diet interaction analysis of the *PPARγ* Pro12Ala polymorphism, there is an inverse association between the PUFA to saturated FA (SFA) ratio (P : S) and BMI/insulin levels in Ala carriers. Because the mean P : S ratio varies by more than 10-fold, for example, from 0.11 in Hungary to 1.2 in Portugal, this ratio may be a more effective stimulator of adipogenesis in Pro carriers than in Ala carriers [175]. This study suggested that when the dietary P : S ratio is low, the BMI in Ala carriers is greater than that in Pro homozygotes. Moreover, although consumption of a PUFA-containing diet does not affect *PPARγ2* mRNA expression, individuals with the Pro12Pro genotype are more

likely to benefit from consumption of a PUFA-containing diet [176]. Similarly, intake of monounsaturated FAs has been shown to have this effect in Ala12 allele carriers. A study in Québec, Canada, showed that total fat and saturated fat intake are positively correlated with body mass change in Pro12 homozygotes, whereas Ala12 allele carriers are protected from this change [177]. Moreover, the Ala12Ala genotype also associated with higher expression of *PPARγ2*, *LPIN1*, and sterol regulatory element-binding protein-1c mRNA compared with that in participants harboring the Pro12Pro genotype. Thus, it is possible that different dietary patterns between ethnic groups could modulate the relationship between BMI and this particular SNP.

Adiponectin, an adipocyte-derived hormone, is encoded by the adipocyte C1q and collagen domain-containing (*ACDC*) gene located in chromosome 3q27. Many studies have shown that adiponectin is reciprocally associated with central and peripheral fat distribution, IR, inflammation, and atherogenic lipid metabolites [178]. In a Danish study, several *ACDC* polymorphisms were found to be associated with body fat distribution, whereas Pro12Ala was found to be associated with body fat accumulation (overall adiposity). Additionally, the CC genotype of SNP-11377, an SNP in the promoter of the *ACDC* gene, was shown to interact with the homozygous Ala12Ala genotype to mediate BMI [179]. Cooperative interactions between the *ACDC* and *PPARγ* genes in the modulation of insulin sensitivity have also been demonstrated in a recent family-based association study, revealing significant interactions between SNP+45T/G of the *ACDC* gene and the Ala12 allele in a Taiwanese population; however, there was no evidence for this associated in the Italian population [180].

Among the SNPs rs10865710 (C-681G), rs7649970 (C-689T), and rs1801282 (C34G, Pro12Ala), the G allele of rs10865710 in the *PPARγ* gene is frequently observed and has been shown to be associated with increased susceptibility to nonalcoholic fatty liver disease (NAFLD) [181]. Despite ethnic differences in the prevalence of NAFLD, the incidence of NAFLD is known to primarily depend on lifestyle, dietary habits, and hepatic metabolic syndrome. Many genetic variations related to the obesogenic environment, including oxidative stress, inflammation, fibrogenic mediators, dyslipidemia, and IR, are involved in the pathogenesis of NAFLD [182]. The A12 allele is associated with lower fasting plasma glucose but does not affect blood pressure, BMI, or other metabolic parameters in Palestinian individuals. However, in obese patients, the 12Ala allele was associated with elevated total plasma cholesterol levels and a tendency toward increased low-density lipoprotein (LDL) cholesterol [183]. The *PPARγ* Pro12Ala polymorphism is associated with a reduced risk of myocardial infarction (MI) according to the Physician's Health Study but confers an increased risk of MI or cardiac death according to the Health Professionals Follow-Up Study [184]. Additionally, we found that the 12Ala variant of PPARγ2 may influence CVD risk by affecting lipid metabolism in obese Palestinian individuals with type II diabetes [184]. Therefore, additional studies of the *PPARγ* Pro12Ala polymorphism are necessary to fully elucidate the role of *PPAR* genetics in obesity independent of CVD, particularly with regard to available pharmacological PPAR-targeted agents.

4.3. The Common C1431T Polymorphism in PPARγ and Obesity. The C1431T polymorphism, also referred to as His447His, His447His, C161T, or CAC478CAT, is a silent mutation located in exon 6 of *PPARγ* and is considered a better predictor of fasting insulin levels and IR than Pro12Ala. The polymorphism C1431T has been shown to be associated with susceptibility to CVDs, diabetes, abnormal leptin concentrations, obesity, and metabolic syndrome and is associated with BMI [185, 186]. Although the C1431T polymorphism has not been extensively studied, the rare T allele has also been inconsistently linked to increases in weight. Because the Pro12Ala and C1431T polymorphisms are in linkage disequilibrium, both rare alleles are associated with increased body weight, and the overall effect is additive when these alleles occur together [187]. In Chinese patients with diabetes, the Pro12Ala and C1431T polymorphisms may not be major etiological factors for type 2 diabetes; however, the C1431T polymorphism is associated with overweightness or obesity, despite the observation that there are no differences in the frequencies of C1431T, Pro12Ala, and their haplotypes between patients with type 2 diabetes and control subjects [188]. Notably, the Ala12 allele is consistently associated with a lower BMI, whereas the T1431 allele is consistently associated with higher BMI in the Scottish nondiabetic population [186]. In contrast, the heterogenotype and Ala homogenotype of *PPARγ* Pro12Ala are significantly associated with higher risk of obesity, whereas the C1431T polymorphism is not significantly associated in individuals from northern India. None of the haplotypes are associated with morbid obesity [189]. In the Korean population, the Pro12Ala and C1431T SNPs have been shown to be associated with some parameters of metabolic syndrome in women [190]. In the EDEN mother-child cohort study, mothers homozygous for the T allele of C1431T were also more obese (24% versus 9%, resp.; $P = 0.035$), and three times more mothers had gestational diabetes (18% versus 6%, resp.; $P = 0.044$). Moreover, the Pro-T haplotype conferred the highest risk of gestational diabetes (odds ratio = 1.89, 95% confidence interval [CI] = 1.05–3.40), whereas the Ala-C haplotype was associated with the lowest risk of gestational diabetes (odds ratio = 0.12, 95% CI = 0.52–1.70) [191]. Additionally, one study showed that both the Pro12Ala and C1431T variants of PPARγ are not associated with metabolic syndrome or obesity in a population from southern India [192]. However, in UK and Chinese individuals with coronary artery disease (CAD), the *PPARγ* C1431T polymorphism is significantly associated with CVD risk factors, such as fasting serum lipid profiles, in the context of variant genotypes (CT + TT) [193, 194]. Angiogram-positive patients carrying the T allele have significantly higher TGs, serum C-reactive protein, and fasting blood glucose levels, and obese patients harboring at least one CAT478 allele have higher leptin levels than other obese patients with similar BMIs, suggesting that the *PPARγ* gene may influence the levels of plasma leptin in obese individuals [195]. Finnish women with both Ala and 478CAT alleles have significantly more fat mass than women with

other alleles. Thus, the CAC478CAT polymorphism is not associated with BMI or other variables related to obesity in different ethnic population. Previous studies on isoflavones have shown their potential antiobesity effects, although the mechanisms are not clear; accordingly, foods containing high levels of isoflavones, such as Korean fermented soy food (*Doenjang*), have been used as functional foods for the treatment or prevention of obesity in Korea [196]. In a clinical study of *Doenjang*, visceral fat area was significantly decreased by *Doenjang* supplementation in individuals with a mutant T allele of *PPARγ2* compared with those harboring a C allele [197], suggesting that *Doenjang* interacted with mutant alleles of *PPARγ2* to exert antiobesity and antioxidative effects in obese individuals.

4.4. Rare PPARγ Polymorphisms and Obesity. The Pro115Gln polymorphism, a very rare gain-of-function mutation in *PPARγ*, is associated with obesity but not IR. Because fibroblasts containing the Pro115Gln mutation accumulate 2.5 times more TGs than the corresponding wild-type cell line, we expected individuals with the Pro115Gln mutation would tend to be obese in field studies. A variant of rare Pro115Gln has been shown to be associated with increased BMI among obese individuals, an effect attributed to constitutive activation of the PPARγ protein, which results in accelerated cell differentiation. Dominant-negative *PPARγ* mutations are associated with severe IR, hypertension, and alterations in lipid profiles (low high-density lipoprotein [HDL], high TGs) [198]. These studies implied that the Pro115Gln polymorphism has pathophysiological relevance in obesity; however, in the nationwide German Epidemiological Field Study, the Pro115Gln polymorphism was shown to have no relevant impact on morbid obesity [199]. The Val290Met and Pro467Leu polymorphisms are the best-characterized dominant-negative mutations of *PPARγ2* and have been shown to dramatically reduce the transcriptional activity of *PPARγ2 in vitro*, resulting in severe IR with increasing fat accumulation, hypertension, and reduced adiponectin levels [165].

Based on these interesting findings from previous studies, we plan to investigate the association of rare or unknown polymorphisms in the *PPARγ2* gene with BMI, obesity, and basal metabolic rates in obese individuals in the future.

5. Conclusion

The modulation of the PPAR activities poses significant impacts on metabolism, irrespective of the modifications that originated from external factors, such as hormones, temperature, excess nutrition, and PPAR-targeted drugs, or from genetic alternations such as polymorphism. Too much activation and too little activation of PPARs are both associated with improper fatty acid handling and maldistribution of fat, which leads to pathogenesis of metabolic diseases. In this review, we intend to provide an integrative view of PPAR regulation by summarizing the recent updates in PPAR regulation in white and brown fat, dietary ligands of PPARs and by incorporating common and rare PPAR polymorphism. We would like to emphasize that PPARs' unique function of depositing extra energy into white adipose tissue and burning out fats in brown/beige adipose tissue and muscle should be balanced for maintaining metabolic health. To reach this goal, wise and prudent usage of natural PPAR ligands through diet could be an option. Also, keen understanding in tissue- and subtype-specific regulation of PPARs is perquisite for the development of drugs to treat metabolic syndrome utilizing PPAR biology. With the advent of "omics era," our knowledge in individual variation in metabolic susceptibility has been tremendously progressed. Therefore, the individual genetic modification of PPARs should be taken into consideration with their environmental modifiers for an innovative approach to prevent obesity such as precision or personalized medicine.

Abbreviations

AA:	Arachidonic acid
ACDC:	Adipocyte C1q and collagen domain containing
ADRB3:	$\beta 3$-Adrenergic receptor
AE:	Acylethanolamide
AEA:	Anandamide
APC:	Adipogenic progenitor cell
BAT:	Brown adipose tissue
BMI:	Body mass index
C/EBP:	CCAAT/enhancer-binding protein
CLA:	Conjugated linoleic acid
CREB:	cAMP-response element-binding protein
CVD:	Cardiovascular disease
DHA:	Docosahexaenoic acid
EPA:	Eicosapentaenoic acid
FA:	Fatty acid
FAS:	Fatty acid synthase
FGF:	Fibroblast growth factor
GR:	Glucocorticoid receptor
IR:	Insulin resistance
IL:	Interleukin
LA:	Linoleic acid
LDL:	Low-density lipoprotein
LNA:	Linolenic acid
LPL:	Lipoprotein lipase
MI:	Myocardial infarction
NAD:	Nicotinamide adenine dinucleotide
NAFLD:	Nonalcoholic fatty liver disease
NF-κB:	Nuclear factor-kappa B
NR:	Nuclear receptor
OEA:	Oleoylethanolamide
PEA:	Palmitoylethanolamide
PGC-1α:	PPARγ coactivator-1 alpha
PPAR:	Peroxisome proliferator-activated receptor
PRDM16:	PR domain-containing protein 16
PUFA:	Polyunsaturated fatty acids
ROS:	Reactive oxygen species
SFA:	Saturated fatty acid
SIRT:	Sir2 homolog
SNP:	Single nucleotide polymorphism
STAT5A:	Signal transducer and activator of transcription 5A
TF:	Transcription factor
TNF-α:	Tumor necrosis factor-α
TZD:	Thiazolidinedione
UCP1:	Uncoupling protein-1
VFA:	Visceral fat area
WAT:	White adipose tissue.

Competing Interests

The authors declare no conflict of interests.

Acknowledgments

This study was funded by National Research Foundation of Korea grant (MSIP: 2014R1A2A1A11049611/1).

References

[1] R. M. Evans, G. D. Barish, and Y.-X. Wang, "PPARs and the complex journey to obesity," *Nature Medicine*, vol. 10, no. 4, pp. 355–361, 2004.

[2] M. Ahmadian, J. M. Suh, N. Hah et al., "PPARγ signaling and metabolism: the good, the bad and the future," *Nature Medicine*, vol. 19, no. 5, pp. 557–566, 2013.

[3] F. A. Monsalve, R. D. Pyarasani, F. Delgado-Lopez, and R. Moore-Carrasco, "Peroxisome proliferator-activated receptor targets for the treatment of metabolic diseases," *Mediators of Inflammation*, vol. 2013, Article ID 549627, 18 pages, 2013.

[4] P. Tontonoz and B. M. Spiegelman, "Fat and beyond: the diverse biology of PPARγ," *Annual Review of Biochemistry*, vol. 77, pp. 289–312, 2008.

[5] J. Yan, Y. Zhao, and B. Zhao, "Green tea catechins prevent obesity through modulation of peroxisome proliferator-activated receptors," *Science China Life Sciences*, vol. 56, no. 9, pp. 804–810, 2013.

[6] D. W. Shin, S. N. Kim, S. M. Lee et al., "(−)-Catechin promotes adipocyte differentiation in human bone marrow mesenchymal stem cells through PPARγ transactivation," *Biochemical Pharmacology*, vol. 77, no. 1, pp. 125–133, 2009.

[7] Y. Sakamoto, A. Naka, N. Ohara, K. Kondo, and K. Iida, "Daidzein regulates proinflammatory adipokines thereby improving obesity-related inflammation through PPARγ," *Molecular Nutrition and Food Research*, vol. 58, no. 4, pp. 718–726, 2014.

[8] K. W. Cho, O.-H. Lee, W. J. Banz, N. Moustaid-Moussa, N. F. Shay, and Y.-C. Kim, "Daidzein and the daidzein metabolite, equol, enhance adipocyte differentiation and PPARγ transcriptional activity," *The Journal of Nutritional Biochemistry*, vol. 21, no. 9, pp. 841–847, 2010.

[9] K. Morikawa, C. Ikeda, M. Nonaka et al., "Epigallocatechin gallate-induced apoptosis does not affect adipocyte conversion of preadipocytes," *Cell Biology International*, vol. 31, no. 11, pp. 1379–1387, 2007.

[10] T. Jin, O. Y. Kim, M.-J. Shin et al., "Fisetin up-regulates the expression of adiponectin in 3t3-L1 adipocytes via the activation of silent mating type information regulation 2 homologue 1 (SIRT1)-deacetylase and peroxisome proliferator-activated receptors (PPARs)," *Journal of Agricultural and Food Chemistry*, vol. 62, no. 43, pp. 10468–10474, 2014.

[11] T. Saito, D. Abe, and K. Sekiya, "Flavanone exhibits PPARγ ligand activity and enhances differentiation of 3T3-L1 adipocytes,"

Biochemical and Biophysical Research Communications, vol. 380, no. 2, pp. 281–285, 2009.

[12] K. Gamo, H. Miyachi, K. Nakamura, and N. Matsuura, "Hesperetin glucuronides induce adipocyte differentiation via activation and expression of peroxisome proliferator-activated receptor-γ," *Bioscience, Biotechnology, and Biochemistry*, vol. 78, no. 6, pp. 1052–1059, 2014.

[13] Q. Sun and G. Chou, "Isoflavonoids from *Crotalaria albida* inhibit adipocyte differentiation and lipid accumulation in 3T3-L1 cells via suppression of PPAR-γ pathway," *PLoS ONE*, vol. 10, no. 8, Article ID e0135893, 2015.

[14] X.-K. Fang, J. Gao, and D.-N. Zhu, "Kaempferol and quercetin isolated from Euonymus alatus improve glucose uptake of 3T3-L1 cells without adipogenesis activity," *Life Sciences*, vol. 82, no. 11-12, pp. 615–622, 2008.

[15] H.-Y. Quan, N. I. Baek, and S. H. Chung, "Licochalcone a prevents adipocyte differentiation and lipogenesis via suppression of peroxisome proliferator-activated receptor γ and sterol regulatory element-binding protein pathways," *Journal of Agricultural and Food Chemistry*, vol. 60, no. 20, pp. 5112–5120, 2012.

[16] H.-S. Park, S.-H. Kim, Y. S. Kim et al., "Luteolin inhibits adipogenic differentiation by regulating PPARc activation," *BioFactors*, vol. 35, no. 4, pp. 373–379, 2009.

[17] L. Chen, T. He, Y. Han et al., "Pentamethylquercetin improves adiponectin expression in differentiated 3T3-L1 cells via a mechanism that implicates PPARγ together with TNF-α and IL-6," *Molecules*, vol. 16, no. 7, pp. 5754–5768, 2011.

[18] S. Wein, N. Behm, R. K. Petersen, K. Kristiansen, and S. Wolfram, "Quercetin enhances adiponectin secretion by a PPAR-γ independent mechanism," *European Journal of Pharmaceutical Sciences*, vol. 41, no. 1, pp. 16–22, 2010.

[19] L. Yang, X.-F. Li, L. Gao, Y.-O. Zhang, and G.-P. Cai, "Suppressive effects of quercetin-3-O-(6″-feruloyl)-β-D- galactopyranoside on adipogenesis in 3T3-L1 preadipocytes through downregulation of PPARγ and C/EBPα expression," *Phytotherapy Research*, vol. 26, no. 3, pp. 438–444, 2012.

[20] T. Saito, D. Abe, and K. Sekiya, "Sakuranetin induces adipogenesis of 3T3-L1 cells through enhanced expression of PPARγ2," *Biochemical and Biophysical Research Communications*, vol. 372, no. 4, pp. 835–839, 2008.

[21] Y. F. He, F. Y. Liu, and W. X. Zhang, "Tangeritin inhibits adipogenesis by down-regulating C/EBPα, C/EBPβ, and PPARγ expression in 3T3-L1 fat cells," *Genetics and Molecular Research*, vol. 14, no. 4, pp. 13642–13648, 2015.

[22] R. Siersbæk, R. Nielsen, and S. Mandrup, "Transcriptional networks and chromatin remodeling controlling adipogenesis," *Trends in Endocrinology & Metabolism*, vol. 23, no. 2, pp. 56–64, 2012.

[23] D. J. Steger, G. R. Grant, M. Schupp et al., "Propagation of adipogenic signals through an epigenomic transition state," *Genes & Development*, vol. 24, no. 10, pp. 1035–1044, 2010.

[24] R. M. Cowherd, R. E. Lyle, and R. E. McGehee Jr., "Molecular regulation of adipocyte differentiation," *Seminars in Cell and Developmental Biology*, vol. 10, no. 1, pp. 3–10, 1999.

[25] E. D. Rosen, P. Sarraf, A. E. Troy et al., "PPARγ is required for the differentiation of adipose tissue in vivo and in vitro," *Molecular Cell*, vol. 4, no. 4, pp. 611–617, 1999.

[26] Z. Wu, E. D. Rosen, R. Brun et al., "Cross-regulation of C/EBPα and PPARγ controls the transcriptional pathway of adipogenesis and insulin sensitivity," *Molecular Cell*, vol. 3, no. 2, pp. 151–158, 1999.

[27] R. P. Brun, P. Tontonoz, B. M. Forman et al., "Differential activation of adipogenesis by multiple PPAR isoforms," *Genes and Development*, vol. 10, no. 8, pp. 974–984, 1996.

[28] P. Tontonoz, E. Hu, and B. M. Spiegelman, "Stimulation of adipogenesis in fibroblasts by PPARγ2, a lipid-activated transcription factor," *Cell*, vol. 79, no. 7, pp. 1147–1156, 1994.

[29] Y. Barak, M. C. Nelson, E. S. Ong et al., "PPARγ is required for placental, cardiac, and adipose tissue development," *Molecular Cell*, vol. 4, no. 4, pp. 585–595, 1999.

[30] S. F. Schmidt, M. Jørgensen, Y. Chen, R. Nielsen, A. Sandelin, and S. Mandrup, "Cross species comparison of C/EBPα and PPARγ profiles in mouse and human adipocytes reveals interdependent retention of binding sites," *BMC Genomics*, vol. 12, article 152, 2011.

[31] M. S. Madsen, R. Siersbæk, M. Boergesen, R. Nielsen, and S. Mandrup, "Peroxisome proliferator-activated receptor γ and C/EBPα synergistically activate key metabolic adipocyte genes by assisted loading," *Molecular and Cellular Biology*, vol. 34, no. 6, pp. 939–954, 2014.

[32] W. Tang, D. Zeve, J. Seo, A.-Y. Jo, and J. M. Graff, "Thiazolidinediones regulate adipose lineage dynamics," *Cell Metabolism*, vol. 14, no. 1, pp. 116–122, 2011.

[33] W. Tang, D. Zeve, J. M. Suh et al., "White fat progenitor cells reside in the adipose vasculature," *Science*, vol. 322, no. 5901, pp. 583–586, 2008.

[34] T. Imai, R. Takakuwa, S. Marchand et al., "Peroxisome proliferator-activated receptor γ is required in mature white and brown adipocytes for their survival in the mouse," *Proceedings of the National Academy of Sciences of the United States of America*, vol. 101, no. 13, pp. 4543–4547, 2004.

[35] K. Tomita, Y. Oike, T. Teratani et al., "Hepatic AdipoR2 signaling plays a protective role against progression of nonalcoholic steatohepatitis in mice," *Hepatology*, vol. 48, no. 2, pp. 458–473, 2008.

[36] A. Tsuchida, T. Yamauchi, S. Takekawa et al., "Peroxisome proliferator-activated receptor (PPAR)α activation increases adiponectin receptors and reduces obesity-related inflammation in adipose tissue: comparison of activation of PPARα, PPARγ, and their combination," *Diabetes*, vol. 54, no. 12, pp. 3358–3370, 2005.

[37] A. N. Hollenberg, V. S. Susulic, J. P. Madura et al., "Functional antagonism between CCAAT/enhancer binding protein-α and peroxisome proliferator-activated receptor-γ on the leptin promoter," *Journal of Biological Chemistry*, vol. 272, no. 8, pp. 5283–5290, 1997.

[38] J. W. Jonker, J. M. Suh, A. R. Atkins et al., "A PPARγ-FGF1 axis is required for adaptive adipose remodelling and metabolic homeostasis," *Nature*, vol. 485, no. 7398, pp. 391–394, 2012.

[39] T. Coskun, H. A. Bina, M. A. Schneider et al., "Fibroblast growth factor 21 corrects obesity in mice," *Endocrinology*, vol. 149, no. 12, pp. 6018–6027, 2008.

[40] P. A. Dutchak, T. Katafuchi, A. L. Bookout et al., "Fibroblast growth factor-21 regulates PPARγ activity and the antidiabetic actions of thiazolidinediones," *Cell*, vol. 148, no. 3, pp. 556–567, 2012.

[41] T. Tomaru, D. J. Steger, M. I. Lefterova, M. Schupp, and M. A. Lazar, "Adipocyte-specific expression of murine resistin is mediated by synergism between peroxisome proliferator-activated receptor γ and CCAAT/enhancer-binding proteins," *Journal of Biological Chemistry*, vol. 284, no. 10, pp. 6116–6125, 2009.

[42] Y. Hou, F. Moreau, and K. Chadee, "PPARγ is an E3 ligase that induces the degradation of NFκB/p65," *Nature Communications*, vol. 3, article 1300, 2012.

[43] J. Ye, "Regulation of PPARγ function by TNF-α," *Biochemical and Biophysical Research Communications*, vol. 374, no. 3, pp. 405–408, 2008.

[44] A. Okuno, H. Tamemoto, K. Tobe et al., "Troglitazone increases the number of small adipocytes without the change of white adipose tissue mass in obese Zucker rats," *Journal of Clinical Investigation*, vol. 101, no. 6, pp. 1354–1361, 1998.

[45] P. Arner, "The adipocyte in insulin resistance: key molecules and the impact of the thiazolidinediones," *Trends in Endocrinology and Metabolism*, vol. 14, no. 3, pp 137–145, 2003.

[46] P. G. Blanchard, V. Turcotte, M. Cote et al., "Peroxisome proliferator-activated receptor γ activation favours selective subcutaneous lipid deposition by coordinately regulating lipoprotein lipase modulators, fatty acid transporters and lipogenic enzymes," *Acta Physiologica*, vol. 217, no. 3, pp. 227–239, 2016.

[47] M. Laplante, W. T. Festuccia, G. Soucy et al., "Tissue-specific postprandial clearance is the major determinant of PPARγ-induced triglyceride lowering in the rat," *American Journal of Physiology—Regulatory Integrative and Comparative Physiology*, vol. 296, no. 1, pp. R57–R66, 2009.

[48] S. Chatterjee, A. Majumder, and S. Ray, "Observational study of effects of saroglitazar on glycaemic and lipid parameters on indian patients with type 2 diabetes," *Scientific Reports*, vol. 5, article 7706, 2015.

[49] R. H. Jani, V. Pai, P. Jha et al., "A multicenter, prospective, randomized, double-blind study to evaluate the safety and efficacy of Saroglitazar 2 and 4 mg compared with placebo in type 2 diabetes mellitus patients having hypertriglyceridemia not controlled with atorvastatin therapy (PRESS VI)," *Diabetes Technology & Therapeutics*, vol. 16, no. 2, pp. 63–71, 2014.

[50] S. G. Kim, D. M. Kim, J.-T. Woo et al., "Efficacy and safety of lobeglitazone monotherapy in patients with type 2 diabetes mellitus over 24-weeks: a multicenter, randomized, double-blind, parallel-group, placebo controlled trial," *PLoS ONE*, vol. 9, no. 4, Article ID e92843, 2014.

[51] S. H. Kim, S. G. Kim, D. M. Kim et al., "Safety and efficacy of lobeglitazone monotherapy in patients with type 2 diabetes mellitus over 52 weeks: an open-label extension study," *Diabetes Research and Clinical Practice*, vol. 110, no. 3, pp. e27–e30, 2015.

[52] J. Wu, P. Boström, L. M. Sparks et al., "Beige adipocytes are a distinct type of thermogenic fat cell in mouse and human," *Cell*, vol. 150, no. 2, pp. 366–376, 2012.

[53] B. B. Lowell and B. M. Spiegelman, "Towards a molecular understanding of adaptive thermogenesis," *Nature*, vol. 404, no. 6778, pp. 652–660, 2000.

[54] A. M. Cypess, A. P. White, C. Vernochet et al., "Anatomical localization, gene expression profiling and functional characterization of adult human neck brown fat," *Nature Medicine*, vol. 19, no. 5, pp. 635–639, 2013.

[55] P. Seale, B. Bjork, W. Yang et al., "PRDM16 controls a brown fat/skeletal muscle switch," *Nature*, vol. 454, no. 7207, pp. 961–967, 2008.

[56] P. Seale, S. Kajimura, W. Yang et al., "Transcriptional control of brown fat determination by PRDM16," *Cell Metabolism*, vol. 6, no. 1, pp. 38–54, 2007.

[57] M. Rosenwald, A. Perdikari, T. Rülicke, and C. Wolfrum, "Bi-directional interconversion of brite and white adipocytes," *Nature Cell Biology*, vol. 15, no. 6, pp. 659–667, 2013.

[58] M. Rosenwald and C. Wolfrum, "The origin and definition of brite versus white and classical brown adipocytes," *Adipocyte*, vol. 3, no. 1, pp. 4–9, 2014.

[59] L. Z. Sharp, K. Shinoda, H. Ohno et al., "Human BAT possesses molecular signatures that resemble beige/brite cells," *PLoS ONE*, vol. 7, no. 11, Article ID e49452, 2012.

[60] W. D. Van Marken Lichtenbelt, J. W. Vanhommerig, N. M. Smulders et al., "Cold-activated brown adipose tissue in healthy men," *The New England Journal of Medicine*, vol. 360, no. 15, pp. 1500–1508, 2009.

[61] L. Ye, J. Wu, P. Cohen et al., "Fat cells directly sense temperature to activate thermogenesis," *Proceedings of the National Academy of Sciences of the United States of America*, vol. 110, no. 30, pp. 12480–12485, 2013.

[62] B. K. Pedersen and M. A. Febbraio, "Muscles, exercise and obesity: skeletal muscle as a secretory organ," *Nature Reviews Endocrinology*, vol. 8, no. 8, pp. 457–465, 2012.

[63] I. B. Sears, M. A. MacGinnitie, L. G. Kovacs, and R. A. Graves, "Differentiation-dependent expression of the brown adipocyte uncoupling protein gene: regulation by peroxisome proliferator-activated receptor gamma," *Molecular and Cellular Biology*, vol. 16, no. 7, pp. 3410–3419, 1996.

[64] S. L. Gray, E. Dalla Nora, E. C. Backlund et al., "Decreased brown adipocyte recruitment and thermogenic capacity in mice with impaired peroxisome proliferator-activated receptor (P465L PPARγ) function," *Endocrinology*, vol. 147, no. 12, pp. 5708–5714, 2006.

[65] S. Rajakumari, J. Wu, J. Ishibashi et al., "EBF2 determines and maintains brown adipocyte identity," *Cell Metabolism*, vol. 17, no. 4, pp. 562–574, 2013.

[66] M. S. Siersbæk, A. Loft, M. M. Aagaard et al., "Genome-wide profiling of peroxisome proliferator-activated receptor γ in primary epididymal, inguinal, and brown adipocytes reveals depot-selective binding correlated with gene expression," *Molecular and Cellular Biology*, vol. 32, no. 17, pp. 3452–3463, 2012.

[67] S. Bartesaghi, S. Hallen, L. Huang et al., "Thermogenic activity of UCP1 in human white fat-derived beige adipocytes," *Molecular Endocrinology*, vol. 29, no. 1, pp. 130–139, 2015.

[68] L. Wilson-Fritch, A. Burkart, G. Bell et al., "Mitochondrial biogenesis and remodeling during adipogenesis and in response to the insulin sensitizer rosiglitazone," *Molecular and Cellular Biology*, vol. 23, no. 3, pp. 1085–1094, 2003.

[69] L. Wilson-Fritch, S. Nicoloro, M. Chouinard et al., "Mitochondrial remodeling in adipose tissue associated with obesity and treatment with rosiglitazone," *Journal of Clinical Investigation*, vol. 114, no. 9, pp. 1281–1289, 2004.

[70] J. X. Rong, Y. Qiu, M. K. Hansen et al., "Adipose mitochondrial biogenesis is suppressed in db/db and high-fat diet-fed mice and improved by rosiglitazone," *Diabetes*, vol. 56, no. 7, pp. 1751–1760, 2007.

[71] N. Petrovic, I. G. Shabalina, J. A. Timmons, B. Cannon, and J. Nedergaard, "Thermogenically competent nonadrenergic recruitment in brown preadipocytes by a PPARγ agonist," *American Journal of Physiology: Endocrinology and Metabolism*, vol. 295, no. 2, pp. E287–E296, 2008.

[72] N. Petrovic, T. B. Walden, I. G. Shabalina, J. A. Timmons, B. Cannon, and J. Nedergaard, "Chronic peroxisome proliferator-activated receptor γ (PPARγ) activation of epididymally derived white adipocyte cultures reveals a population of thermogenically competent, UCP1-containing adipocytes molecularly

distinct from classic brown adipocytes," *The Journal of Biological Chemistry*, vol. 285, no. 10, pp. 7153–7164, 2010.

[73] Y. Fukui, S.-I. Masui, S. Osada, K. Umesono, and K. Motojima, "A new thiazolidinedione, NC-2100, which is a weak PPAR-γ activator, exhibits potent antidiabetic effects and induces uncoupling protein 1 in white adipose tissue of KKAy obese mice," *Diabetes*, vol. 49, no. 5, pp. 759–767, 2000.

[74] H. Ohno, K. Shinoda, B. M. Spiegelman, and S. Kajimura, "PPARγ agonists induce a white-to-brown fat conversion through stabilization of PRDM16 protein," *Cell Metabolism*, vol. 15, no. 3, pp. 395–404, 2012.

[75] W. T. Festuccia, P.-G. Blanchard, V. Turcotte et al., "The PPARγ agonist rosiglitazone enhances rat brown adipose tissue lipogenesis from glucose without altering glucose uptake," *American Journal of Physiology—Regulatory Integrative and Comparative Physiology*, vol. 296, no. 5, pp. R1327–R1335, 2009.

[76] W. T. Festuccia, S. Oztezcan, M. Laplante et al., "Peroxisome proliferator-activated receptor-γ-mediated positive energy balance in the rat is associated with reduced sympathetic drive to adipose tissues and thyroid status," *Endocrinology*, vol. 149, no. 5, pp. 2121–2130, 2008.

[77] E. Bakopanos and J. E. Silva, "Thiazolidinediones inhibit the expression of β3-adrenergic receptors at a transcriptional level," *Diabetes*, vol. 49, no. 12, pp. 2108–2115, 2000.

[78] L. Qiang, L. Wang, N. Kon et al., "Brown remodeling of white adipose tissue by SirT1-dependent deacetylation of Pparγ," *Cell*, vol. 150, no. 3, pp. 620–632, 2012.

[79] T. L. Rachid, A. Penna-de-Carvalho, I. Bringhenti, M. B. Aguila, C. A. Mandarim-de-Lacerda, and V. Souza-Mello, "Fenofibrate (PPARalpha agonist) induces beige cell formation in subcutaneous white adipose tissue from diet-induced male obese mice," *Molecular and Cellular Endocrinology*, vol. 402, pp. 86–94, 2015.

[80] P. Boström, J. Wu, M. P. Jedrychowski et al., "A PGC1-α-dependent myokine that drives brown-fat-like development of white fat and thermogenesis," *Nature*, vol. 481, no. 7382, pp. 463–468, 2012.

[81] A. Fredenrich and P. A. Grimaldi, "PPAR delta: an uncompletely known nuclear receptor," *Diabetes and Metabolism*, vol. 31, no. 1, pp. 23–27, 2005.

[82] Q. A. Wang and P. E. Scherer, "The AdipoChaser mouse: a model tracking adipogenesis in vivo," *Adipocyte*, vol. 3, no. 2, pp. 146–150, 2014.

[83] Q. A. Wang, C. Tao, R. K. Gupta, and P. E. Scherer, "Tracking adipogenesis during white adipose tissue development, expansion and regeneration," *Nature Medicine*, vol. 19, no. 10, pp. 1338–1344, 2013.

[84] J. R. Brestoff, B. S. Kim, S. A. Saenz et al., "Group 2 innate lymphoid cells promote beiging of white adipose tissue and limit obesity," *Nature*, vol. 519, no. 7542, pp. 242–246, 2015.

[85] M.-W. Lee, J. I. Odegaard, L. Mukundan et al., "Activated type 2 innate lymphoid cells regulate beige fat biogenesis," *Cell*, vol. 160, no. 1-2, pp. 74–87, 2015.

[86] K. D. Nguyen, Y. Qiu, X. Cui et al., "Alternatively activated macrophages produce catecholamines to sustain adaptive thermogenesis," *Nature*, vol. 480, no. 7375, pp. 104–108, 2011.

[87] Y. Qiu, K. D. Nguyen, J. I. Odegaard et al., "Eosinophils and type 2 cytokine signaling in macrophages orchestrate development of functional beige fat," *Cell*, vol. 157, no. 6, pp. 1292–1308, 2014.

[88] A. Bartelt, O. T. Bruns, R. Reimer et al., "Brown adipose tissue activity controls triglyceride clearance," *Nature Medicine*, vol. 17, no. 2, pp. 200–205, 2011.

[89] P. A. Kern, B. S. Finlin, B. Zhu et al., "The effects of temperature and seasons on subcutaneous white adipose tissue in humans: evidence for thermogenic gene induction," *The Journal of Clinical Endocrinology & Metabolism*, vol. 99, no. 12, pp. E2772–E2779, 2014.

[90] M. Matsushita, T. Yoneshiro, S. Aita, T. Kameya, H. Sugie, and M. Saito, "Impact of brown adipose tissue on body fatness and glucose metabolism in healthy humans," *International Journal of Obesity*, vol. 38, no. 6, pp. 812–817, 2014.

[91] T. Yoneshiro, S. Aita, M. Matsushita et al., "Age-related decrease in cold-activated brown adipose tissue and accumulation of body fat in healthy humans," *Obesity*, vol. 19, no. 9, pp. 1755–1760, 2011.

[92] J. Bae, J. Chen, and L. Zhao, "Chronic activation of pattern recognition receptors suppresses brown adipogenesis of multipotent mesodermal stem cells and brown pre-adipocytes," *Biochemistry and Cell Biology*, vol. 93, no. 3, pp. 251–261, 2015.

[93] M. d. Ibarra-Lara, M. Sánchez-Aguilar, E. Soria et al., "Peroxisome proliferator-activated receptors (PPAR) downregulate the expression of pro-inflammatory molecules in an experimental model of myocardial infarction," *Canadian Journal of Physiology and Pharmacology*, vol. 94, no. 6, pp. 634–642, 2016.

[94] E. L. Schiffrin and P. Paradis, "Suppression of peroxisome proliferator-activated receptor-γ activity by angiotensin II in vascular smooth muscle involves Bcr kinase: the fire that drowns the water," *Circulation Research*, vol. 104, no. 1, pp. 4–6, 2009.

[95] A. H. V. Remels, R. C. J. Langen, H. R. Gosker et al., "PPARγ inhibits NF-κB-dependent transcriptional activation in skeletal muscle," *American Journal of Physiology—Endocrinology and Metabolism*, vol. 297, no. 1, pp. E174–E183, 2009.

[96] M. Okla, W. Wang, I. Kang, A. Pashaj, T. Carr, and S. Chung, "Activation of Toll-like receptor 4 (TLR4) attenuates adaptive thermogenesis via endoplasmic reticulum stress," *The Journal of Biological Chemistry*, vol. 290, no. 44, pp. 26476–26490, 2015.

[97] T. Goto, S. Naknukool, R. Yoshitake et al., "Proinflammatory cytokine interleukin-1β suppresses cold-induced thermogenesis in adipocytes," *Cytokine*, vol. 77, pp. 107–114, 2016.

[98] S. Hirai, N. Takahashi, T. Goto et al., "Functional food targeting the regulation of obesity-induced inflammatory responses and pathologies," *Mediators of Inflammation*, vol. 2010, Article ID 367838, 8 pages, 2010.

[99] T. Varga, Z. Czimmerer, and L. Nagy, "PPARs are a unique set of fatty acid regulated transcription factors controlling both lipid metabolism and inflammation," *Biochimica et Biophysica Acta (BBA)—Molecular Basis of Disease*, vol. 1812, no. 8, pp. 1007–1022, 2011.

[100] H. Martin, "Role of PPAR-gamma in inflammation. Prospects for therapeutic intervention by food components," *Mutation Research*, vol. 669, no. 1-2, pp. 1–7, 2009.

[101] B. M. Forman, J. Chen, and R. M. Evans, "Hypolipidemic drugs, polyunsaturated fatty acids, and eicosanoids are ligands for peroxisome proliferator-activated receptors α and δ," *Proceedings of the National Academy of Sciences of the United States of America*, vol. 94, no. 9, pp. 4312–4317, 1997.

[102] S. A. Kliewer, S. S. Sundseth, S. A. Jones et al., "Fatty acids and eicosanoids regulate gene expression through direct interactions with peroxisome proliferator-activated receptors α and γ," *Proceedings of the National Academy of Sciences of the United States of America*, vol. 94, no. 9, pp. 4318–4323, 1997.

[103] V. R. Narala, R. K. Adapala, M. V. Suresh, T. G. Brock, M. Peters-Golden, and R. C. Reddy, "Leukotriene B4 is a

physiologically relevant endogenous peroxisome proliferator-activated receptor-α agonist," *Journal of Biological Chemistry*, vol. 285, no. 29, pp. 22067–22074, 2010.

[104] G. Krey, O. Braissant, F. L'Horset et al., "Fatty acids, eicosanoids, and hypolipidemic agents identified as ligands of peroxisome proliferator-activated receptors by coactivator-dependent receptor ligand assay," *Molecular Endocrinology*, vol. 11, no. 6, pp. 779–791, 1997.

[105] G. M. Reaven and A. Laws, "Insulin resistance, compensatory hyperinsulinaemia, and coronary heart disease," *Diabetologia*, vol. 37, no. 9, pp. 948–952, 1994.

[106] M. Y. Abeywardena and R. J. Head, "Longchain n-3 polyunsaturated fatty acids and blood vessel function," *Cardiovascular Research*, vol. 52, no. 3, pp. 361–371, 2001.

[107] R. De Caterina and A. Zampolli, "n-3 fatty acids: antiatherosclerotic effects," *Lipids*, vol. 36, supplement, pp. S69–S78, 2001.

[108] S. A. Khan and J. P. Vanden Heuvel, "Role of nuclear receptors in the regulation of gene expression by dietary fatty acids," *The Journal of Nutritional Biochemistry*, vol. 14, no. 10, pp. 554–567, 2003.

[109] G. Schmitz and J. Ecker, "The opposing effects of n-3 and n-6 fatty acids," *Progress in Lipid Research*, vol. 47, no. 2, pp. 147–155, 2008.

[110] J. R. Marszalek and H. F. Lodish, "Docosahexaenoic acid, fatty acid-interacting proteins, and neuronal function: breastmilk and fish are good for you," *Annual Review of Cell and Developmental Biology*, vol. 21, pp. 633–657, 2005.

[111] W. Wahli and L. Michalik, "PPARs at the crossroads of lipid signaling and inflammation," *Trends in Endocrinology and Metabolism*, vol. 23, no. 7, pp. 351–363, 2012.

[112] C. Couet, J. Delarue, P. Ritz et al., "Effect of dietary fish oil on body fat mass and basal fat oxidation in healthy adults," *International Journal of Obesity and Related Metabolic Disorders*, vol. 21, no. 8, pp. 637–643, 1997.

[113] T. A. Mori, D. Q. Bao, V. Burke, I. B. Puddey, G. F. Watts, and L. J. Beilin, "Dietary fish as a major component of a weight-loss diet: effect on serum lipids, glucose, and insulin metabolism in over-weight hypertensive subjects," *American Journal of Clinical Nutrition*, vol. 70, no. 5, pp. 817–825, 1999.

[114] G. W. Power and E. A. Newsholme, "Dietary fatty acids influence the activity and metabolic control of mitochondrial carnitine palmitoyltransferase I in rat heart and skeletal muscle," *Journal of Nutrition*, vol. 127, no. 11, pp. 2142–2150, 1997.

[115] P. R. Devchand, H. Keller, J. M. Peters, M. Vazquez, F. J. Gonzalez, and W. Wahli, "The PPARα-leukotriene B4 pathway to inflammation control," *Nature*, vol. 384, no. 6604, pp. 39–43, 1996.

[116] K. Yu, W. Bayona, C. B. Kallen et al., "Differential activation of peroxisome proliferator-activated receptors by eicosanoids," *The Journal of Biological Chemistry*, vol. 270, no. 41, pp. 23975–23983, 1995.

[117] F. Borrelli and A. A. Izzo, "Role of acylethanolamides in the gastrointestinal tract with special reference to food intake and energy balance," *Best Practice and Research: Clinical Endocrinology and Metabolism*, vol. 23, no. 1, pp. 33–49, 2009.

[118] S. E. O'Sullivan, "Cannabinoids go nuclear: evidence for activation of peroxisome proliferator-activated receptors," *British Journal of Pharmacology*, vol. 152, no. 5, pp. 576–582, 2007.

[119] T. Waku, T. Shiraki, T. Oyama et al., "Structural insight into PPARγ activation through covalent modification with endogenous fatty acids," *Journal of Molecular Biology*, vol. 385, no. 1, pp. 188–199, 2009.

[120] J. Huber, M. Löffler, M. Bilban et al., "Prevention of high-fat diet-induced adipose tissue remodeling in obese diabetic mice by n-3 polyunsaturated fatty acids," *International Journal of Obesity*, vol. 31, no. 6, pp. 1004–1013, 2007.

[121] J. Todoric, M. Löffler, J. Huber et al., "Adipose tissue inflammation induced by high-fat diet in obese diabetic mice is prevented by n-3 polyunsaturated fatty acids," *Diabetologia*, vol. 49, no. 9, pp. 2109–2119, 2006.

[122] M. W. Pariza and Y. L. Ha, "Conjugated dienoic derivatives of linoleic acid: a new class of anticarcinogens," *Medical Oncology and Tumor Pharmacotherapy*, vol. 7, no. 2-3, pp. 169–171, 1990.

[123] Y. Park, K. J. Albright, W. Liu, J. M. Storkson, M. E. Cook, and M. W. Pariza, "Effect of conjugated linoleic acid on body composition in mice," *Lipids*, vol. 32, no. 8, pp. 853–858, 1997.

[124] Y. Park, J. M. Storkson, K. J. Albright, W. Liu, and M. W. Pariza, "Evidence that the trans-10,cis-12 isomer of conjugated linoleic acid induces body composition changes in mice," *Lipids*, vol. 34, no. 3, pp. 235–241, 1999.

[125] S. Y. Moya-Camarena, J. P. Vanden Heuvel, S. G. Blanchard, L. A. Leesnitzer, and M. A. Belury, "Conjugated linoleic acid is a potent naturally occurring ligand and activator of PPARα," *Journal of Lipid Research*, vol. 40, no. 8, pp. 1426–1433, 1999.

[126] Y. Yu, P. H. Correll, and J. P. Vanden Heuvel, "Conjugated linoleic acid decreases production of pro-inflammatory products in macrophages: evidence for a PPARγ-dependent mechanism," *Biochimica et Biophysica Acta (BBA)—Molecular and Cell Biology of Lipids*, vol. 1581, no. 3, pp. 89–99, 2002.

[127] A. Truitt, G. McNeill, and J. Y. Vanderhoek, "Antiplatelet effects of conjugated linoleic acid isomers," *Biochimica et Biophysica Acta—Molecular and Cell Biology of Lipids*, vol. 1438, no. 2, pp. 239–246, 1999.

[128] C. Ip, Y. Dong, H. J. Thompson, D. E. Bauman, and M. M. Ip, "Control of rat mammary epithelium proliferation by conjugated linoleic acid," *Nutrition and Cancer*, vol. 39, no. 2, pp. 233–238, 2001.

[129] A. Kennedy, S. Chung, K. LaPoint, O. Fabiyi, and M. K. McIntosh, "Trans-10, cis-12 conjugated linoleic acid antagonizes ligand-dependent PPARγ activity in primary cultures of human adipocytes," *Journal of Nutrition*, vol. 138, no. 3, pp. 455–461, 2008.

[130] D. B. Jump, "Dietary polyunsaturated fatty acids and regulation of gene transcription," *Current Opinion in Lipidology*, vol. 13, no. 2, pp. 155–164, 2002.

[131] D. B. Jump and S. D. Clarke, "Regulation of gene expression by dietary fat," *Annual Review of Nutrition*, vol. 19, pp. 63–90, 1999.

[132] M. A. Zulet, A. Marti, M. D. Parra, and J. A. Martínez, "Inflammation and conjugated linoleic acid: mechanisms of action and implications for human health," *Journal of Physiology and Biochemistry*, vol. 61, no. 3, pp. 483–494, 2005.

[133] C. E. Loscher, E. Draper, O. Leavy, D. Kelleher, K. H. G. Mills, and H. M. Roche, "Conjugated linoleic acid suppresses NF-kappa B activation and IL-12 production in dendritic cells through ERK-mediated IL-10 induction," *The Journal of Immunology*, vol. 175, no. 8, pp. 4990–4998, 2005.

[134] M. Luongo, B. Knotek, and L. Biel, "Peritoneal dialysis nurse resource guide," *Nephrology Nursing Journal*, vol. 30, no. 5, pp. 535–564, 2003.

[135] B. Winkel-Shirley, "Flavonoid biosynthesis. A colorful model for genetics, biochemistry, cell biology, and biotechnology," *Plant Physiology*, vol. 126, no. 2, pp. 485–493, 2001.

[136] M. Ferrali, C. Signorini, B. Caciotti et al., "Protection against oxidative damage of erythrocyte membrane by the flavonoid quercetin and its relation to iron chelating activity," *FEBS Letters*, vol. 416, no. 2, pp. 123–129, 1997.

[137] L. G. Korkina and I. B. Afanas'ev, "Antioxidant and chelating properties of flavonoids," *Advances in Pharmacology*, vol. 38, pp. 151–163, 1996.

[138] R. Hirano, W. Sasamoto, A. Matsumoto, H. Itakura, O. Igarashi, and K. Kondo, "Antioxidant ability of various flavonoids against DPPH radicals and LDL oxidation," *Journal of Nutritional Science and Vitaminology*, vol. 47, no. 5, pp. 357–362, 2001.

[139] A. J. Elliott, S. A. Scheiber, C. Thomas, and R. S. Pardini, "Inhibition of glutathione reductase by flavonoids. A structure-activity study," *Biochemical Pharmacology*, vol. 44, no. 8, pp. 1603–1608, 1992.

[140] K. E. Heim, A. R. Tagliaferro, and D. J. Bobilya, "Flavonoid antioxidants: chemistry, metabolism and structure-activity relationships," *Journal of Nutritional Biochemistry*, vol. 13, no. 10, pp. 572–584, 2002.

[141] J. Sastre, F. V. Pallardö, and J. Viña, "Mitochondrial oxidative stress plays a key role in aging and apoptosis," *IUBMB Life*, vol. 49, no. 5, pp. 427–435, 2000.

[142] W. Takabe, E. Niki, K. Uchida, S. Yamada, K. Satoh, and N. Noguchi, "Oxidative stress promotes the development of transformation: Involvement of a potent mutagenic lipid peroxidation product, acrolein," *Carcinogenesis*, vol. 22, no. 6, pp. 935–941, 2001.

[143] S. Kawanishi, Y. Hiraku, and S. Oikawa, "Mechanism of guanine-specific DNA damage by oxidative stress and its role in carcinogenesis and aging," *Mutation Research*, vol. 488, no. 1, pp. 65–76, 2001.

[144] K. Kondo, R. Hirano, A. Matsumoto, O. Igarashi, and H. Itakura, "Inhibition of LDL oxidation by cocoa," *The Lancet*, vol. 348, no. 9040, p. 1514, 1996.

[145] A. Mazur, D. Bayle, C. Lab, E. Rock, and Y. Rayssiguier, "Inhibitory effect of procyanidin-rich extracts on LDL oxidation in vitro," *Atherosclerosis*, vol. 145, no. 2, pp. 421–422, 1999.

[146] M. A. Khan and A. Baseer, "Increased malondialdehyde levels in coronary heart disease," *Journal of the Pakistan Medical Association*, vol. 50, no. 8, pp. 261–264, 2000.

[147] R. M. Facino, M. Carini, G. Aldini et al., "Diet enriched with procyanidins enhances antioxidant activity and reduces myocardial post-ischaemic damage in rats," *Life Sciences*, vol. 64, no. 8, pp. 627–642, 1999.

[148] P. Chantre and D. Lairon, "Recent findings of green tea extract AR25 (exolise) and its activity for the treatment of obesity," *Phytomedicine*, vol. 9, no. 1, pp. 3–8, 2002.

[149] S. Wang, S. K. Noh, and S. I. Koo, "Green tea catechins inhibit pancreatic phospholipase A_2 and intestinal absorption of lipids in ovariectomized rats," *The Journal of Nutritional Biochemistry*, vol. 17, no. 7, pp. 492–498, 2006.

[150] A. G. Dulloo, C. Duret, D. Rohrer et al., "Efficacy of a green tea extract rich in catechin polyphenols and caffeine in increasing 24-h energy expenditure and fat oxidation in humans," *American Journal of Clinical Nutrition*, vol. 70, no. 6, pp. 1040–1045, 1999.

[151] M. L. Bertoia, E. B. Rimm, K. J. Mukamal et al., "Dietary flavonoid intake and weight maintenance: three prospective cohorts of 124,086 US men and women followed for up to 24 years," *BMJ*, vol. 352, article i17, 2016.

[152] E. D. Rosen, C.-H. Hsu, X. Wang et al., "C/EBPα induces adipogenesis through PPARγ: a unified pathway," *Genes and Development*, vol. 16, no. 1, pp. 22–26, 2002.

[153] R. M. Lago, P. P. Singh, and R. W. Nesto, "Congestive heart failure and cardiovascular death in patients with prediabetes and type 2 diabetes given thiazolidinediones: a meta-analysis of randomised clinical trials," *The Lancet*, vol. 370, no. 9593, pp. 1129–1136, 2007.

[154] S. Mudaliar, A. R. Chang, and R. R. Henry, "Thiazolidinediones, peripheral edema, and type 2 diabetes: incidence, pathophysiology, and clinical implications," *Endocrine Practice*, vol. 9, no. 5, pp. 406–416, 2003.

[155] R. W. Nesto, D. Bell, R. O. Bonow et al., "Thiazolidinedione use, fluid retention, and congestive heart failure: a consensus statement from the American Heart Association and American Diabetes Association," *Diabetes Care*, vol. 27, no. 1, pp. 256–263, 2004.

[156] C. Weidner, J. C. de Groot, A. Prasad et al., "Amorfrutins are potent antidiabetic dietary natural products," *Proceedings of the National Academy of Sciences of the United States of America*, vol. 109, no. 19, pp. 7257–7262, 2012.

[157] L. Wang, B. Waltenberger, E.-M. Pferschy-Wenzig et al., "Natural product agonists of peroxisome proliferator-activated receptor gamma (PPARγ): a review," *Biochemical Pharmacology*, vol. 92, no. 1, pp. 73–89, 2014.

[158] Y. Zhang, L. Yu, W. Cai et al., "Protopanaxatriol, a novel PPAR γ antagonist from Panax ginseng, alleviates steatosis in mice," *Scientific Reports*, vol. 4, article 7375, 2014.

[159] R. H. Houtkooper and J. Auwerx, "Obesity: new life for antidiabetic drugs," *Nature*, vol. 466, no. 7305, pp. 443–444, 2010.

[160] A. V. Contreras, N. Torres, and A. R. Tovar, "PPAR-α as a key nutritional and environmental sensor for metabolic adaptation," *Advances in Nutrition*, vol. 4, no. 4, pp. 439–452, 2013.

[161] R. Stienstra, C. Duval, M. Müller, and S. Kersten, "PPARs, obesity, and inflammation," *PPAR Research*, vol. 2007, Article ID 95974, 10 pages, 2007.

[162] W. He, "Polymorphism and human health," *PPAR Research*, vol. 2009, Article ID 849538, 15 pages, 2009.

[163] I. Barroso, M. Gurnell, V. E. F. Crowley et al., "Dominant negative mutations in human PPARγ associated with severe insulin resistance, diabetes mellitus and hypertension," *Nature*, vol. 402, no. 6764, pp. 880–883, 1999.

[164] M. Laakso, "Mutations in PPARr gene relevant for the diabetes and the metabolic syndrome," in *Nutritional Genomics: Impact on Health and Disease*, H. G. J. R. Brigelius-Flohe, Ed., pp. 195–205, Wiley-VCH, New York, NY, USA, 2006.

[165] M. Ristow, D. Müller-Wieland, A. Pfeiffer, W. Krone, and C. R. Kahn, "Obesity associated with a mutation in a genetic regulator of adipocyte differentiation," *The New England Journal of Medicine*, vol. 339, no. 14, pp. 953–959, 1998.

[166] M. Stumvoll and H. Häring, "The peroxisome proliferator-activated receptor-γ2 Pro12Ala polymorphism," *Diabetes*, vol. 51, no. 8, pp. 2341–2347, 2002.

[167] D. Altshuler, J. N. Hirschhorn, M. Klannemark et al., "The common PPARγ Pro12Ala polymorphism is associated with decreased risk of type 2 diabetes," *Nature Genetics*, vol. 26, no. 1, pp. 76–80, 2000.

[168] V. Radha, K. S. Vimaleswaran, H. N. S. Babu et al., "Role of genetic polymorphism peroxisome proliferator-activated receptor-γ2 Pro12Ala on ethnic susceptibility to diabetes in South-Asian and Caucasian subjects: evidence for heterogeneity," *Diabetes Care*, vol. 29, no. 5, pp. 1046–1051, 2006.

[169] E. S. Tai, D. Corella, M. Deurenberg-Yap et al., "Differential effects of the C1431T and Pro12Ala PPARγ gene variants on plasma lipids and diabetes risk in an Asian population," *Journal of Lipid Research*, vol. 45, no. 4, pp. 674–685, 2004.

[170] M. K. Moon, Y. M. Cho, H. S. Jung et al., "Genetic polymorphisms in peroxisome proliferator-activated receptor γ are associated with Type 2 diabetes mellitus and obesity in the Korean population," *Diabetic Medicine*, vol. 22, no. 9, pp. 1161–1166, 2005.

[171] R. Meshkani, M. Taghikhani, B. Larijani et al., "Pro12Ala polymorphism of the peroxisome proliferator-activated receptor-γ2 (PPARγ2) gene is associated with greater insulin sensitivity and decreased risk of type 2 diabetes in an Iranian population," *Clinical Chemistry and Laboratory Medicine*, vol. 45, no. 4, pp. 477–482, 2007.

[172] A. Mansoori, M. Amini, F. Kolahdooz, and E. Seyedrezazadeh, "Obesity and Pro12Ala polymorphism of peroxisome proliferator-activated receptor-gamma gene in healthy adults: a systematic review and meta-analysis," *Annals of Nutrition and Metabolism*, vol. 67, no. 2, pp. 104–118, 2015.

[173] J. Ma, Y. Li, F. Zhou, X. Xu, G. Guo, and Y. Qu, "Meta-analysis of association between the Pro12Ala polymorphism of the peroxisome proliferator-activated receptor- γ2 gene and diabetic retinopathy in Caucasians and Asians," *Molecular Vision*, vol. 18, pp. 2352–2360, 2012.

[174] A. Passaro, E. Dalla Nora, C. Marcello et al., "PPARγ Pro12Ala and ACE ID polymorphisms are associated with BMI and fat distribution, but not metabolic syndrome," *Cardiovascular Diabetology*, vol. 10, article 112, 2011.

[175] J. Luan, P. O. Browne, A.-H. Harding et al., "Evidence for gene-nutrient interaction at the PPARγ locus," *Diabetes*, vol. 50, no. 3, pp. 686–689, 2001.

[176] J. Pihlajamäki, U. Schwab, D. Kaminska et al., "Dietary polyunsaturated fatty acids and the Pro12Ala polymorphisms of PPARG regulate serum lipids through divergent pathways: a randomized crossover clinical trial," *Genes & Nutrition*, vol. 10, no. 6, article 43, 2015.

[177] J. Robitaille, J.-P. Després, L. Pérusse, and M.-C. Vohl, "The PPAR-gamma P12A polymorphism modulates the relationship between dietary fat intake and components of the metabolic syndrome: results from the Québec Family Study," *Clinical Genetics*, vol. 63, no. 2, pp. 109–116, 2003.

[178] N. Ouchi, S. Kihara, T. Funahashi, Y. Matsuzawa, and K. Walsh, "Obesity, adiponectin and vascular inflammatory disease," *Current Opinion in Lipidology*, vol. 14, no. 6, pp. 561–566, 2003.

[179] L. B. Tankó, A. Siddiq, C. Lecoeur et al., "ACDC/adiponectin and PPAR-γ gene polymorphisms: implications for features of obesity," *Obesity Research*, vol. 13, no. 12, pp. 2113–2121, 2005.

[180] W.-S. Yang, C. A. Hsiung, L.-T. Ho et al., "Genetic epistasis of adiponectin and PPARγ2 genotypes in modulation of insulin sensitivity: a family-based association study," *Diabetologia*, vol. 46, no. 7, pp. 977–983, 2003.

[181] C.-Y. Cao, Y.-Y. Li, Y.-J. Zhou, Y.-Q. Nie, and Y.-J. Y. Wan, "The C 681G polymorphism of the PPAR-γ gene is associated with susceptibility to non-alcoholic fatty liver disease," *Tohoku Journal of Experimental Medicine*, vol. 227, no. 4, pp. 253–262, 2012.

[182] Z. Yang, J. Wen, Q. Li et al., "PPARG gene Pro12Ala variant contributes to the development of non-alcoholic fatty liver in middle-aged and older Chinese population," *Molecular and Cellular Endocrinology*, vol. 348, no. 1, pp. 255–259, 2012.

[183] S. Ereqat, A. Nasereddin, K. Azmi, Z. Abdeen, and R. Amin, "Impact of the pro12Ala polymorphism of the PPAR-gamma 2 gene on metabolic and clinical characteristics in the palestinian type 2 diabetic patients," *PPAR Research*, vol. 2009, Article ID 874126, 5 pages, 2009.

[184] L. Gallicchio, B. Kalesan, H. Huang, P. Strickland, S. C. Hoffman, and K. J. Helzlsouer, "Genetic polymorphisms of peroxisome proliferator-activated receptors and the risk of cardiovascular morbidity and mortality in a community-based cohort in Washington County, Maryland," *PPAR Research*, vol. 2008, Article ID 276581, 9 pages, 2008.

[185] T.-H. Chao, Y.-H. Li, J. H. Chen et al., "The 161TT genotype in the exon 6 of the peroxisome-proliferator-activated receptor γ gene is associated with premature acute myocardial infarction and increased lipid peroxidation in habitual heavy smokers," *Clinical Science*, vol. 107, no. 5, pp. 461–466, 2004.

[186] A. Doney, B. Fischer, D. Frew et al., "Haplotype analysis of the PPARγ Pro12Ala and C1431T variants reveals opposing associations with body weight," *BMC Genetics*, vol. 3, article 21, 2002.

[187] A. Meirhaeghe, L. Fajas, N. Helbecque et al., "Impact of the peroxisome proliferator activated receptor γ2 Pro12Ala polymorphism on adiposity, lipids and non-insulin-dependent diabetes mellitus," *International Journal of Obesity and Related Metabolic Disorders*, vol. 24, no. 2, pp. 195–199, 2000.

[188] G.-P. Dong, L. He, J.-N. Li, F. Ye, M. He, and Y. Wang, "Association of the Pro12Ala and C1431T polymorphism of the PPAR gamma2 gene and their haplotypes with obesity and type 2 diabetes," *Chinese Journal of Medical Genetics*, vol. 25, no. 4, pp. 447–451, 2008.

[189] J. Prakash, N. Srivastava, S. Awasthi et al., "Association of PPAR-γ gene polymorphisms with obesity and obesity-associated phenotypes in north indian population," *American Journal of Human Biology*, vol. 24, no. 4, pp. 454–459, 2012.

[190] E. J. Rhee, K. W. Oh, W. Y. Lee et al., "Effects of two common polymorphisms of peroxisome proliferator-activated receptor-γ gene on metabolic syndrome," *Archives of Medical Research*, vol. 37, no. 1, pp. 86–94, 2006.

[191] B. Heude, V. Pelloux, A. Forhan et al., "Association of the Pro12Ala and C1431T variants of PPARγ and their haplotypes with susceptibility to gestational diabetes," *Journal of Clinical Endocrinology and Metabolism*, vol. 96, no. 10, pp. E1656–E1660, 2011.

[192] A. Haseeb, M. Iliyas, S. Chakrabarti et al., "Single-nucleotide polymorphisms in peroxisome proliferator-activated receptor γ and their association with plasma levels of resistin and the metabolic syndrome in a South Indian population," *Journal of Biosciences*, vol. 34, no. 3, pp. 405–414, 2009.

[193] M. Oladi, M. Nohtani, A. Avan et al., "Impact of the C1431T polymorphism of the peroxisome proliferator activated receptor-gamma (PPAR-γ) gene on fasted serum lipid levels in patients with coronary artery disease," *Annals of Nutrition and Metabolism*, vol. 66, no. 2-3, pp. 149–154, 2015.

[194] X. Zhou, J. Chen, and W. Xu, "Association between C1431T polymorphism in peroxisome proliferator-activated receptor-γ gene and coronary artery disease in Chinese Han population," *Molecular Biology Reports*, vol. 39, no. 2, pp. 1863–1868, 2012.

[195] R. Valve, K. Sivenius, R. Miettinen et al., "Two polymorphisms in the peroxisome proliferator-activated receptor-γ gene are associated with severe overweight among obese women," *Journal of Clinical Endocrinology and Metabolism*, vol. 84, no. 10, pp. 3708–3712, 1999.

[196] J. W. Yun, "Possible anti-obesity therapeutics from nature—a review," *Phytochemistry*, vol. 71, no. 14-15, pp. 1625–1641, 2010.

[197] Y.-S. Cha, Y. Park, M. Lee et al., "Doenjang, a korean fermented soy food, exerts antiobesity and antioxidative activities in overweight subjects with the PPAR-γ2 C1431T polymorphism; 12-week, double-blind randomized clinical trial," *Journal of Medicinal Food*, vol. 17, no. 1, pp. 119–127, 2014.

[198] M. M. Swarbrick, C. M. L. Chapman, B. M. McQuillan, J. Hung, P. L. Thompson, and J. P. Beilby, "A Pro12Ala polymorphism in the human peroxisome proliferator-activated receptor-γ2 is associated with combined hyperlipidaemia in obesity," *European Journal of Endocrinology*, vol. 144, no. 3, pp. 277–282, 2001.

[199] O. W. Hamer, D. Forstner, I. Ottinger et al., "The pro115Gln polymorphism within the PPAR γ2 gene has no epidemiological impact on morbid obesity," *Experimental and Clinical Endocrinology and Diabetes*, vol. 110, no. 5, pp. 230–234, 2002.

4

Portulaca Extract Attenuates Development of Dextran Sulfate Sodium Induced Colitis in Mice through Activation of PPARγ

Rui Kong [ID],[1,2] Hui Luo,[1] Nan Wang [ID],[1] Jingjing Li [ID],[1] Shizan Xu,[1,3] Kan Chen [ID],[1] Jiao Feng,[1] Liwei Wu,[1] Sainan Li,[1] Tong Liu,[1] Xiya Lu,[1] Yujing Xia [ID],[1] Yanhong Shi,[1] Yingqun Zhou [ID],[1] Weigang He [ID],[4] Qi Dai [ID],[5] Yuejuan Zheng [ID],[4] and Jie Lu [ID][1]

[1]*Department of Gastroenterology, Shanghai Tenth People's Hospital, Tongji University School of Medicine, Shanghai 200072, China*
[2]*The School of Medicine, Soochow University, Suzhou 215006, China*
[3]*Department of Gastroenterology, Shanghai Tenth Hospital, School of Clinical Medicine, Nanjing Medical University,*
Shanghai 200072, China
[4]*Department of Immunology and Microbiology, Shanghai University of Traditional Chinese Medicine, Shanghai 201203, China*
[5]*The Eye Hospital, Wenzhou Medical University, Wenzhou City, Zhejiang 325027, China*

Correspondence should be addressed to Qi Dai; dq@mail.eye.ac.cn, Yuejuan Zheng; 13641776412@163.com,
and Jie Lu; kennisren@hotmail.com

Academic Editor: Yuewen Gong

Portulaca oleracea L. is a traditional Chinese medicine, which has been used as adjuvant therapy for inflammatory bowel disease (IBD). However, the mechanism of its activity in IBD still remains unclear. Since previous studies have documented the anti-inflammatory effect of peroxisome proliferator activated receptors-γ (PPAR-γ), *Portulaca* regulation of PPAR-γ in inflammation was examined in current study. Ulcerative colitis (UC) was generated by 5% dextran sulfate sodium (DSS) in mice and four groups were established as normal control, DSS alone, DSS plus mesalamine, and DSS plus *Portulaca*. Severity of UC was evaluated by body weight, stool blood form, and length of colorectum. Inflammation was examined by determination of inflammatory cytokines (TNF-a, IL-6, and IL-1a). *Portulaca* extract was able to attenuate development of UC in DSS model similar to the treatment of mesalazine. Moreover, *Portulaca* extract inhibited proinflammatory cytokines release and reduced the level of DSS-induced NF-κB phosphorylation. Furthermore, *Portulaca* extract restored PPAR-γ level, which was reduced by DSS. In addition, *Portulaca* extract protected DSS induced apoptosis in mice. In conclusion, *Portulaca* extract can alleviate colitis in mice through regulation of inflammatory reaction, apoptosis, and PPAR-γ level; therefore, *Portulaca* extract can be a potential candidate for the treatment of IBD.

1. Introduction

Inflammatory bowel disease (IBD) consists of Crohn's disease and ulcerative colitis and has been considered as a global health threat to children and adults [1]. The distribution of IBD varies in geographical regions with high incidence rate in North American and Northern Europe; however, the morbidity remains stable in these regions. In the developing regions in the world such as Asia, the incidence and morbidity are increased every year [2]. Enormous efforts have been made to find an effective therapy for IBD although current drugs including sulfasalazine, mesalamine, and corticosteroids taken alone or in combination contribute to

decelerating disease progression [3]. However, with current treatments and medications, some patients suffer from side effects and complications of these drugs such as weakened immunity, infectious diseases, or increased malignant potentiality. Therefore, a promising medication with no or mild side effects is needed for IBD treatment.

Portulaca oleracea L. (*Portulaca*) is a traditional Chinese herb praised with rich multiminerals, proteins, α-amyrin, β-carotene, terpenoids, vitamins, and fatty acids [4]. The medicinal properties and usage of *Portulaca* have been recorded in many ancient Chinese books [5]. Moreover, current researches reveal that *Portulaca* has several biological functions such as antibacteria, neuroprotection, anti-inflammation, antiatherosclerosis, and antitumor [6–10]. Furthermore, decoction of *Portulaca* has been used as a remedy for inflammatory bowel disease to alleviate symptoms of bloody stools, diarrhea, and abdominal pain in clinic. Several clinical trials have been conducted on the safety and effectiveness of *Portulaca*, which showed no adverse effects of *Portulaca*. Reports from animal studies also indicate low toxicity of *Portulaca* with LD_{50} value of 1853 mg/kg and high therapeutic index [11].

Peroxisome proliferator-activated receptor-γ (PPAR-γ) is an important member of the nuclear receptor superfamily. The essential role of PPAR-γ in acute inflammation [12], adipogenesis [13], and several carcinomas has been identified [14–16]. Moreover, PPAR-γ activation was found in various types of immune cells, including primary peritoneal macrophages, dendritic cells, and T cells [17]. Several studies have shown that activation of PPAR-γ could downregulate some vital proinflammatory cytokines, such as IL-1β, IL-2, IL-6, and TNF-α [18] as well as inhibition of NF-κB phosphorylation in monocyte and other types of cells. Therefore, activation of PPAR-γ exerts a direct anti-inflammatory effect in IBD, while the mechanism of PPAR-γ activation remains to be further explored [19].

In the current study, the anti-inflammatory activity and mechanism of *Portulaca* in dextran sulfate sodium (DSS) induced UC animal model were explored.

2. Materials and Methods

2.1. Plant Material and Preparation of the Extracts. The *Portulaca* material was obtained from the Department of Traditional Chinese Medicine Pharmacy of the Shanghai Tenth People's Hospital. The herb was triturated into powder and water-soluble substance was extracted as described previously [20]. Briefly, the prepared powder was boiled in distilled water (80°C, 25 g/120 ml water, w/v) for 60 min and then smashed via ultrasonic concussion (3 cycles of 15 sec). The mixture of water and concussion was filtered using 2 mm pores strainer and the resultant material was lyophilized under vacuum.

2.2. Animals and Acute Colitis Induction. Forty adult female mice weighting 18–22 g were purchased from the Shanghai Laboratory Animal Co., Ltd. (Shanghai, China), and maintained in an environment of 25°C with controlled 12 h light/dark cycle. Mice were permitted free access to water and standard mouse chow. The animal protocol was approved by the Ethics Committee of the Tongji University, which meets the recommendations in the Guide for Care and Use of Laboratory Animals of the National Institutes of Health. The dextran sulfate sodium reagent (molecular weight: 36,000–50,000 from MP Biochemicals Solon, OH, USA) was diluted with drinking water to make final concentration of 3%.

The mice were divided into 4 groups at random:

(1) Normal control: given normal food and water for 7 days

TABLE 1: DAI assessment (disease activity index).

Weight loss %	Shape of stool	FOBT[*]/blood stool	Score
0	Normal	Normal	0
1–5	Shapeless stool	FOBT positive	1
6–10			2
11–15	Loose stool	Gross blood stool	3
>16			4

[*]FOBT: fecal occult blood test.

(2) DSS group: 3% DSS + saline by gavage for 7 days

(3) Mesalamine positive control group: 3% DSS + 7.4 mg/kg mesalamine daily by gavage for 7 days

(4) *Portulaca* group: 3% DSS + 100 mg/kg daily by gavage for 7 days

During the period of modeling, mice weight, stool form, and stool occult blood were recorded every day to assess the disease activity index (DAI) of acute colitis; the evaluative criteria were clarified in Table 1.

2.3. Serum Cytokine Analysis. The serum levels of TNF-α, IL-1β, and IL-6 concentrations were determined by using ELISA Kits (Elabscience, Wuhan, China), respectively, according to the manufacturer's instruction. The OD values of absorbance at 450 nm were examined by ThermoMax microplate reader.

2.4. Determination of MPO (Myeloperoxidase) Activity in Serum Sample. Myeloperoxidase is found in activated neutrophils and macrophages, which plays a defensive role during inflammatory response via catalyzing hydrogen peroxide into hypochlorous acid. The serum samples reacted with the mixed solution including 3,3'-dimethoxybiphenyl-4,4'-diamine and hydrogen peroxide, pH 6.0, according to the MPO assay kit (Nanjing Jiancheng Bioengineering Institute, A044, China). The absorbance of control well and testing well at 460 nm was determined by microplate reader. The activity of MPO was calculated as the following formula:

$$\text{MPO performance (U/L)} = \frac{(\text{testing OD values} - \text{control OD values})}{11.3} \times \text{sample volume (L)} . \tag{1}$$

2.5. Fecal Occult Blood Testing. The form of stool was recorded and the severity of stool occult blood was analyzed by urine fecal occult blood test kit (Nanjing Jiancheng Bioengineering Institute, C027, China). A small amount of feces samples was picked and smeared on the slides. Add orthotolidine and hydrogen peroxide reagent on the surface of stool samples. The results were analyzed according to the indications: negative (−): the samples do not show color within 3 minutes; weakly positive (+): the samples show blue within 30 to 60 seconds; positive (++): the samples appear

TABLE 2: The sequence of primers used in experiments.

Gene	Primer sequence (5′ 3′)	Annealing temperature (°C)
GADPH		
F	GGACCTCATGGCCTACATGG	57.6
R	TAGGGCCTCTCTTGCTCAGT	
IL-6		
F	GGCGGATCGGATGTTGTGAT	57.3
R	GGACCCCAGACAATCGGTTG	
IL 1β		
F	CTTTGAAGTTGACGGACCC	53.1
R	TGAGTGATACTGCCTGCCTG	
TNF-α		
F	CACCACCATCAAGGACTCAA	54.5
R	AGGCAACCTGACCACTCTCC	
PPAR-γ		
F	CCCAATGGTTGCTGATTACA	54.4
R	GGACGCAGGCTCTACTTTGA	
NFκBp65		
F	TGCGATTCCGCTATAAATGCG	60.2
R	ACAAGTTCATGTGGATGAGGC	
Bax		
F	AGACAGGGGCCTTTTTGCTAC	57.3
R	AATTCGCCGGAGACACTCG	
Bcl-2		
F	GAGCCTGTGAGAGACGTGG	57.3
R	CGAGTCTGTGTATAGCAATCCCA	

bluish green; strongly positive (+++): samples show mazarine immediately.

2.6. Gene Expression Analysis by Real-Time Reverse Transcriptase Polymerase Chain Reaction. Total RNA was extracted from fresh colorectum tissues by the Trizol reagent from the Thermo Fisher Scientific (Waltham, MA, USA) and washed by 75% ethanol. One microgram total RNA was transcribed into cDNA using reverse transcription kit (Takara Biotechnology, Dalian, China). The first transcribed cDNA was diluted ten times and applied to real-time polymerase chain reaction (SYBR Premix EX Taq, Takara Biotechnology) with the following cycle of denaturing at 94°C for 30 seconds, annealing at different temperature according to the primers for 30 seconds and elongation at 72°C for 45 seconds using a 7900HT Fast Real-Time PCR System (Thermo Fisher Scientific). All primers used in experiments were listed in Table 2.

2.7. Hematoxylin and Eosin Staining. Fresh colorectum tissues were fixed in formalin and embedded in paraffin. The tissue blot was cut into 4 μm thick section for histological examination using hematoxylin and eosin (H&E). The injury index of histology was evaluated according to three aspects:

the destructive degree of the intestine epithelium, the presence of the immune cell infiltration in intestine mucosa, and the infiltration degree of immune cell in submucosa. The histology score was depicted in Table 3. Two experienced pathologists made the assessment independently.

2.8. Western Blotting Analysis. Total protein was extracted from fresh colorectum tissue by cell lysis buffer with protease and phosphatase inhibitor mixture (New Cell & Molecular Biotech Co., Ltd., China). The protein quantification was determined by BCA methods (Beyotime, Shanghai, China). Equal amount of protein (25 ng) from each sample was loaded on to 12% SDS-PAGE. After separation through electrophoresis, the proteins were transferred onto PVDF membranes (Millipore Corp, Billerica, MA, USA). The membranes were then incubated with 5% nonfat milk in tris-buffered saline (TBS) to block nonspecific binding with antibody. The membranes were then incubated with primary antibodies at 4°C overnight. The primary antibodies used in experiments were as follows: β-actin, PPAR-γ, NF-κB, pNF-κB (all from Cell Signaling Technology, Danvers, MA, USA), Bcl-2, Bax (all from Proteintech Group, Inc., Chicago, IL, USA), and caspase 3 (Cell Signaling Technology, Danvers, MA, USA) with dilution of 1 : 1000, 1 : 1000, 1 : 1000, 1 : 500, 1 : 500, and 1 : 1000, respectively. After incubation with primary antibody, the membranes were washed three times with TBST and then incubated with the appropriate horseradish peroxidase-conjugated secondary antibodies. The signals were detected and the intensity of bands was analyzed by Odyssey.

2.9. Immunohistochemical Staining. Tissue specimen collected from mice was fixed in 4% paraformaldehyde overnight and embedded in paraffin. Sections (4 μm) were dewaxed and hydrated through serial graded xylene ethanol. After being washed with phosphate-buffered saline (PBS) solution three times, antigen retrieval was performed using a microwave with heating to 95°C and cooling to room temperature (four times). Primary antibody PPAR-γ (Cell Signaling Technology, Danvers, MA, USA) was diluted into working concentration and then incubated with the slices at 4°C overnight. Following incubation of secondary antibody, DAB substrate was used as the chromogen. Positive expression areas were observed under microscope.

2.10. Statistical Analysis. The statistical analysis was performed using the SPSS 20.0 software package (IBM Corporation, Armonk, NY, USA). All values were expressed with the mean ± standard deviation using the Student–Newman–Keuls test or one-way analysis of variance. A p value < 0.05 was considered statistically significant. The positively stained areas of IHC were evaluated and analyzed using Image-Pro Plus 6.0 software (Media Cybernetics, Silver Spring, MD, USA).

3. Results

3.1. Portulaca Extract Decreases the Disease Activity Index, the Length of Colorectum, and Myeloperoxidase Activity of Dextran Sulfate Sodium Induced Colitis. Since severity of

TABLE 3: Histology scoring.

Lesions of colonic epithelium	Granulocyte infiltration of intestine mucosa	Granulocyte infiltration of submucosa	Score
Normal	Normal	Normal	0
Cellular proliferation/anomalous crypt/absence of goblet cell	Mild	Mild to moderate	1
Absence of intestinal crypt (10%–50%)	Moderate	Severe	2
Absence of intestinal crypt (50%–90%)	Severe		3
Entire absence of intestinal crypt with integral epithelia			4
Mild to moderate ulceration epithelia			5
Severe ulceration			6

colitis is evaluated by the DAI, MPO, and the length of colorectum, the effects of *Portulaca* extract on these parameters were examined. As shown in Figure 1(b), mice in DSS group have significant higher DAI than those in all other groups starting from day 3 ($p < 0.05$). Mice in *Portulaca* extract and mesalamine groups showed higher DAI starting from day 3 and reaching to the peak at day 5 compared to those in normal control. After day 5, DAI was gradually decreased although they were still higher than that in normal control. Since DAI consists of three aspects including weight loss, diarrhea, and the bloody stool scores. The weight loss and bloody stool scores were further evaluated and shown in Figures 1(c) and 1(d). DSS induced ulcerative colitis and significantly reduced body weight of the mice in DSS group ($p < 0.01$). However, the treatment of *Portulaca* extract and mesalamine significantly restored the body weights as shown in the *Portulaca* and mesalamine groups. In addition, there was a higher bloody stool score in DSS group than all other groups. Treatment of *Portulaca* and mesalamine reduced the score (Figure 1(d)).

The length of colorectum was an evaluation content of colitis, which means the total length from cecum to anus of mice. Compared with that of control group, there was a significant decrease in the length of colorectum in DSS group ($p < 0.0001$). But the length of colorectum in mesalamine and *Portulaca* group was longer than that in DSS group (Figure 1(e)). Moreover, myeloperoxidase (MPO) serves as an independent predictor for oxidative stress and inflammatory reactions. The average MPO activity in mice of control group was $0.56 \pm 0.05 \times 10^{-3}$ U/ml, while DSS exposure increased the MPO activity to $2.19 \pm 0.82 \times 10^{-3}$ U/ml. The treatment of mesalamine and *Portulaca* group reduced the MPO activity to $0.84 \pm 0.11 \times 10^{-3}$ U/ml and $0.71 \pm 0.04 \times 10^{-3}$ U/ml respectively (Figure 1(f)).

3.2. Effect of Portulaca Extract on Proinflammatory Cytokines Expression and Colorectum Injury. Since DSS induced ulcerative colitis, the expressions of three proinflammatory cytokines (TNF-α, IL-6, and IL-1β) were examined in the serum and colorectum tissue. As shown in Figures 2(a) and 2(b), there were significant increases in all three proinflammatory cytokines at both mRNA and protein levels ($p < 0.05$). Moreover, treatment of *Portulaca* and mesalamine significantly reduced the DSS-induced cytokine expression

at both mRNA and protein levels ($p < 0.05$). Two independent experienced pathologists examined the tissue injury of colorectum. The injury score resulted from the evaluation of enterocyte lessons and inflammatory cell infiltration in mucosa and submucosa regions. Figure 2(c) showed HE staining of colorectum tissues from mice of four different groups with magnification of 200x in the upper row and different magnification of colorectum in DSS mice. There was a significant increase in tissue injury score in DSS mice compared to all other mice ($p < 0.0001$). Treatment of *Portulaca* extract and mesalamine resulted in lesser enterocyte lesions and inflammatory cell infiltration in mucosa and submucosa (Figures 2(c) and 2(d)).

3.3. Regulation of NF-κB and PPAR-γ by Portulaca Extracts in Colorectum. Both NF-κB and PPAR-γ play an important role in inflammation, activation of NF-κB is the critical step to increase the expression of different inflammatory cytokines such as TNF-α. Moreover, previous studies documented that PPAR-γ could antagonize inflammatory responses through inhibition of transcriptional activation of inflammatory response genes such as transcriptional factor NF-κB. Therefore, the expressions of NF-κB and PPAR-γ were examined in the study. Figure 3(a) showed the staining of PPAR-γ in colorectum tissues from mice of four different groups. Significant reduction of PPAR-γ staining was observed in the colorectum of mice in DSS groups, while treatment of either *Portulaca* extract or mesalamine restored back the staining of PPAR-γ in the colorectum. Figure 3(b) displayed both NF-kBp65 and PPAR-γ proteins by western blot and Figure 3(c) showed the mRNA levels of both NF-kB and PPAR-γ. There was significant decrease in PPAR-γ expression at both mRNA and protein levels in DSS group compared to that in normal control group ($p < 0.05$). Both *Portulaca* extract and mesalamine restored PPAR-γ levels back to that in normal control group. DSS treatment significantly induced NF-kB expression at both mRNA and protein levels ($p < 0.05$), while treatments of either *Portulaca* extract or mesalamine brought NF-kB levels back to that in normal control group.

3.4. Regulation of Apoptosis Protein in Colorectum by Portulaca Extract. Inflammatory reaction usually results in cell death; however whether it is through apoptosis or necrosis remains to be explored. In the current study, three apoptotic proteins were examined including proapoptotic proteins (Bax

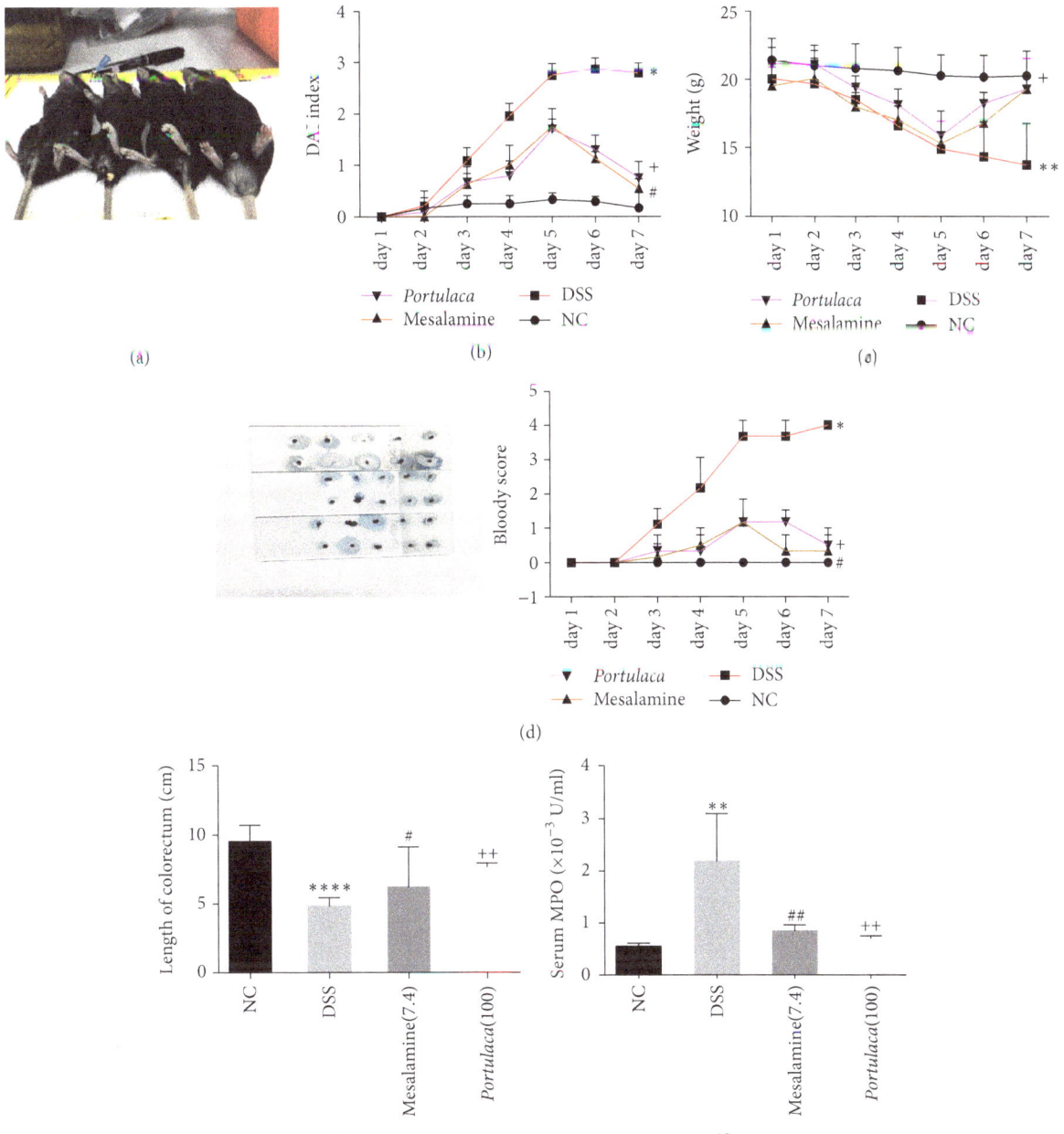

FIGURE 1: Effect of *Portulaca* treatment on disease severity of DSS-induced UC model. Panel (a) shows the appearance of representative mice from four experiment groups from left to right: control group, DSS-induced group, mesalamine group, and *Portulaca* group. Panel (b) displays the graph of disease activity index (DAI) of four groups at different days of the experiment. Panel (c) represents the weight of mice daily in different group. Panel (d) shows the image of fecal occult blood testing at 8th day with the darker color and more severe bloody stool and shows the score of bloody stool at different days of each group. Panel (e) represents the length of colorectum from four groups at 8th day after DSS administration. Panel (f) indicates the MPO activity in serum. (Data were presented as mean ± SD from six rats. * indicates comparison between DSS and NC; # indicates comparison between mesalamine and DSS; + indicates the comparison between *Portulaca* and DSS. The number of symbols indicates significance of difference; for example, four symbols indicate $p < 0.0001$; three symbols indicate $p < 0.001$; two symbols indicate $p < 0.01$; and one symbol indicates $p < 0.05$.)

and cleaved caspase 3) and antiapoptotic protein (Bcl-2). As shown in Figure 4, abundance of Bcl-2, Bax, and caspase 3 was documented by western blot analyses. There was significant decrease in Bcl-2 level ($p < 0.001$) but significant increase in Bax level in colorectum of mice in DSS group compared to all other groups ($p < 0.0001$). Although whole caspase 3 showed no change in the colorectum of mice in DSS group, the cleaved form of caspase 3 was significantly increased ($p < 0.01$). All these changes were corrected after treatment of either *Portulaca* extract or mesalazine. Moreover, mRNA levels of Bcl-2 and Bax showed the same changes as their proteins in the four different groups of mice.

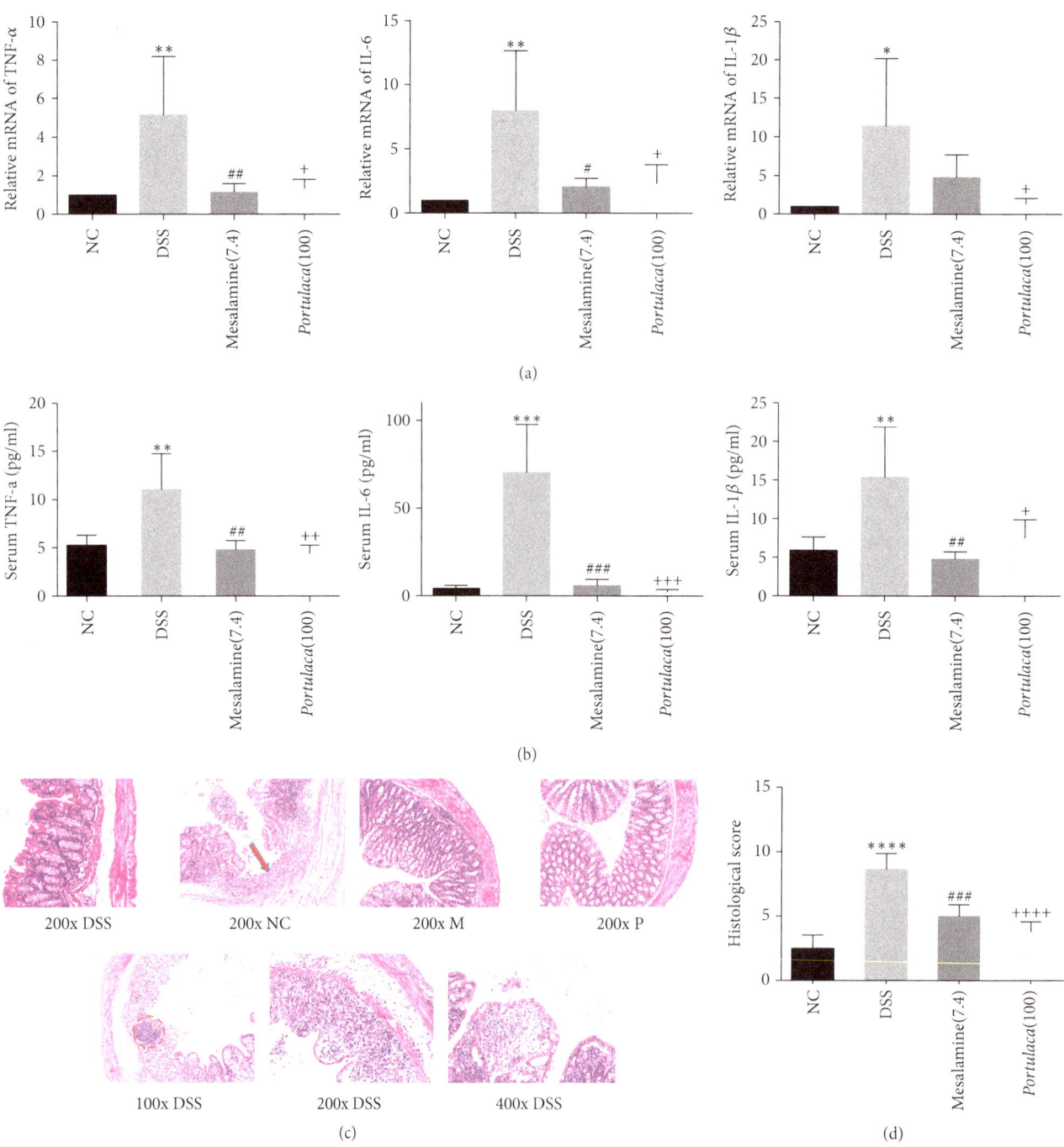

FIGURE 2: Effect of *Portulaca* extract on serum cytokines and tissue injury scores of DSS-induced acute colitis. Panel (a) indicates that the mRNA expressions of TNF-α, IL-6, and IL-1β were evaluated in each group with qRT- PCR. Panel (b) shows that the levels of TNF-α, IL-6, and IL-1β in serum were detected via ELISA assay. Panel (c) displays the H&E stained colon images (NC refers to negative control; DSS refers to DSS alone group; M refers to mesalamine group; P refers to *Portulaca* group). The dotted potion indicated the hyperplasia of lymphoid follicle; red arrow pointed the infiltration of inflammatory cells. Panel (d) indicates the histological scores of H&E stained colorectum images. (Data were presented as mean ± SD from six rats. ∗ indicates comparison between DSS and NC; # indicates comparison between mesalamine and DSS; + indicates the comparison between *Portulaca* and DSS. The number of symbols indicates significance of difference; for example, four symbols indicate $p < 0.0001$; three symbols indicate $p < 0.001$; two symbols indicate $p < 0.01$; and one symbol indicates $p < 0.05$.)

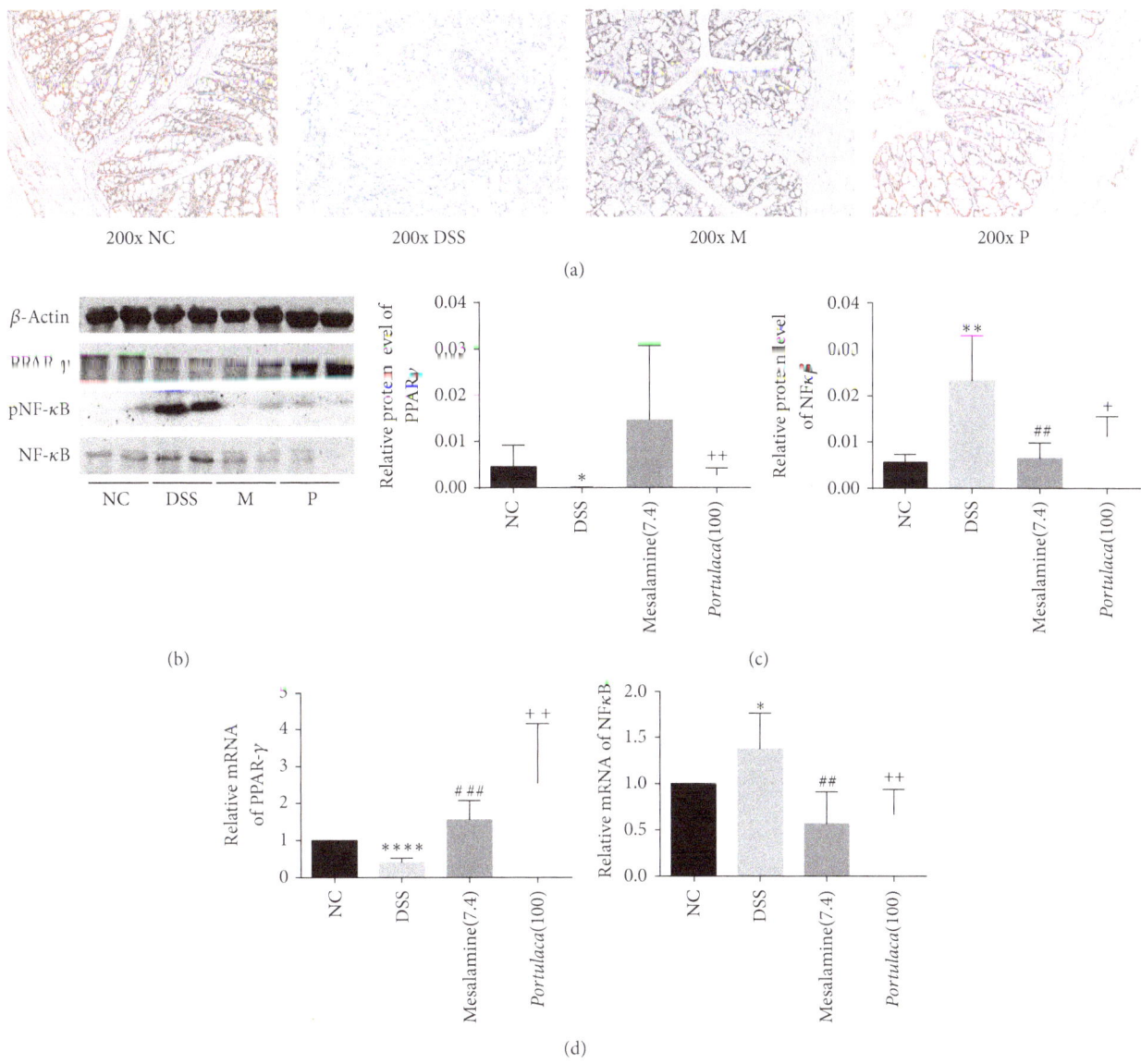

FIGURE 3: Effect of *Portulaca* extracts on NF-κB and PPAR-γ expression in colonic tissue. Panel (a) represents the immunohistochemistry staining of PPAR-γ. (NC refers to negative control; DSS refers to DSS alone group; M refers to mesalamine group; P refers to *Portulaca* group, original magnification: ×200). Panel (b) shows the expression of PPAR-γ, NF-κB, and pNF-κB in colorectum tissues from western blot. Panel (c) shows the histograms of grey intensity for PPAR-γ and NF-κB relative to β-actin. Panel (d) shows the relative mRNA expression of PPAR-γ and NF-κB from quantitative real-time PCR. (Data are presented as mean ± SD from six experiments. ∗ indicates comparison between DSS and NC; # indicates comparison between mesalamine and DSS; + indicates the comparison between *Portulaca* and DSS. The number of symbols indicates significance of difference; for example, four symbols indicate $p < 0.0001$; three symbols indicate $p < 0.001$; two symbols indicate $p < 0.01$; and one symbol indicates $p < 0.05$.)

4. Discussion

Inflammatory bowel disease commonly presents with intestine and extraintestine manifestations [21]. The typical symptom of IBD clinically is the blood and mucus mixed with stool. Other symptoms may include fevers, weight loss, arthritis, mucocutaneous lesions, and extraintestine presentations, which are useful for diagnosis, evaluating patient's condition and drug selection [22]. In the current study, weight loss and feces changes accompanied by blood and mucus mixed with stool were recorded daily to estimate the DAI (disease activity index) of the colitis. Significant high index of DAI in DSS induced UC mice in the current study indicates successful establishment of UC model in mice. Moreover, with this model, therapeutic activity of *Portulaca* extract was also demonstrated showing that mice with treatment of *Portulaca* extract had significant lower DAI index than that without *Portulaca* treatment. Furthermore, with this successful model of UC, the effect of *Portulaca* extract on the length of colorectum was also documented.

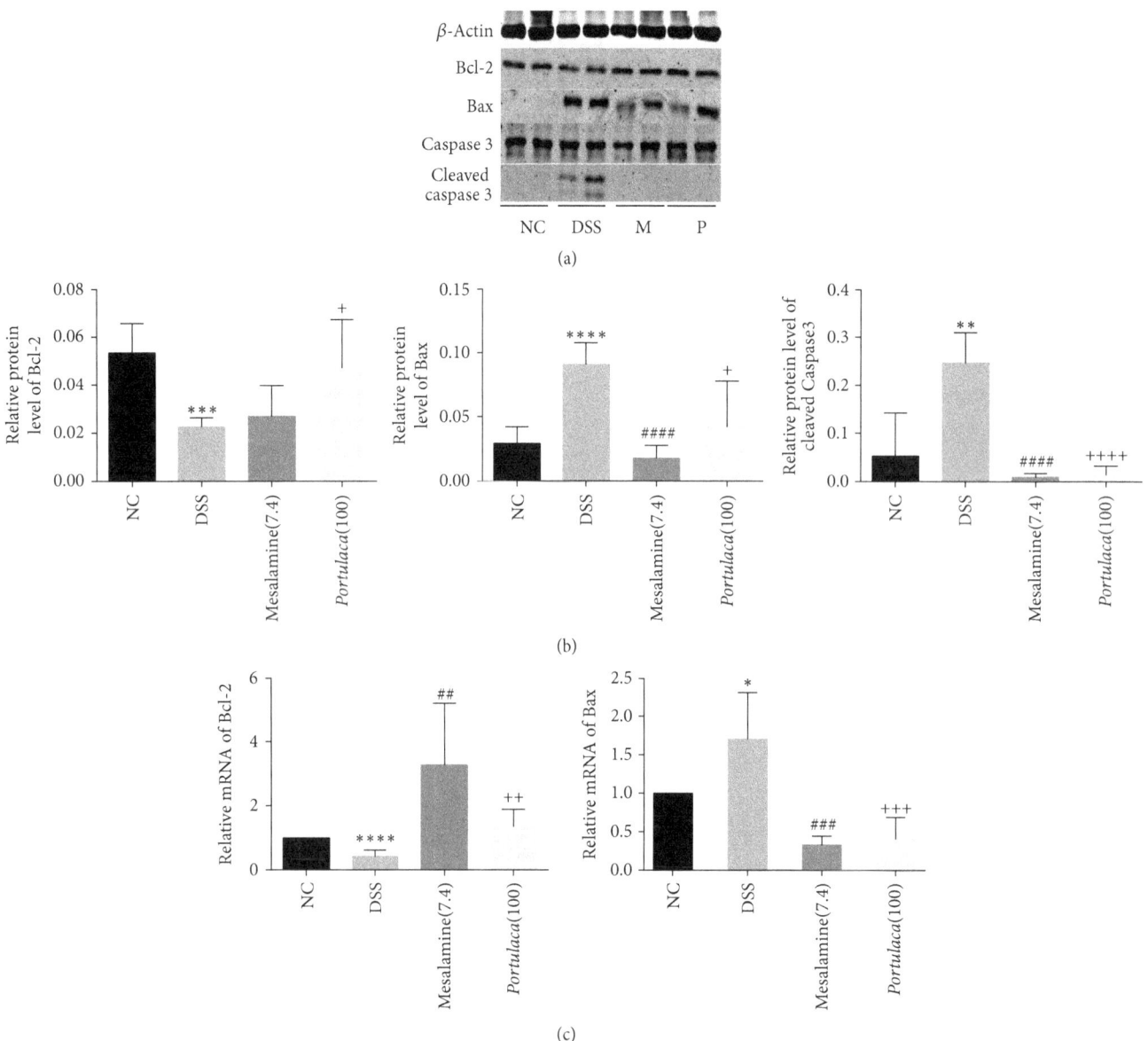

FIGURE 4: Effects of *Portulaca* extract on apoptosis in mice on inflammatory bowel disease. Panel (a) shows the protein level of Bcl-2, Bax, caspase 3, and cleaved caspase 3 in each group. Panel (b) represents the histogram of density for Bcl-2, Bax, and cleaved caspase 3. Panel (c) represents the relative mRNA level of Bcl-2 and Bax from quantitative real-time PCR, respectively. (Data are presented as mean ± SD from six experiments. ∗ indicates comparison between DSS and NC; # indicates comparison between mesalamine and DSS; + indicates the comparison between *Portulaca* and DSS. The number of symbols indicates significance of difference; for example, four symbols indicate $p < 0.0001$; three symbols indicate $p < 0.001$; two symbols indicate $p < 0.01$; and one symbol indicates $p < 0.05$.)

Mice with DSS-induced UC showed shorter colorectum than normal mice, which is consistent with the report of UC [23]. Treatment of *Portulaca* extract could also increase the length of colorectum in rats with DSS-induced colitis. The findings indicate that *Portulaca* extract could ameliorate general symptoms of IBD.

Currently, myeloperoxidase activity is considered as an independent indicator of inflammation and oxidative stress. This enzyme in leukocyte usually has the capacity to catalyze the hydrogen peroxide [24]. Clinically, myeloperoxidase activity has been used to predict inflammation and oxidative stress in renal failure [25], myocardial infarction [26],

inflammatory vascular disease [27], and so on. Consistent with these reports, higher level of MPO was observed in mice of DSS treatment, which induces inflammation and ulcerative colitis in the intestine [28]. This elevation of MPO in serum is also consistent with intestine injury score observed in the colorectum tissues especially the infiltration of inflammatory cells in the mucosa and submucosa. These findings suggest that MPO could be an indicator for either DSS-induced colitis or clinical presentation of IBD.

Several immune cells and immune-regulatory proteins participated in the disturbance of intestine immune system, which account for activation and augmentation of inflammation cascade in IBD. The intestinal epithelial cells usually act as the first barrier for any intestinal disorders [29]. Once the epithelial cells are injured by external stress, intestine pathogens may enter the intestine, which triggers antigen-presenting cells and transform naive T cells into effector T cells such as Th1, Th17, Th2, and natural killer T cells. These cells are responsible for generating multiple types of proinflammatory cytokines [30]. Moreover, these cells could secret interferon γ, interleukin 1β, and other cytokines to activate macrophages, which in turn could secrete large amounts of cytokines including tumor necrosis factor α, interleukin 1, and interleukin 6. Furthermore, several cell types in the process such as dendritic cells, mast cells, and leucocytes can also promote the dysfunction of innate and adaptive immune response of inflammatory disease [31]. In current study, we found application of Portulaca could significantly reduce the expression levels of these cytokines including TNF-α, IL-6, and IL-1β. These findings suggested that Portulaca may affect T cell activation and participate in inflammation to some extent.

In present study, three proinflammatory cytokines (TNF-α, IL-6, and IL-1β) were examined. These cytokines are mainly released by macrophages and differentiated T cells [32]. In addition, TNF-α could also exert its inflammation response through upregulation of IL-1β and IL-6 and induce tissue damage through necrosis and apoptosis [33] and activate NF-κB [34]. Moreover, all three cytokines are able to exert other functions by interacting with other molecules through different pathway. The findings of TNF-α, IL-1β, and IL-6 in the current study are in line with the reports in patients with either UC or CD [35, 36].

Except cytokines, transcriptional factors are also important in regulation of inflammation. The transcriptional factor NF-κB is known to regulate the level of TNF-α, IL-6, and IL-1β during the progression of inflammatory bowel disease [37]. Moreover, NF-κB can facilitate cell apoptosis through the upregulation of c-FLIP level while lowering the expression of antiapoptotic proteins such as Bcl-2, Bcl-xl, c-IAP1/2, and x-IAP [38]. In the present study, overexpressed TNF-α, IL-6, IL-1β, and pNF-κB were observed in DSS treated mice, which indicate an enhanced inflammatory process and aggravated tissue damage. On the contrary, the addition of Portulaca extract reduced inflammation response and tissue damage indicating a role of Portulaca extract in prevention and treatment of inflammatory bowel disease.

PPAR-γ is another transcription factor, which plays an important role in adipogenesis, glucose metabolism [39], and anti-inflammatory reaction. Several reports suggest that PPAR-γ agonists may have beneficial effects for the inflammatory diseases, including mastitis, IBD, and arthritis [40–42]. Jiang et al. observed that PPAR agonist (15d-PGJ$_2$) could abrogate the production of proinflammatory cytokines TNF-α and interleukin-6 [43]. Moreover, the NF-κB activation is inhibited after PPAR-γ agonist due to changes of conformation in NF-kB subunits. The findings from the current study also observed that PPAR-γ level was increased in DSS-induced group following Portulaca extract intervention together with suppressed cytokines and NF-κB.

The mechanism of apoptosis in IBD remains controversial. Some studies observed an increased apoptosis in lamina propria (LP) and epithelium, which contributed to the severity of UC [44]. Moreover, activation of PPAR-γ could attenuate the cascade of apoptosis [45]. In the current study, antiapoptosis protein (Bcl-2) was decreased and proapoptosis proteins (Bax and cleaved caspase 3) were increased in UC mice. However, treatment of Portulaca extract reverses apoptosis in the colorectum. This finding suggests further investigation of apoptosis and Portulaca in inflammatory bowel disease.

5. Conclusion

With the successful model of inflammatory bowel disease, Portulaca extract was demonstrated to reduce severity of the disease. The mechanism of Portulaca extract in alleviation of inflammatory bowel disease could be related to its regulation of inflammatory cytokines (TNF-α, IL-6, and IL-1β), transcription factors (NF-kB and PPAR-γ), and apoptosis. Therefore, Portulaca extract might be a potential agent for the treatment of patients with inflammatory bowel disease.

Conflicts of Interest

The authors declare that there are no conflicts of interest regarding the publication of this paper.

Authors' Contributions

Rui Kong makes main contribution to this work.

Acknowledgments

The authors would like to sincerely thank Dr. Jie Lu, Professor Yuejuan Zheng, and Dr. Qi Dai and the staff of the Central Laboratory of Shanghai Tenth People's Hospital for their technical assistance. This study was supported by the National Nature Science Foundation of China (81300340; 81471537).

References

[1] M. D. Kappelman, S. L. Rifas-Shiman, C. Q. Porter et al., "Direct health care costs of Crohn's disease and ulcerative colitis in US children and adults," Gastroenterology, vol. 135, no. 6, pp. 1907–1913, 2008.

[2] S. C. Ng, C. N. Bernstein, M. H. Vatn et al., "Geographical variability and environmental risk factors in inflammatory bowel disease," Gut, vol. 62, no. 4, pp. 630–649, 2013.

[3] B. A. Hendrickson, R. Gokhale, and J. H. Cho, "Clinical aspects and pathophysiology of inflammatory bowel disease," Clinical Microbiology Reviews, vol. 15, no. 1, pp. 79–94, 2002.

[4] M. K. Uddin, A. S. Juraimi, M. E. Ali, and M. R. Ismail, "Evaluation of antioxidant properties and mineral composition of purslane (Portulaca oleracea L.) at different growth stages," International Journal of Molecular Sciences, vol. 13, no. 8, pp. 10257–10267, 2012.

[5] C.-J. Chen, W.-Y. Wang, X.-L. Wang et al., "Anti-hypoxic activity of the ethanol extract from *Portulaca oleracea* in mice," *Journal of Ethnopharmacology*, vol. 124, no. 2, pp. 246–250, 2009.

[6] L. F. Hu, X. Y. Xu, and B. Q. Wang, "Research and utilization situation of PortulacaOleracea L. in China," *Journal of Pharmacy Practice and Community Medicine*, vol. 20, pp. 315-316, 2003.

[7] L. Xiang, D. Xing, W. Wang, R. Wang, Y. Ding, and L. Du, "Alkaloids from *Portulaca oleracea* L.," *Phytochemistry*, vol. 66, no. 21, pp. 2595–2601, 2005.

[8] A. N. Rashed, F. U. Afifi, and A. M. Disi, "Simple evaluation of the wound healing activity of a crude extract of *Portulaca oleracea* L. (growing in Jordan) in Mus musculus JVI-1," *Journal of Ethnopharmacology*, vol. 88, no. 2-3, pp. 131–136, 2003.

[9] X. J. Zhang, Y. B. Ji, QuZh Y., and et al., "Experimental studies on antibiotic functions of Portulacaoleracea L. in vitro," *Chinese Journal of Microbiology and Immunology*, vol. 14, pp. 277–280, 2002.

[10] W. Wang, L. Gu, L. Dong, X. Wang, C. Ling, and M. Li, "Protective effect of Portulacaoleracea extracts on hypoxic nerve tissue and its mechanism," *Asia Pacific Journal of Clinical Nutrition*, pp. 227–233, 2007.

[11] K. Y. Musa, A. Ahmed, G. Ibrahim et al., "Toxicity studies on the methanolic extract of *Portulaca oleracea* L. (Fam. Portulacaceae)," *Journal of Biological Sciences*, vol. 7, no. 7, pp. 1293–1295, 2007.

[12] A. T. Reddy, S. P. Lakshmi, and R. C. Reddy, "PPAR γ in Bacterial Infections: A Friend or Foe?" *PPAR Research*, vol. 2016, Article ID 7963540, 2016.

[13] T. D. Hinds, K. John, L. McBeth, C. J. Trabbic, and E. R. Sanchez, "Timcodar (VX-853) Is a Non-FKBP12 Binding Macrolide Derivative That Inhibits PPAR γ and Suppresses Adipogenesis," *PPAR Research*, vol. 2016, Article ID 6218637, 2016.

[14] G. D. Demetri, C. D. Fletcher, E. Mueller et al., "Induction of solid tumor differentiation by the peroxisome proliferator-activated receptor-γ ligand troglitazone in patients with liposarcoma," *Proceedings of the National Acadamy of Sciences of the United States of America*, vol. 96, no. 7, pp. 3951–3956, 1999.

[15] T. Kubota, K. Koshizuka, E. A. Williamson, and et al., "Ligand for peroxisome proliferator-activated receptor gamma (troglitazone) has potent antitumor effect against human prostate cancer both in vitro and in vivo," *Cancer Research*, vol. 58, no. 15, pp. 3344–3352, 1998.

[16] S. P. Lakshmi, A. T. Reddy, A. Banno, and R. C. Reddy, "PPAR Agonists for the Prevention and Treatment of Lung Cancer," *PPAR Research*, vol. 2017, pp. 1–8, 2017.

[17] G. Chinetti, S. Lestavel, V. Bocher, and et al., "PPAR-alpha and PPAR-gamma activators induce cholesterol removal from human macrophage foam cells through stimulation of the ABCA1 pathway," *Nature Medicine*, vol. 7, no. 1, pp. 53–58, 2001.

[18] L. F. da Rocha Junior, A. T. Dantas, Â. L. B. P. Duarte, M. J. B. de Melo Rego, I. D. R. Pitta, and M. G. D. R. Pitta, "PPARγ agonists in adaptive immunity: what do immune disorders and their models have to tell us?" *PPAR Research*, vol. 2013, Article ID 519724, 9 pages, 2013.

[19] M. Ricote, A. C. Li, T. M. Willson, C. J. Kelly, and C. K. Glass, "The peroxisome proliferator-activated receptor-gamma is a negative regulator of macrophage activation," *Nature*, vol. 391, no. 6662, pp. 79–82, 1998.

[20] W. Hozayen, M. Bastawy, and H. Elshafeey, "Effects of Aqueous Purslane (PortulacaOleracea) Extractand Fish Oil on Gentamicin Nephrotoxicity in Albino Rats," *Natural Sciences*, vol. 9, pp. 47–62, 2011.

[21] A. N. Ananthakrishnan, E. L. McGinley, and D. G. Binion, "Does it matter where you are hospitalized for inflammatory bowel disease? A nationwide analysis of hospital volume," *American Journal of Gastroenterology*, vol. 103, no. 11, pp. 2789–2798, 2008.

[22] D. Bojic, Z. Radojicic, M. Nedeljkovic-Protic, M. Al-Ali, D. P. Jewell, and S. P. L. Travis, "Long-term outcome after admission for acute severe ulcerative colitis in Oxford: The 1992-1993 cohort," *Inflammatory Bowel Diseases*, vol. 15, no. 6, pp. 823–828, 2009.

[23] S. Kang, Y. Jeon, K. Moon et al., *Journal of Medicinal Food*, vol. 20, no. 7, pp. 667–675, 2017.

[24] D. Ristovski-Kornic, A. Stefanović, J. Kotur-Stevuljević et al., "Association of Myeloperoxidase and the Atherogenic Index of Plasma in Children with End-Stage Renal Disease," *Journal of Medical Biochemistry*, vol. 36, no. 1, pp. 23–31, 2017.

[25] A. Ece, F. Gürkan, M. Kervancıoğlu et al., "Oxidative stress, inflammation and early cardiovascular damage in children with chronic renal failure," *Pediatric Nephrology*, vol. 21, no. 4, pp. 545–552, 2006.

[26] E. Cavusoglu, C. Ruwende, C. Eng et al., "Usefulness of baseline plasma myeloperoxidase levels as an independent predictor of myocardial infarction at two years in patients presenting with acute coronary syndrome," *American Journal of Cardiology*, vol. 99, no. 10, pp. 1364–1368, 2007.

[27] D. Lau and S. Baldus, "Myeloperoxidase and its contributory role in inflammatory vascular disease," *Pharmacology & Therapeutics*, vol. 111, no. 1, pp. 16–26, 2006.

[28] L. Zhang, Y. Zhang, W. Zhong, C. Di, X. Lin, and Z. Xia, "Heme oxygenase-1 ameliorates dextran sulfate sodium-induced acute murine colitis by regulating Th17/Treg cell balance," *The Journal of Biological Chemistry*, vol. 289, no. 39, pp. 26847–26858, 2014.

[29] D. C. Baumgart and A. U. Dignass, "Intestinal barrier function," *Current Opinion in Clinical Nutrition & Metabolic Care*, vol. 5, no. 6, pp. 685–694, 2002.

[30] M. A. Degli-Esposti and M. J. Smyth, "Close encounters of different kinds: dendritic cells and NK cells take centre stage," *Nature Reviews Immunology*, vol. 5, no. 2, pp. 112–124, 2005.

[31] D. Gómez, N. Muñoz, R. Guerrero, O. Acosta, and C. A. Guerrero, "PPAR γ agonists as an anti-inflammatory treatment inhibiting rotavirus infection of small intestinal villi," *PPAR Research*, vol. 2016, Article ID 4049373, 2016.

[32] H. Baumann and J. Gauldie, "The acute phase response," *Trends in Immunology*, vol. 15, no. 2, pp. 74–80, 1994.

[33] B. Begue, H. Wajant, J.-C. Bambou et al., "Implication of TNF-related apoptosis-inducing ligand in inflammatory intestinal epithelial lesions," *Gastroenterology*, vol. 130, no. 7, pp. 1962–1974, 2006.

[34] M. N. Ince and D. E. Elliott, "Immunologic and Molecular Mechanisms in Inflammatory Bowel Disease," *Surgical Clinics of North America*, vol. 87, no. 3, pp. 681–696, 2007.

[35] J. Bauditz, S. Wedel, and H. Lochs, "Thalidomide reduces tumour necrosis factor-α and interleukin 12 production in patients with chronic active Crohn's disease," *Gut*, vol. 50, no. 2, pp. 196–200, 2002.

[36] S. C. Ng, S. Plamondon, M. A. Kamm et al., "Immunosuppressive effects via human intestinal dendritic cells of probiotic bacteria and steroids in the treatment of acute ulcerative colitis," *Inflammatory Bowel Diseases*, vol. 16, no. 8, pp. 1286–1298, 2010.

[37] Y. Liu, J. Peng, T. Sun, and et al., "Epithelial EZH2 serves as an epigenetic determinant in experimental colitis by inhibiting

TNFalpha-mediated inflammation and apoptosis," in *Proceedings of the National Academy of Sciences*, pp. E3796–E3805, 2017.

[38] R. Ravi, G. C. Bedi, L. W. Engstrom et al., "Regulation of death receptor expression and TRAIL/Apo2L-induced apoptosis by NF-κB," *Nature Cell Biology*, vol. 3, no. 4, pp. 409–416, 2001.

[39] Y. Chen, H. Ma, D. Zhu et al., "Discovery of Novel Insulin Sensitizers: Promising Approaches and Targets," *PPAR Research*, vol. 2017, pp. 1–13, 2017.

[40] F. Rosa, J. S. Osorio, E. Trevisi, F. Yanqui-Rivera, C. T. Estill, and M. Bionaz, "2,4-Thiazolidinedione Treatment Improves the Innate Immune Response in Dairy Goats with Induced Subclinical Mastitis," *PPAR Research*, vol. 2017, pp. 1–22, 2017.

[41] L. Dubuquoy, C. Bourdon, M. Peuchmaur, and et al., "Peroxisome proliferator-activated receptor (PPAR) gamma: a new target for the treatment of inflammatory bowel disease," *Gastroenterologie Clinique Et Biologique*, vol. 24, no. 8-9, pp. 719–724, 2000.

[42] Y. Kawahito, M. Kondo, Y. Tsubouchi et al., "15-deoxy-Δ12,14-PGJ2 induces synoviocyte apoptosis and suppresses adjuvant-induced arthritis in rats," *The Journal of Clinical Investigation*, vol. 106, no. 2, pp. 189–197, 2000.

[43] C. Jiang, A. T. Ting, and B. Seed, "PPAR-γ agonists inhibit production of monocyte inflammatory cytokines," *Nature*, vol. 391, no. 6662, pp. 82–86, 1998.

[44] H. S. P. Souza, C. J. A. Tortori, M. T. L. Castelo-Branco et al., "Apoptosis in the intestinal mucosa of patients with inflammatory bowel disease: evidence of altered expression of FasL and perforin cytotoxic pathways," *International Journal of Colorectal Disease*, vol. 20, no. 3, pp. 277–286, 2005.

[45] R. Sreedhar, S. Arumugam, V. Karuppagounder et al., "Jumihaidokuto effectively inhibits colon inflammation and apoptosis in mice with acute colitis," *International Immunopharmacology*, vol. 29, no. 2, pp. 957–963, 2015.

5

Vascular Remodeling, Oxidative Stress, and Disrupted PPARγ Expression in Rats of Long-Term Hyperhomocysteinemia with Metabolic Disturbance

Yajing Huo [ID],[1] Xuqing Wu,[1] Jing Ding,[1] Yang Geng,[1] Weiwei Qiao,[2] Anyan Ge,[1] Cen Guo,[1] Jianing Lv,[1] Haifeng Bao,[1] and Wei Fan [ID] [1]

[1]Department of Neurology, Zhongshan Hospital, Fudan University, Shanghai 200032, China
[2]Department of Laboratory Animal Science, Fudan University, Shanghai 200032, China

Correspondence should be addressed to Wei Fan; fan.wei@zs-hospital.sh.cn

Academic Editor: Lingyan Xu

Hyperhomocysteinemia, a risk factor for vascular disease, is associated with metabolic syndrome. Our study was aimed at exploring the effect of long-term hyperhomocysteinemia with metabolic disturbances on vascular remodeling. We also studied oxidative stress and expression of PPARγ in the coronary arteriole as a possible mechanism underlying vascular remodeling. Rats were treated with standard rodent chow (Control) or diet enriched in methionine (Met) for 48 weeks. Plasma homocysteine, blood glucose, serum lipids, malondialdehyde (MDA), superoxide dismutase (SOD), and nitric oxide (NO) levels were measured. Coronary arteriolar and carotid arterial remodeling was assessed by histomorphometric techniques and the expression of PPARγ in vessel wall was investigated. In Met group, an increase in the level of fasting blood glucose, serum triglyceride, total cholesterol, MDA, and NO, a decline in the serum SOD level, and increased collagen deposition in coronary and carotid arteries were found. Moreover, we detected decreased expression of PPARγ in the coronary arterioles in Met group. In summary, our study revealed metabolic disturbances in this model of long-term hyperhomocysteinemia together with vascular remodeling and suggested that impaired oxidative stress, endothelium dysfunction, and decreased PPARγ expression in the vessel wall could be underlying mechanisms.

1. Introduction

Hyperhomocysteinemia is an important risk factor for atherosclerosis [1]. Several clinical studies have shown that hyperhomocysteinemia was independently associated with increased vascular disease risk [2–4]. The previous study from our group has also demonstrated that elevated homocysteine correlated with severity and prognosis in patients with atherothrombotic stroke [5]. However, the precise mechanism of hyperhomocysteinemia with atherosclerosis has not been well elucidated [6].

Several animal studies have demonstrated that hyperhomocysteinemia could induce vascular remodeling [7–9]. Some clinical studies also showed that hyperhomocysteinemia was associated with increased carotid artery wall thickness in human beings [10, 11]. It has been implicated that possible mechanisms involved in homocysteine-mediated vascular remodeling could be oxidative stress and decreased NO bioavailability [9, 12]; however, the mechanisms have not been well described.

Several studies indicated that hyperhomocysteinemia may be a possible component of the metabolic syndrome [13, 14]. Previous studies showed that hyperhomocysteinemia might induce insulin resistance [15]. Hyperhomocysteinemia may lead to altered cellular redox reactions [16, 17]. It may also affect NO bioproduction and NO bioavailability [18]. Oxidative stress and NO may be involved in the activation of matrix metalloproteinases (MMPs) [9, 19]. Hyperhomocysteinemia could cause increased deposition of collagen by the activation of MMPs [20, 21]. In addition, oxidative stress might be involved in disturbances of lipid and glucose metabolism in hyperhomocysteinemia [22].

Peroxisome proliferator activated receptor gamma (PPARγ) is a nuclear receptor superfamily member, which may mitigate vascular complications. Homocysteine has been shown to antagonize PPARγ and be inversely related to the expression of PPARγ [23, 24], which could promote the synthesis of superoxide dismutase (SOD) and decrease oxidative stress [25, 26].

Because cardiovascular disease is a chronic disease, we used a rat model of long-term hyperhomocysteinemia to learn the long-term effect of hyperhomocysteinemia on metabolic parameters and vascular remodeling. Moreover, we studied oxidative stress and expression of PPARγ in the coronary arteriole as a possible mechanism underlying vascular remodeling. In our study, the methionine supplementation was chosen to reflect the upper range that may be consumed additionally during overnutrition in human beings.

2. Materials and Methods

2.1. Animals and Treatments. All experiments were conducted in accordance with the National Institutes of Health Guide for the Care and Use of Laboratory Animals and approved by the Animal Care and Use Committee of Fudan University. Seven-week-old male Wistar rats from Shanghai Experimental Animal Center, Chinese Academy of Sciences, China, were used in the study. The rats were housed in polyethylene cages with a 12 h light-dark cycle and kept in a room at a constant temperature of $22 \pm 3°C$. Food and water were provided ad libitum. Body weight, food consumption, and water intake were monitored periodically. L-Methionine was purchased from Sigma-Aldrich (St. Louis, MO, USA).

After 7 days of acclimatization to the facility, the animals were randomized into two groups ($n = 6$ in each group): (1) the control-diet group was fed with standard rodent chow; (2) the Met-diet group was fed with the diet enriched in methionine (3%; wt/wt). All rats were killed after 48 weeks. Fasted blood glucose was measured upon the 48th week of diet following 6 h of fasting. Tail blood glucose concentrations were measured using a handheld glucometer (AccuCheck performa meter).

2.2. Serum, Spleen, and Heart Collection and Storage. After 48 weeks of diet, the animals were sacrificed under 10% chloral hydrate (350 mg/Kg, intraperitoneal injection) anesthesia. Abdominal aorta blood was collected, immediately cooled on ice, and centrifuged at 3000 rpm for 10 min at $+4°C$. Aliquots of serum layer were stored at $-80°C$ until analysis. Then, the spleen, the heart, and carotid artery were removed. The spleen was weighed.

2.3. Measurement of Plasma Homocysteine. At the 48th week, the fasting animals were bled from the retroorbital plexus under aether anesthesia. Blood samples were obtained in chilled EDTA-containing microtubes and immediately centrifuged at 3000 rpm for 10 minutes at 4°C to limit the release of homocysteine (Hcy) from blood cells. Plasma was then stored at $-80°C$. Plasma Hcy concentration was measured by enzymatic cycling assay by Hitachi Model 7600 Series Automatic Analyzer (Hitachi High-Technologies Corporation, Japan).

2.4. Oral Glucose Tolerance Test (OGTT). After 48 weeks of diet, OGTT was performed in rats after being fasted overnight. Glucose (3 g/Kg bodyweight glucose 500 g/l) solution was given orally to rats. Tail blood glucose concentration was determined at 0, 30, 50, 90, 120 minutes after administration.

2.5. Measurement of Serum Triglycerides, Total Cholesterol, High Density Lipoprotein, and Low Density Lipoprotein. The serum triglycerides, total cholesterol, high density lipoprotein (HDL), and low density lipoprotein (LDL) were measured using enzymatic assay kits (Nanjing Jiancheng Bioengineering Institute, Nanjing, China). All assays were performed according to the manufacturers' instructions.

2.6. Determination of Lipid Peroxidation and Superoxide Dismutase Activity. The degree of MDA in the serum was determined by measuring thiobarbituric acid reactive substances (TBARS) [27, 28]. A Malondialdehyde (MDA) Detection Kit (A003; Nanjing Jiancheng Bioengineering Institute, Nanjing, China) was used to determine the MDA level as a marker of lipid peroxidation. The Superoxide Dismutase Detection Kit (A001; Nanjing Jiancheng Bioengineering Institute, Nanjing, China) was used for SOD measurement. Both assays were conducted according to the manufacturer's instruction.

2.7. Measurement of Serum Nitric Oxide (NO). The serum NO levels were detected by nitrate reductase method. The nitric oxide (NO) assay kit (A001; Nanjing Jiancheng Bioengineering Institute, Nanjing, China) was selected for NO measurement. The assay was conducted according to the manufacturer's instruction.

2.8. Histological Analysis. Coronal sections of ventricular myocardium and carotid artery were fixed in 10% neutral buffered formalin. The tissue sections (5 um) were stained with hematoxylin and eosin (H&E). Masson's trichrome stain was used for collagen and proteoglycans. Optical light microscopy was performed at 10x and 40x magnification. The coronary arteriolar wall-to-lumen ratio was analyzed in 50 to 200 um vessels. Percentages of collagen area of the carotid artery were calculated by dividing the area marked positive for collagen by the total tissue area.

2.9. Immunohistochemistry. The slices were dewaxed in xylene and hydrated in graded ethanol. Microwaves antigen retrieval was performed with citrate buffer for 10 min. Sections were washed in dH2O three times for 5 min each, incubated in 3% hydrogen peroxide for 10 min, washed in dH2O two times for 5 min each, and washed in wash buffer for 5 min. Then, each section was blocked with preferred blocking solution for 1 hour at room temperature. After blocking solution was removed, PPARγ (Cell Signaling Technology, USA) diluted in antibody diluent was added as the primary antibody and incubated overnight at 4°C.

TABLE 1: Parameter values in Wistar rats after 48 weeks of treatment with control and methionine-supplemented diets (n = 6/group).

Parameters	Control-diet group	Met-diet group	p
Water intake (ml/d)	23.75 ± 1.69	31.29 ± 1.87*	0.014
Food intake (g/d)	17.59 ± 0.65	16.10 ± 1.10	0.142
Spleen weight/body weight (mg/100 g)	111.51 ± 4.24	169.04 ± 7.53*	0.001
Fasting blood glucose (mmol/L)	4.23 ± 0.08	4.93 ± 0.08*	<0.001
Serum triglyceride (mmol/L)	0.29 ± 0.02	0.71 ± 0.03*	<0.001
Serum total cholesterol (mmol/L)	1.37 ± 0.08	1.81 ± 0.04*	<0.001
Serum high density lipoprotein (mmol/L)	0.73 ± 0.07	0.76 ± 0.05	0.753
Serum low density lipoprotein (mmol/L)	0.68 ± 0.07	0.77 ± 0.09	0.423
Serum NO (umol/L)	22.46 ± 1.05	8.22 ± 1.16*	<0.001
Serum MDA (umol/L)	27.05 ± 4.51	137.18 ± 16.01*	<0.001
Serum SOD (umol/L)	71.74 ± 1.64	20.31 ± 1.78*	<0.001
Plasma homocysteine (umol/L)	3.00 ± 0.35	10.75 ± 0.80*	<0.001

Met, methionine. Data are presented as mean ± SEM. *Significantly different from corresponding values in the control group.

Then antibody solution was removed and washed with wash buffer three times for 5 min each. Section was covered with horseradish peroxidase (HRP, Rabbit) as needed, incubated in a humidified chamber for 30 min at room temperature, and washed three times with wash buffer for 5 min each. DAB was applied to each section. The slides were washed with dH2O. Hematoxylin restaining, dehydration, transparent, sheet sealing, and microscopic examination were performed.

2.10. Statistical Analysis. Data were expressed as mean with standard errors (SEM) and statistical analysis was performed by SPSS 22.0 statistical software. All data were tested for normality prior to further analysis. Student's unpaired t-test was used to compare differences between groups. A p value of <0.05 was considered statistically significant.

3. Results

3.1. Plasma Homocysteine Levels. To confirm whether methionine administration induced an increase in plasma homocysteine, the plasma homocysteine level was measured. The plasma homocysteine level in the Met-diet group at the 48th week was significantly increased compared with the control-diet group at the same time (Table 1).

3.2. Physiological Variables after Methionine Loading. In the feeding period, the average water intake in Met-loaded rats was significantly increased compared with control animals (p < 0.05) (Table 1). There was no significant difference in the food consumption between the two groups (p > 0.05) (Table 1). The weight gain in Met-supplemented rats was slower than that in control rats (p < 0.05) (Figure 1). At the 48th week, the spleen weight/body weight in Met-supplemented rats was higher than that in control rats (p < 0.05) (Table 1).

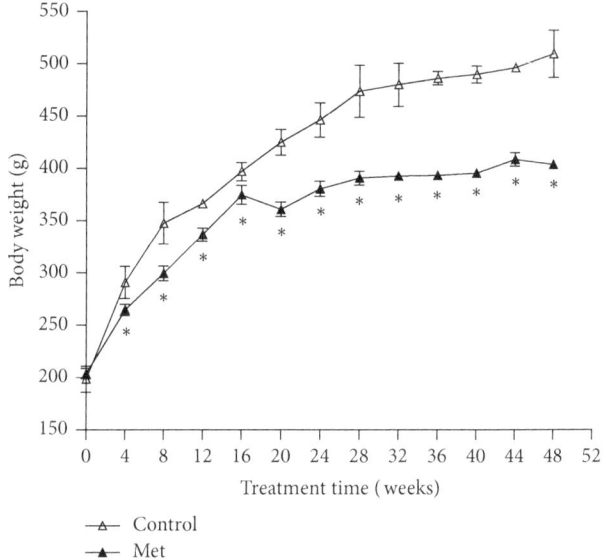

FIGURE 1: Effect of a control or methionine- (Met-) supplemented diet on change in body weight in Met-diet group (n = 6) and control-diet group (n = 6). Values are mean ± SEM. Mean values for the Met-diet group were significantly different from those of the control-diet group. *P < 0.05.

3.3. Oral Glucose Tolerance Test. We determined glucose tolerance by OGTT in each group at the 48th week. The glucose level rose to significantly higher concentrations in the Met-diet group compared with the control-diet group at 0 min, 30 min, 60 min, 90 min, and 120 min after glucose administration (p < 0.05) (Figure 2).

3.4. Metabolic Parameters. The results for metabolic measurements are shown in Table 1. At the 48th week, Met-supplemented rats showed an increase in the fasting blood glucose compared with control rats (p < 0.05). At the 48th week, the serum triglyceride level and the serum total

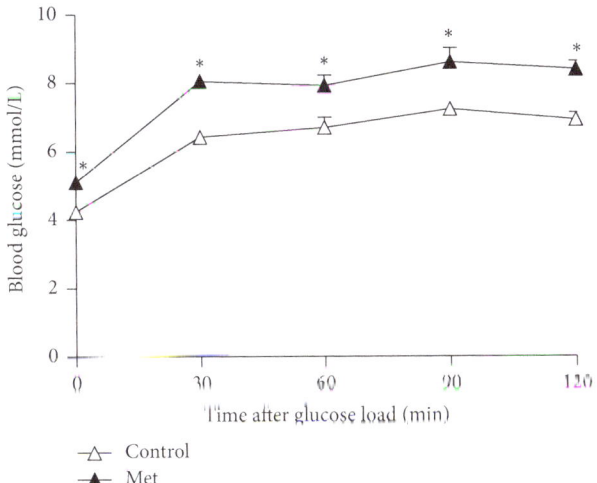

FIGURE 2: Glucose concentrations during the oral glucose tolerance test (OGTT) in the control-diet group ($n = 6$) and the Met-diet group ($n = 6$) at the 48th week. Values are mean ± SEM. $^*p < 0.005$ versus the control-diet group.

cholesterol level in the Met-diet group were higher than those in the control-diet group ($p < 0.05$). However, there was no significant difference in the levels of the serum HDL and LDL between the two groups at the 48th week ($p > 0.05$).

3.5. Serum Malondialdehyde (MDA) and Superoxide Dismutase (SOD) Levels. Forty-eight weeks after methionine administration, the serum MDA levels were significantly increased and the serum SOD levels were significantly decreased in the Met-diet group compared with the control-diet group ($p < 0.05$) (Table 1).

3.6. Serum Nitrates (NO) Levels. The serum NO levels were significantly decreased in the control-diet group at the 48th week ($p < 0.05$) (Table 1).

3.7. Effect of Homocysteine on Carotid Arterial Remodeling. Carotid artery was stained with trichrome stain to detect the collagen deposition. Our result suggested that collagen content was significantly higher in the Met-diet group than the control-diet group, demonstrating arterial remodeling (Figure 3).

3.8. Effect of Homocysteine on Coronary Arteriolar Remodeling. To determine structural alteration by homocysteine, histological analysis was performed. Coronary arteriole was stained with H&E and trichrome (Figure 3). Coronary arteriolar wall thickness was increased in the Met-diet group compared with the control-diet group at the 48th week. The wall-to-lumen ratios of coronary arterioles in the Met-diet group were higher than those in the control-diet group ($p < 0.05$). The collagen deposition was increased in coronary arterioles of the Met-diet group compared with the control-diet group (Figure 4).

3.9. Effect of Homocysteine on PPARγ Expression in the Coronary Arteriole. As shown in Figure 5, PPARγ expression was found in the coronary arteriole of the control-diet group; PPARγ expression decreased in the coronary arteriole of the Met-diet group ($p < 0.05$).

4. Discussion

In the current study, we found that long-term hyperhomocysteinemia could cause carotid arterial and coronary arteriolar remodeling due to collagen deposition in the vessels. We also found that PPARγ expression decreased in the coronary arteriole. Moreover, our results showed that homocysteine could lead to disturbances of lipid and glucose metabolism, impaired oxidative stress, and endothelium dysfunction.

Results from our study showed disturbances of glucose metabolism after 48 weeks of administration of methionine diet. We speculated the disturbances of glucose metabolism may be associated with insulin resistance. Some studies suggested that hyperhomocysteinemia may induce insulin resistance [15, 29]. However, other studies showed that hyperinsulinemia can cause elevated plasma Hcy by impairing the activity of Hcy metabolizing enzymes [30, 31]. After 48 weeks of administration of methionine, the rats had significantly increased levels of plasma cholesterol and triglycerides. Previous studies also indicated that cholesterol and triglycerides were not significantly elevated in the plasma but significantly elevated in the livers of mice fed hyperhomocysteinemic diets for 10 to 20 weeks [32]. So hyperhomocysteinemia may cause ectopic accumulation of fat in liver at an early stage and disturbances of plasma lipid in the long run. The mechanisms between hyperhomocysteinemia and disturbances of lipid and glucose metabolism are not fully elucidated and may be associated with methyl group [33] and oxidative stress [22].

The present study demonstrated that plasma MDA levels were increased and SOD activity was decreased in the hyperhomocysteinemic rats. Our findings were consistent with previous studies [6, 34–36]. Oxidative radicals may be responsible for decreased production and bioavailability of endothelial-derived NO which may result in impaired endothelial-dependent vascular reactivity [37]. Hcy indirectly diminishes NO bioavailability by generating superoxide which rapidly reacts with NO causing the generation of peroxynitrite [38]. In this study, we demonstrated that hyperhomocysteinemia was associated with decreased NO levels, lower SOD activity, and increased MDA levels, suggesting that oxidative stress caused by Hcy may be related to the decreased NO bioavailability.

Oxidative stress may regulate the quantity and quality of extracellular matrix by activating matrix metalloproteinases (MMPs) [19]. Hcy can promote oxidative stress, thereby triggering the activation of MMPs [39]. NO may also have a role in the activation of MMPs [9]. The increased activity of MMPs can result in the degradation of extracellular matrix (ECM) components. Hence, Hcy may cause MMP-mediated degradation of ECM components and increased deposition of

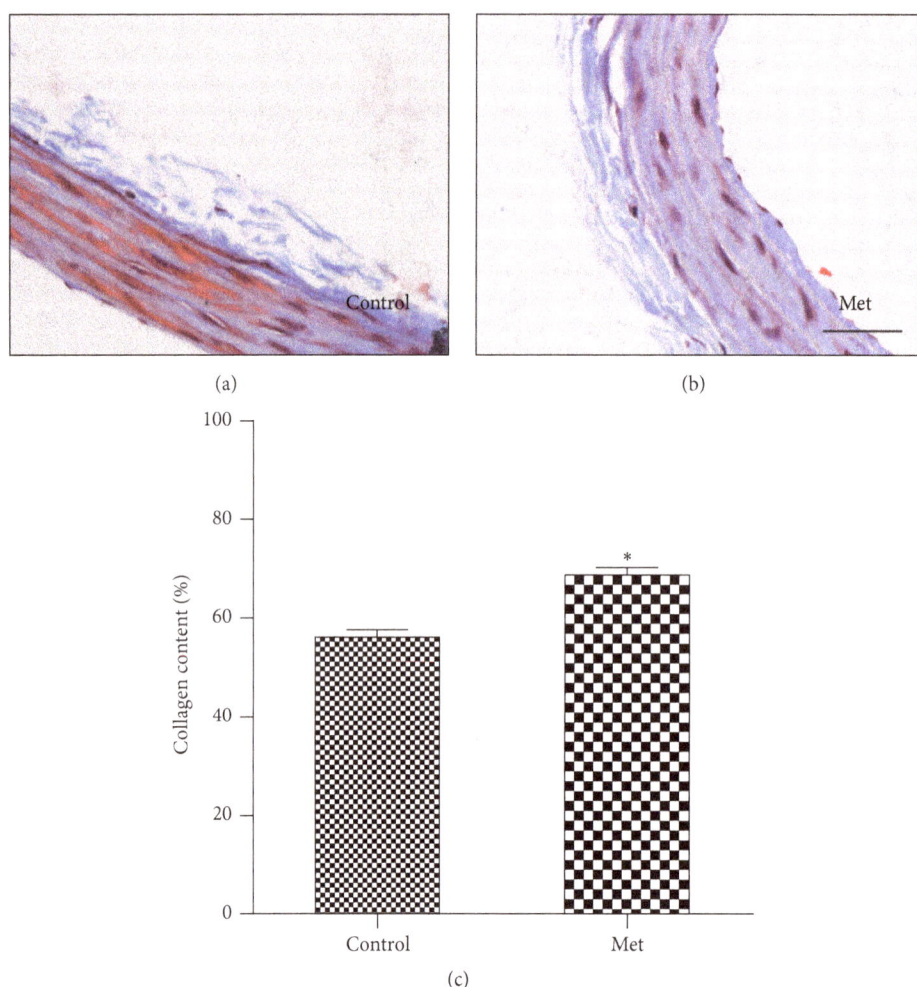

(a)

(b)

(c)

FIGURE 3: Histological analysis of carotid artery in the control-diet group and the Met-diet group. Tissue sections were labeled with trichrome (blue) for collagen. The staining showed hyperhomocysteinemia induced collagen accumulation in carotid artery in the Met-diet group (b) compared with representative vessels from the control-diet group (a). Collagen content was significantly increased in the Met-diet group ($^*p < 0.05$) (c). Original magnification was ×400 for (a)-(b) and the scale bar = 50 um. Values are mean ± SEM.

collagen, leading to the remodeling of the vessel wall [20, 21]. Some clinical studies indicated that hyperhomocysteinemia was a risk factor for increased carotid wall thickness [10, 11]. Our results indicated that Hcy caused the remodeling of the carotid artery after a long term of methionine-enriched diet, which may be related to the collagen deposition in the vessels, and so was the coronary arteriole.

In the present study, PPARγ expression decreased in the coronary arteriole of the Met-diet group compared with the control group. It is known that PPARγ induces SOD and decreases oxidative stress [25, 26]. On the other hand, previous study has suggested that homocysteine might induce vascular constrictive remodeling by antagonizing PPAR [40]. So we postulated that oxidative stress might activate MMPs leading to vascular remodeling by antagonizing PPARγ. Our study may suggest a potential benefit of PPARγ agonists on reversing the Hcy-mediated vascular remodeling in patients with hyperhomocysteinemia.

In our study, the spleens were enlarged after 48 weeks of feeding 3% methionine diets. The mechanism of which excessive methionine diet causes spleen hypertrophy is probably by changes in iron metabolism [41, 42].

There are some limitations in this study. First, we did not measure markers of oxidative stress (SOD, MDA) and MMPs in the carotid and coronary arteries. Second, the mechanisms of vascular remodeling remained unclear. Impaired oxidative stress, endothelium dysfunction, and decreased PPARγ expression in the vessel wall may be involved, but further studies are needed to elucidate the underlying mechanisms.

5. Conclusion

In conclusion, the results of this study suggested that chronic hyperhomocysteinemia caused metabolic disturbances together with vascular remodeling and suggested that impaired oxidative stress, endothelium dysfunction, and

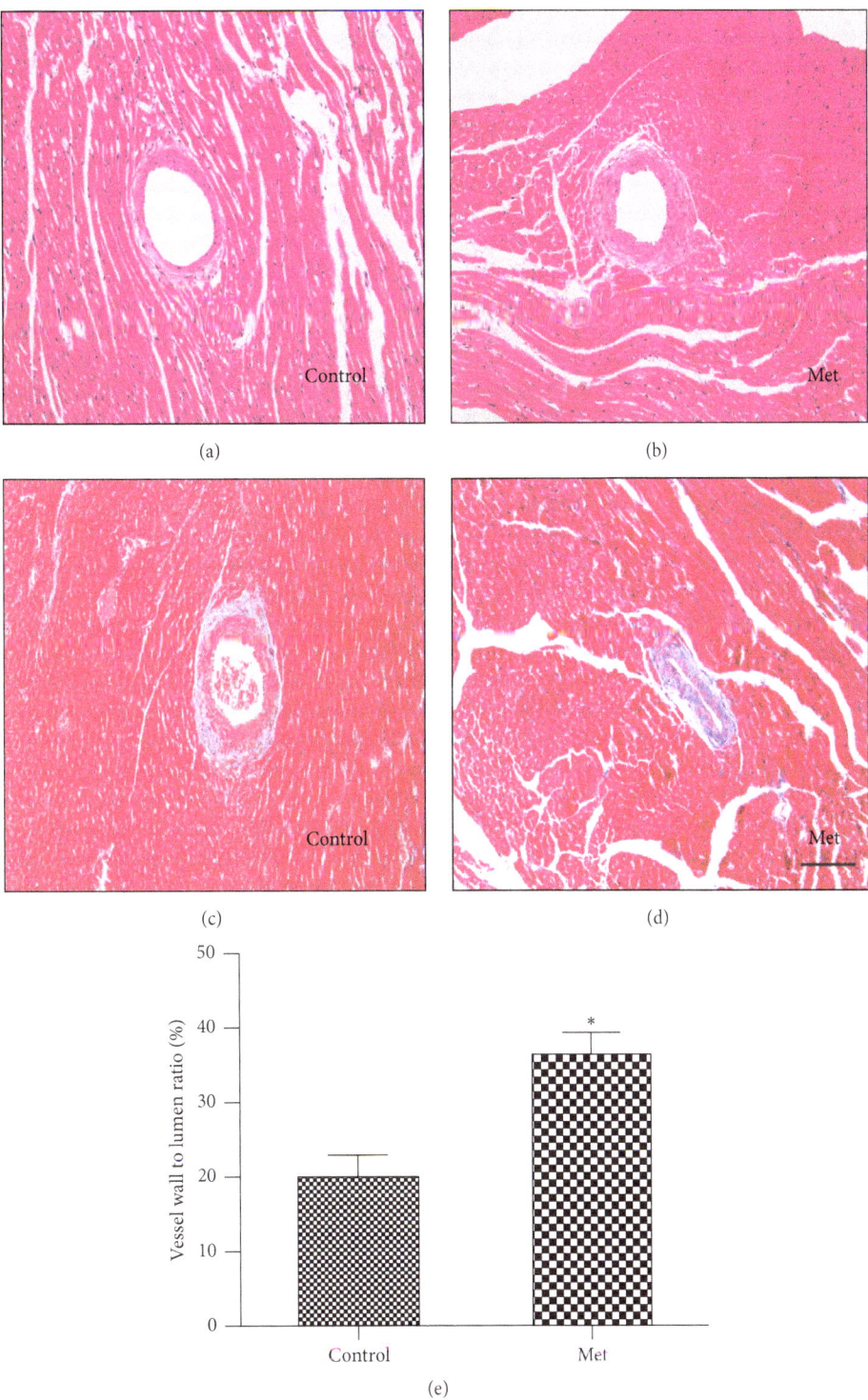

FIGURE 4: Representative images of stained heart sections. H&E stained sections from the control-diet group (a) and the Met-diet group (b) showed hyperhomocysteinemia induced coronary arteriolar wall thickening. Masson's trichrome staining showed hyperhomocysteinemia induced collagen accumulation in coronary arterioles in the Met-diet group (d) compared with vessels from the control-diet group (c). The wall-to-lumen ratios of coronary arterioles in the Mct-diet group were increased compared with the control-diet group ($^*p < 0.05$) (e). Original magnification was ×100 for (a)–(d) and the scale bar = 100 um. Values are mean ± SEM.

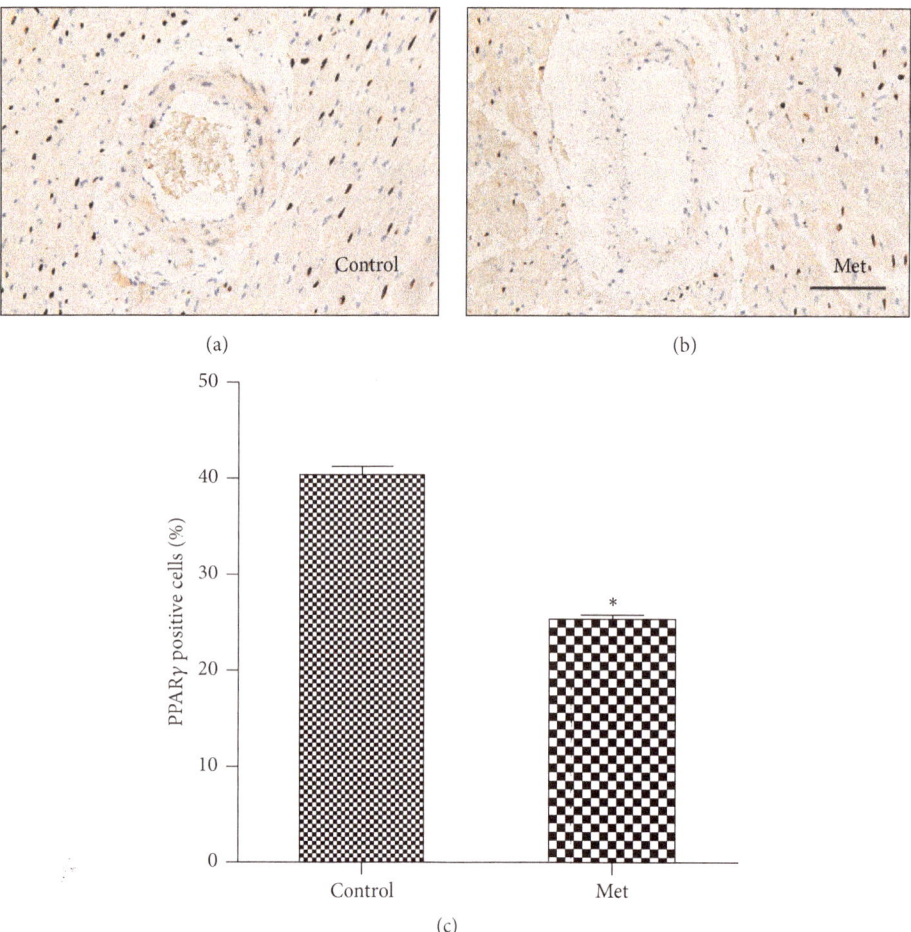

Figure 5: Representative immunohistochemical images of PPARγ in the coronary arteriole in the control-diet group (a) and the Met-diet group (b). Positive staining of PPARγ was found in the nuclei of the cells. The Met-diet group had significantly fewer PPARγ positive cells ($^*p < 0.05$) (c). Original magnification was ×200 for (a)-(b) and the scale bar = 100 um. Values are mean ± SEM.

decreased PPARγ expression in the vessel wall could be underlying mechanisms.

Conflicts of Interest

The authors declare no conflicts of interest.

Authors' Contributions

Yajing Huo and Xuqing Wu contributed equally to this article.

Acknowledgments

This work was supported by the Shanghai Municipal Science and Technology Commission (Grant no. 12140903300).

References

[1] K. S. McCully, "Homocysteine metabolism, atherosclerosis, and diseases of aging," *Comprehensive Physiology*, vol. 6, no. 1, pp. 471–505, 2015.

[2] W. H. Giles, J. B. Croft, K. J. Greenlund, E. S. Ford, and S. J. Kittner, "Total homocyst(e)ine concentration and the likelihood of nonfatal stroke: Results from the Third National Health and Nutrition Examination Survey, 1988-1994," *Stroke*, vol. 29, no. 12, pp. 2473–2477, 1998.

[3] A. G. Bostom, H. Silbershatz, I. H. Rosenberg et al., "Nonfasting plasma total homocysteine levels and all-cause and cardiovascular disease mortality in elderly Framingham men and women," *JAMA Internal Medicine*, vol. 159, no. 10, pp. 1077–1080, 1999.

[4] H. S. Collaboration, "Homocysteine and risk of ischemic heart disease and stroke: a meta-analysis," *Jama*, vol. 288, no. 16, pp. 2015–2022, 2002.

[5] X.-Q. Wu, J. Ding, A.-Y. Ge, F.-F. Liu, X. Wang, and W. Fan, "Acute phase homocysteine related to severity and outcome of atherothrombotic stroke," *European Journal of Internal Medicine*, vol. 24, no. 4, pp. 362–367, 2013.

[6] J. Kolling, E. B. Scherer, A. A. Da Cunha, M. J. Da Cunha, and A. T. S. Wyse, "Homocysteine induces oxidative-nitrative stress in heart of rats: Prevention by folic acid," *Cardiovascular Toxicology*, vol. 11, no. 1, pp. 67–73, 2011.

[7] J. Joseph, A. Washington, L. Joseph et al., "Hyperhomocysteinemia leads to adverse cardiac remodeling in hypertensive

rats," *American Journal of Physiology Heart And Circulatory Physiology*, vol. 283, no. 6, pp. H2567–H2574, 2002.

[8] M. Kumar, N. Tyagi, K. S. Moshal et al., "Homocysteine decreases blood flow to the brain due to vascular resistance in carotid artery," *Neurochemistry International*, vol. 53, no. 6-8, pp. 214–219, 2008.

[9] C. Munjal, S. Givvimani, N. Qipshidze, N. Tyagi, J. C. Falcone, and S. C. Tyagi, "Mesenteric vascular remodeling in hyperhomocysteinemia," *Molecular and Cellular Biochemistry*, vol. 348, no. 1-2, pp. 99–108, 2011.

[10] H. Adachi, Y. Hirai, Y. Fujiura, H. Matsuoka, A. Satoh, and T. Imaizumi, "Plasma homocysteine levels and atherosclerosis in Japan: Epidemiological study by use of carotid ultrasonography," *Stroke*, vol. 33, no. 9, pp. 2177–2181, 2002.

[11] M. Dietrich, P. F. Jacques, J. F. Polak et al., "Segment-specific association between plasma homocysteine level and carotid artery intima-media thickness in the Framingham Offspring Study," *Journal of Stroke and Cerebrovascular Diseases*, vol. 20, no. 2, pp. 155–161, 2011.

[12] M. M. Steed and S. C. Tyagi, "Mechanisms of cardiovascular remodeling in hyperhomocysteinemia," *Antioxidants & Redox Signaling*, vol. 15, no. 7, pp. 1927–1943, 2011.

[13] J. B. Meigs, P. F. Jacques, J. Selhub et al., "Fasting plasma homocysteine levels in the insulin resistance syndrome: the Framingham offspring study," *Diabetes Care*, vol. 24, no. 8, pp. 1403–1410, 2001.

[14] M. Oron-Herman, T. Rosenthal, and B.-A. Sela, "Hyperhomocysteinemia as a component of syndrome X," *Metabolism - Clinical and Experimental*, vol. 52, no. 11, pp. 1491–1495, 2003.

[15] J. Golbahar, M. A. Aminzadeh, S. E. Kassab, and G. R. Omrani, "Hyperhomocysteinemia induces insulin resistance in male Sprague-Dawley rats," *Diabetes Research and Clinical Practice*, vol. 76, no. 1, pp. 1–5, 2007.

[16] S. Dayal and S. R. Lentz, "Role of redox reactions in the vascular phenotype of hyperhomocysteinemic animals," *Antioxidants & Redox Signaling*, vol. 9, no. 11, pp. 1899–1909, 2007.

[17] N. Weiss, S. J. Heydrick, O. Postea, C. Keller, J. F. Keaney Jr., and J. Loscalzo, "Influence of hyperhomocysteinemia on the cellular redox state - Impact on homocysteine-induced endothelial dysfunction," *Clinical Chemistry and Laboratory Medicine*, vol. 41, no. 11, pp. 1455–1461, 2003.

[18] W. Y. Fu, N. P. B. Dudman, M. A. Perry, and X. L. Wang, "Homocysteine attenuates hemodynamic responses to nitric oxide in vivo," *Atherosclerosis*, vol. 161, no. 1, pp. 169–176, 2002.

[19] D. A. Siwik, P. J. Pagano, and W. S. Colucci, "Oxidative stress regulates collagen synthesis and matrix metalloproteinase activity in cardiac fibroblasts," *American Journal of Physiology Cell Physiology*, vol. 280, no. 1, pp. C53–C60, 2001.

[20] A. V. Ovechkin, N. Tyagi, U. Sen et al., "3-Deazaadenosine mitigates arterial remodeling and hypertension in hyperhomocysteinemic mice," *American Journal of Physiology-Lung Cellular and Molecular Physiology*, vol. 291, no. 5, pp. L905–L911, 2006.

[21] N. Narayanan, S. B. Pushpakumar, S. Givvimani et al., "Epigenetic regulation of aortic remodeling in hyperhomocysteinemia," *The FASEB Journal*, vol. 28, no. 8, pp. 3411–3422, 2014.

[22] C. Matté, F. M. Stefanello, V. Mackedanz et al., "Homocysteine induces oxidative stress, inflammatory infiltration, fibrosis and reduces glycogen/glycoprotein content in liver of rats," *International Journal of Developmental Neuroscience*, vol. 27, no. 4, pp. 337–344, 2009.

[23] S. C. Tyagi, W. Rodriguez, A. M. Patel et al., "Hyperhomocysteinemic diabetic cardiomyopathy: Oxidative stress, remodeling, and endothelial-myocyte uncoupling," *Journal of Cardiovascular Pharmacology and Therapeutics*, vol. 10, no. 1, pp. 1–10, 2005.

[24] N. Tyagi, K. S. Moshal, D. Lominadze, A. V. Ovechkin, and S. C. Tyagi, "Homocysteine-dependent cardiac remodeling and endothelial-myocyte coupling in a 2 kidney, 1 clip Goldblatt hypertension mouse model," *Canadian Journal of Physiology and Pharmacology*, vol. 83, no. 7, pp. 583–594, 2005.

[25] I. Inoue, S.-I. Goto, T. Matsunaga et al., "The ligands/activators for peroxisome proliferator-activated receptor α (PPARα) and PPARγ increase Cu^{2+},Zn^{2+}-superoxide dismutase and decrease p22phox message expressions in primary endothelial cells," *Metabolism Clinical and Experimental*, vol. 50, no. 1, pp. 3–11, 2001.

[26] N. Tyagi, N. Qipshidze, U. Sen, W. Rodriguez, A. Ovechkin, and S. C. Tyagi, "Cystathionine beta synthase gene dose dependent vascular remodeling in murine model of hyperhomocysteinemia," *International Journal of Physiology, Pathophysiology and Pharmacology*, vol. 3, no. 3, pp. 210–222, 2011.

[27] H. Ohkawa, N. Ohishi, and K. Yagi, "Assay for lipid peroxides in animal tissues by thiobarbituric acid reaction," *Analytical Biochemistry*, vol. 95, no. 2, pp. 351–358, 1979.

[28] F. L. Sung, T. Y. Zhu, K. K. W. Au-Yeung, Y. L. Siow, and K. O, "Enhanced MCP-1 expression during ischemia/reperfusion injury is mediated by oxidative stress and NF-κB," *Kidney International*, vol. 62, no. 4, pp. 1160–1170, 2002.

[29] M. Pravenec, V. Kožich, J. Krijt et al., "Folate deficiency is associated with oxidative stress, increased blood pressure, and insulin resistance in spontaneously hypertensive rats," *American Journal of Hypertension*, vol. 26, no. 1, pp. 135–140, 2013.

[30] V. Fonseca, A. Dicker-Brown, S. Ranganathan et al., "Effects of a high-fat-sucrose diet on enzymes in homocysteine metabolism in the rat," *Metabolism - Clinical and Experimental*, vol. 49, no. 6, pp. 736–741, 2000.

[31] A. Dicker-Brown, V. A. Fonseca, L. M. Fink, and P. A. Kern, "The effect of glucose and insulin on the activity of methylene tetrahydrofolate reductase and cystathionine-β-synthase: Studies in hepatocytes," *Atherosclerosis*, vol. 158, no. 2, pp. 297–301, 2001.

[32] G. H. Werstuck, S. R. Lentz, S. Dayal et al., "Homocysteine-induced endoplasmic reticulum stress causes dysregulation of the cholesterol and triglyceride biosynthetic pathways," *The Journal of Clinical Investigation*, vol. 107, no. 10, pp. 1263–1273, 2001.

[33] R. Obeid and W. Herrmann, "Homocysteine and lipids: S-Adenosyl methionine as a key intermediate," *FEBS Letters*, vol. 583, no. 8, pp. 1215–1225, 2009.

[34] R. Lin, J. Liu, W. Gan, and C. Ding, "Protective effect of quercetin on the homocysteine-injured human umbilical vein vascular endothelial cell line (ECV304)," *Basic & Clinical pharmacology & Toxicology*, vol. 101, no. 3, pp. 197–202, 2007.

[35] L. Chang, J. X. Xu, J. Zhao, Y. Z. Pang, C. S. Tang, and Y. F. Qi, "Taurine antagonized oxidative stress injury induced by homocysteine in rat vascular smooth muscle cells," *Acta Pharmacologica Sinica*, vol. 25, no. 3, pp. 341–346, 2004.

[36] F. Derouiche, C. Bôle-Feysot, D. Naïmi, and M. Coëffier, "Hyperhomocysteinemia-induced oxidative stress differentially alters proteasome composition and activities in heart and aorta," *Biochemical and Biophysical Research Communications*, vol. 452, no. 3, pp. 740–745, 2014.

[37] M. R. Hayden and S. C. Tyagi, "Homocysteine and reactive oxygen species in metabolic syndrome, type 2 diabetes mellitus, and atheroscleropathy: The pleiotropic effects of folate supplementation," *Nutrition Journal*, vol. 3, article no. 4, 2004.

[38] F. M. Faraci, "Hyperhomocysteinemia: A million ways to lose control," *Arteriosclerosis, Thrombosis, and Vascular Biology*, vol. 23, no. 3, pp. 371–373, 2003.

[39] S. C. Tyagi, "Homocysteine redox receptor and regulation of extracellular matrix components in vascular cells," *The American Journal of Physiology*, vol. 274, no. 2, pp. C396–C405, 1998.

[40] V. S. Mujumdar, C. M. Tummalapalli, G. M. Aru, and S. C. Tyagi, "Mechanism of constrictive vascular remodeling by homocysteine: role of PPAR," *American Journal of Physiology Cell Physiology*, vol. 282, no. 5, pp. C1009–C1015, 2002.

[41] J. A. Stekol and J. Szaran, "Pathological effects of excessive methionine in the diet of growing rats," *The Journal of Nutrition*, vol. 77, pp. 81–90, 1962.

[42] C. E. Mengel and J. V. Klavins, "Development of hemolytic anemia in rats fed methionine," *The Journal of Nutrition*, vol. 92, no. 1, pp. 104–110, 1967.

6

Quercetin and Quercetin-Rich Red Onion Extract Alter *Pgc-1α* Promoter Methylation and Splice Variant Expression

Prasad P. Devarshi, Aarin D. Jones, Erin M. Taylor, Barbara Stefanska, and Tara M. Henagan

Department of Nutrition Science, Purdue University, West Lafayette, IN, USA

Correspondence should be addressed to Tara M. Henagan; thenagan@purdue.edu

Academic Editor: Rozalyn M. Anderson

Pgc-1α and its various isoforms may play a role in determining skeletal muscle mitochondrial adaptations in response to diet. 8 wks of dietary supplementation with the flavonoid quercetin (Q) or red onion extract (ROE) in a high fat diet (HFD) ameliorates HFD-induced obesity and insulin resistance in C57BL/J mice while upregulating *Pgc-1α* and increasing skeletal muscle mitochondrial number and function. Here, mice were fed a low fat (LF), high fat (HF), high fat plus quercetin (HF + Q), or high fat plus red onion extract (HF + RO) diet for 9 wks and skeletal muscle *Pgc-1α* isoform expression and DNA methylation were determined. Quantification of various *Pgc-1α* isoforms, including isoforms *Pgc-1α-a*, *Pgc-1α-b*, *Pgc-1α-c*, *Pgc-1α4*, total *NT-Pgc-1α*, and *FL-Pgc-1α*, showed that only total *NT-Pgc-1α* expression was increased in LF, HF + Q, and HF + RO compared to HF. Furthermore, Q supplementation decreased *Pgc-1α-a* expression compared to LF and HF, and ROE decreased *Pgc-1α-a* expression compared to LF. *FL-Pgc-1α* was decreased in HF + Q and HF + RO compared to LF and HF. HF exhibited hypermethylation at the −260 nucleotide (nt) in the *Pgc-1α* promoter. Q and ROE prevented HFD-induced hypermethylation. −260 nt methylation levels were associated with *NT-Pgc-1α* expression only. *Pgc-1α* isoform expression may be epigenetically regulated by Q and ROE through DNA methylation.

1. Introduction

Peroxisome proliferator activated-receptor gamma coactivator 1 alpha *(Pgc-1α)* is a transcriptional coactivator that coordinates gene expression from the nuclear and mitochondrial genomes in order to determine mitochondrial biogenesis and function [1–4]. Environmentally induced upregulation of *Pgc-1α* plays a major role in determining skeletal muscle mitochondrial adaptations that are important in attenuating obesity and insulin resistance [1, 4–11]. Energy and nutritional status, such as the obese and diabetic state, and environmental cues, such as cold exposure, exercise training, and various dietary components, determine *Pgc-1α* expression [1, 2, 4–6, 12]. For example, high fat diet (HFD) feeding and palmitate treatment decrease *Pgc-1α* expression [6, 12, 13], whereas antiobesogenic and diabetic dietary supplements increase *Pgc-1α* expression [7, 13]. Traditionally, the molecular mechanisms regulating *Pgc-1α* have focused on posttranslational regulation of the protein affecting protein stability

and its ability to bind target genes to induce transcriptional activation [1, 14]; however, more recent investigations have shown a major role of epigenetic modifications to the *Pgc-1α* promoter to play a role in its transcriptional regulation and mRNA expression in response to environmental and energy/nutritional inputs [5, 6, 13, 15, 16]. Exercise training, dietary fat content, long chain fatty acid exposure, and the presence of diabetes and overweight or obesity have all been shown to epigenetically regulate *Pgc-1α* mRNA expression and downstream mitochondrial adaptations in skeletal muscle [5, 6, 13, 15, 16].

Not only is *Pgc-1α* regulated posttranslationally and transcriptionally, but also several *Pgc-1α* isoforms with novel and specific activities have been identified [17–19]. The various expression patterns of these *Pgc-1α* isoforms are also regulated by environmental stimuli, including cold exposure and exercise training, and by the obese state [15, 17–22]. To date, more than ten isoforms of *Pgc-1α* are known to exist, arising from a combination of distinct promoter start sites and alternative splicing [23]. The most extensively studied isoforms in skeletal muscle are *Pgc-1α-b*, *Pgc-1α-c*, *Pgc-1α4*, the *n*-truncated splice variant *NT-Pgc-1α*, and the full length variant *FL-Pgc-1α* [17–19, 21, 23, 24]. While many isoforms possess overlapping functions, several have been shown to have distinct functions in skeletal muscle [23]. For example, exercise training preferentially upregulates expression of the isoforms arising from the alternative, distal promoter region, including isoforms *Pgc-1α-b*, *Pgc-1α-c*, *Pgc-1α4*, total *NT-Pgc-1α*, and *FL-Pgc-1α* [23]. Additionally, *Pgc-1α-a*, *Pgc-1α-b*, *Pgc-1α-c*, total *NT-Pgc-1α*, and *FL-Pgc-1α* are all known to play a role in exercise-induced mitochondrial adaptations in skeletal muscle [19]. Distinct from the other exercise-induced isoforms, *Pgc-1α4* plays a role in promoting muscle hypertrophy [21]. More recently, various isoforms of *NT-Pgc-1α* (*NT-Pgc-1α-a*, *NT-Pgc-1α-b*, and *NT-Pgc-1α-c*), derived from either the proximal or distal promoters, have been characterized. All *NT-Pgc-1α* isoforms have been shown to be induced during either high intensity (*NT-Pgc-1α-a*) or low intensity (*NT-Pgc-1α-b* and *NT-Pgc-1α-c*) exercise, contributing to upregulation of total *NT-Pgc-1α* that occurs at all intensities of exercise [19]. Additionally, all *NT-Pgc-1α* isoforms and total *NT-Pgc-1α* are upregulated in skeletal muscle in response to AICAR treatment, a pharmacological activator of AMPK known to increase mitochondrial biogenesis and fatty acid oxidation in skeletal muscle [19]. Collectively, the isoforms most notably known to play roles in skeletal muscle mitochondrial adaptations to date include *Pgc-1α-a*, *Pgc-1α-b*, *Pgc-1α-c*, *Pgc-1α4*, total *NT-Pgc-1α*, and *FL-Pgc-1α*. Expression patterns of these various splice variants may have the ability to prevent disease, as overexpression of total *NT-Pgc-1α* is also known to attenuate HFD-induced obesity [25]. Interestingly, recent studies show that epigenetics may play a role in determining mRNA splicing [26] in addition to its role in determining transcription initiation and −1 nucleosome positioning may play a role in determining *FL-Pgc-1α* and total *NT-Pgc-1α* expression in skeletal muscle in relation to cardiovascular disease during overweight and obesity [15]. Thus, *Pgc-1α* isoform expression may be epigenetically regulated during disease and in response to environmental stimuli, including dietary inputs.

Quercetin (Q) is a bioflavanoid that protects against mitochondrial dysfunction and attenuates HFD-induced obesity and insulin resistance when supplemented in a HFD at low concentrations [7, 27–32]. We have recently shown that a low dose (50 ug/day) of dietary Q supplementation or dietary supplementation with red onion extract (ROE), containing equivalent amounts of Q glycosides (50 ug/day), increases skeletal muscle mitochondrial number and function, leading to more complete fatty acid oxidation [7, 32], similar to the effects of exercise training on skeletal muscle. However, the effects of Q or ROE appear to occur through regulation of differential molecular mechanisms at the level of mitochondrial gene transcription [32], a process that may be controlled by the transcriptional coactivation abilities of *Pgc-1α*.

To investigate the role of dietary fat, purified dietary Q, and ROE in determining *Pgc-1α* DNA methylation in skeletal muscle in association with HFD-induced obesity and insulin resistance and elaborate on how these epigenetic effects

associate with splice variant expression, we used diet-induced obese C57BL/6J mice as a model system. We hypothesized that the mitochondrial gene expression patterns previously observed and published [32] would be associated with differential diet-induced methylation patterns in the PGC-1 promoter and regulation of those specific *Pgc-1α* isoforms known to play a role in skeletal muscle mitochondrial adaptations in response to environmental stimuli [17, 18, 21, 25].

2. Materials and Methods

2.1. Animals and Diets. The protocols for animal and diets have been previously published [32]. Briefly, ROE was prepared as previously described [32] and formulated into a purified high fat diet (Research Diets D12451, 45% kcal fat) to yield 17 mg/kg of quercetin equivalents [32]. 5-week-old C57BL/6J mice (Jackson Laboratories, Bar Harbor, MN, USA) were weaned onto low fat diet (LF; Research Diets 12450B, 10% kcal fat) for 1 week and then randomized into 4 dietary treatment groups ($N = 10$/group): LF (Research Diets 12450B, 10% kcal fat); high fat (HF; Research Diets D12451, 45% kcal fat); HF + Q (Research Diets D08072305, 45% kcal fat) with 17 mg/kg quercetin aglycone (Enzo Life Technologies ALX-385-001-G005; Farmingdale, NY, USA); or HF + RO (Research Diets D08072306). Mice were fed respective diets for 9 wks, during which time 48 h food consumption and body weight and composition via nuclear magnetic resonance (Bruker Minispec, Billerica, MA, USA) were assessed weekly. Mice were euthanized after 9 wks of feeding and quadriceps muscle was extracted and snap frozen in liquid nitrogen for further analyses. All experiments were reviewed and approved by the Pennington Biomedical Research Center Institutional Animal Care and Use Committee.

2.2. DNA Isolation and Bisulfite Treatment. To provide a more homogenous sample, frozen quadriceps muscle was ground under liquid nitrogen using a mortar and pestle. Ground muscle was then used for the extraction of genomic DNA with a DNeasy Blood and Tissue Kit (Qiagen 69581) via the manufacturer's protocol. The quantity and quality of the gDNA extracted were determined by spectrophotometry using a NanoDrop (Thermo Scientific, Wilmington, DE, USA). Approximately 200 ng of gDNA was subjected to bisulfite conversion using the EpiTect Bisulfite Kit (Qiagen 59104) via the manufacturer's protocol.

2.3. Bisulfite Sequencing. Bisulfite sequencing was performed on the Qiagen PyroMark Q24 platform (Qiagen 9001514). Bisulfite converted gDNA was PCR amplified using the EpiTect MSP kit (Qiagen) and biotinylated primers targeting the *Pgc-1α* gene. Human primer sequences that amplify the region of the *Pgc-1α* promoter surrounding the −260 nucleotide site have been previously published [6]. Here, primer sequences (IDT) that amplified and biotinylated the corresponding region within the mm10 reference genome that surrounds the methylation site were used with the PyroMark PCR kit (Qiagen 978703) per the manufacturer's

TABLE 1: *Pgc-1α* isoform primer pair sequences are shown for the forward (F) and reverse (R) primers used to measure isoform expression via qRT-PCR. Primer pairs have previously been reported by Miura et al. 2008, Ruas et al. 2012, and Zhang et al. 2009.

Primer target	Primer sequence (5′ to 3′)
Pgc-1α-a F	GCTTGACTGGCGTCATTCG
Pgc-1α-a R	ACAGAGTCTTGGCTGCACATGT
Pgc-1α-b F	GACATGGATGTTGGGATTGTCA
Pgc-1α-b R	ACCAACCAGAGCAGCACATTT
Pgc-1α-c F	AGTGACATGGATGTTGGGATTG
Pgc-1α-c R	GAATGCCTCCGGTTACTCACTT
Pgc-1α4 F	TCACACCAAACCCACAGAAA
Pgc-1α4 R	CTG GAA GAT ATG GCA CAT
*FL-Pgc-1α*F	TGCCATTGTTAAGACCGA
*FL-Pgc-1α*R	CCAGAGTCACCAAATGACC
total *NT-Pgc-1α* F	TGCCATTGTTAAGACCGA
total *NT-Pgc-1α* R	CCATATCTTCCAGTGACC
total *Pgc-1α* F	TGATGTGAATGACTTGGATACAGACA
total *Pgc-1α* R	GCT CAT TGT TGT ACT GGT TGG ATA TG

instructions. Biotinylated DNA then subjected to pyrosequencing on the PyroMark Q24 (Qiagen 9001514) with PyroMark Gold Reagents (Qiagen), following the manufacturer's instructions. PyroMark analysis software was used to determine the DNA methylation percentage at the −260 nucleotide (nt).

2.4. RNA Isolation.
Total RNA was extracted from quadriceps muscle tissue using Tri-Reagent (Molecular Research Center, Cincinnati, OH, USA) followed by further purification with a RNeasy mini kit (Qiagen, Valencia, CA, USA), as previously described [32]. The quantity and quality of the RNA were analyzed by spectrophotometry (NanoDrop, ND-1000, Thermo Scientific, Wilmington, DE, USA). RNA was reverse transcribed into a cDNA library using M-MLV reverse transcriptase (Promega, Madison, WI, USA).

2.5. qRT-PCR.
qRT-PCR was performed using previously published primer pairs that targeted various *Pgc-1α* isoforms [17, 18, 21]. Primer sequences are shown in Table 1. All samples were run in duplicate on the ABI QuantStudio 6 Flex platform (Applied Biosystems, Foster City, CA, USA) using SyBR Green MasterMix (Applied Biosystems, Foster City, CA, USA). Gene expression was analyzed using a standard curve and normalization to cyclophilin B as the endogenous control. Data are expressed as arbitrary units (AU).

2.6. Statistical Analysis.
The data were analyzed with Graph-Pad Prism 5.0 statistical analysis software. Results are expressed as means ± standard error. Food consumption and body weight composition parameters were analyzed by repeated measures ANOVA. All other measurements were analyzed by one-way ANOVA. A Tukey test was used post hoc as necessary. A P value < 0.05 was used to determine significance.

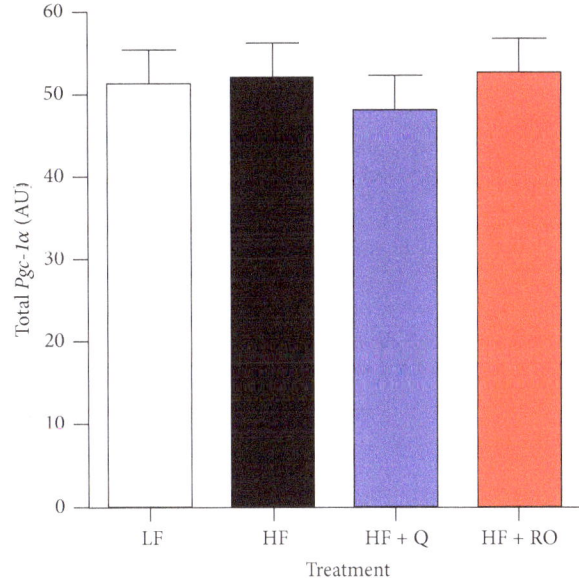

FIGURE 1: *Pgc-1α* mRNA was measured by qRT-PCR in skeletal muscle samples of mice fed a low fat (LF), high fat (HF), high fat plus quercetin (HF + Q), or high fat plus red onion extract (HF + RO) diet for 9 wks. Values are shown as means ± SEM in arbitrary units (AU).

3. Results

3.1. Mouse Dietary Model.
We have previously published the phenotypic data showing that 50 ug/g of dietary quercetin or ROE supplementation attenuates HFD-induced obesity and insulin resistance in C57BL/6J mice [32]. Interestingly, the antiobesogenic and antidiabetic effects of quercetin and ROE occur in association with ~50% increase in skeletal muscle mitochondrial number and more complete beta oxidation in skeletal muscle [32]. In our previous studies, C57BL/6J mice received Q supplementation for 8 wks and this resulted in an increase in skeletal muscle *Pgc-1α* expression in skeletal muscle [32]. Thus, in the present study, we also aimed to determine if ROE acts similarly to Q to upregulate *Pgc-1α* in association with previously observed beneficial mitochondrial adaptations. Contrary to our previous findings, in the present study we found that, after 9 wks of supplementation, neither Q nor ROE altered total *Pgc-1α* expression despite the previously published improvements in skeletal muscle mitochondrial number in these animals (Figure 1).

3.2. Pgc-1α Isoform Expression.
Several splice variants of *Pgc-1α* have recently been described, with some splice variants showing overlapping transcriptional coactivator activities and downstream physiological changes in metabolic and mitochondrial adaptations in response to environmental inputs [17–19, 21]. Due to the lack of change observed in total *Pgc-1α* (Figure 1) despite the significant increase in mitochondrial number, we aimed to determine if Q or ROE may act to upregulate specific splice variants of *Pgc-1α* using our model with known skeletal muscle mitochondrial adaptations [7, 32]. A schematic of the various *Pgc-1α* variants

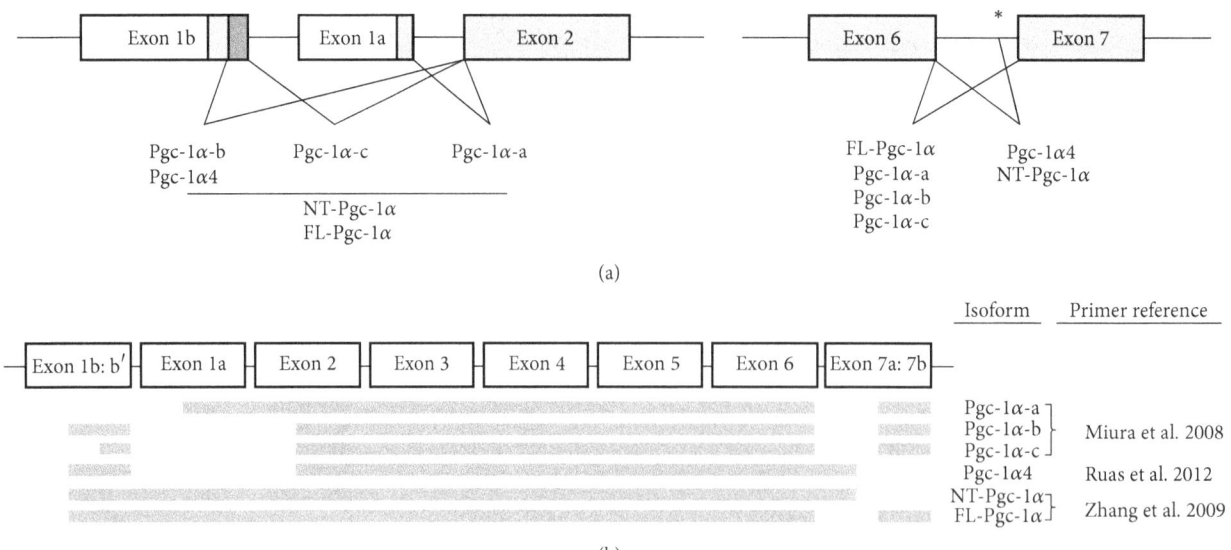

FIGURE 2: (a) Schematic structures of the 5′ and 3′ regions of *Pgc-1α* are shown for each isoform. The 5′ schematic was slightly adapted from Miura et al. 2008. The proximal (exon 1a) or alternate (exon 1b) promoters can be spliced to exon 2. Within exon 1b, upstream (exon 1b) or downstream (exon 1b′) splicing to exon 2 can occur. Splicing also occurs between exons 6 and 7 near the 3′ end of the gene. Exon 6 can be spliced directly to exon 7, at two separate regions, 7a or 7b. Alternatively, exon 6 can be spliced to the intronic region preceding exon 7 to result in a truncated form of *Pgc-1α*. Total *NT-Pgc-1α*, *FL-Pgc-1α*, and total *Pgc-1α* all contain exons 1b:1b′, 1a, and 2 as indicated. Total *Pgc-1α* contains both exons 6 and 7, as indicated. (b) Schematic representation of the start and stop of each *Pgc-1α* isoform is shown. Primer pairs have previously been designed and published, and the corresponding reference for each pair is indicated. ∗ is the alternative splice site between exons 6 and 7.

measured in the present study is shown in Figure 2. *Pgc-1α-a, Pgc-1α-b, Pgc-1α-c,* and *Pgc-1α4* differ in their N-termini due to transcription starting within either the distal, alternate (exon 1b), or proximal (exon 1a) promoters and also due to alternative splicing of exon 1b to produce exon 1b′, whereas *NT-Pgc-1α* and *FL-Pgc-1α* both contain the full exonic regions from 1b, 1b/, 1a, and 2 (Figure 2(a)). In addition to splicing at the 5′ region, *Pgc-1α* may undergo further splicing at the 3′ end, resulting in differential C-termini. As depicted in Figure 2(a), *Pgc-1α-a, Pgc-1α-b, Pgc-1α-c,* and *FL-Pgc-1α* contain exons 6 and 7 within the respective, mature transcripts, whereas *Pgc-1α4* and *NT-Pgc-1α* undergo alternative splicing resulting in an insertion between exons 6 and 7 and subsequent termination of translation before exon 7. Interestingly, both HF + Q and HF + RO exhibited decreases in *FL-Pgc-1α* compared to LF and HF groups (Figure 3(a)). HF + Q and HF + RO also showed a decrease in *Pgc-1α-a* compared to LF and HF, although the decrease in HF + RO compared to HF did not reach statistical significance (Figure 3(b)). HF + RO but not HF + Q showed decreased *Pgc-1α-b* expression compared to LF (Figure 3(c)). No change was observed in any groups for *Pgc-1α-c* or *Pgc-1α4* (Figures 3(d) and 3(e)). Interestingly, the only differences observed between LF and HF occurred with a decrease in total *NT-Pgc-1α* expression (Figure 3(f)). HFD-induced decreases in total *NT-Pgc-1α* were prevented in HF + Q and HF + RO, who showed a significant increase in total *NT-Pgc-1α* expression compared to HF (Figure 3(f)).

3.3. Pgc-1α DNA Methylation at the −260 Nucleotide. *Pgc-1α* has recently been shown to be hypermethylated in the skeletal muscle of type 2 diabetic individuals, in response to palmitate and oleate treatment of myocytes in vitro and by 10 wks of HFD feeding in C57BL/6J mice [6, 13]. Specific DNA methylation at the −260 nt is sufficient to decrease *Pgc-1α* expression and leads to detrimental skeletal muscle mitochondrial adaptations [6, 13]. To determine if Q and RO may work to ameliorate HFD-induced skeletal muscle mitochondrial maladaptations through epigenetic regulation of *Pgc-1α*, bisulfite sequencing of the *Pgc-1α* promoter was performed, specifically measuring the percentage of DNA methylation at the regulatory −260 nt site. The bisulfite converted DNA sequence and location of the pyrosequencing primer and known DNA methylation site are shown in Figure 4(a). *Pgc-1α*−260 nt methylation was significantly increased in HF compared to LF (Figure 4(b)). Q and ROE supplementation at 50 ug/day prevented the HFD-induced increases in DNA methylation, leading to a percentage of methylation in these groups that was similar to that observed in LF animals (Figure 4(b)).

4. Discussion

DNA methylation of the *Pgc-1α* promoter decreases skeletal muscle *Pgc-1α* expression and mitochondrial number and function, both of which may be important in determining insulin sensitivity during obesity [5, 6, 8, 9, 13, 33, 34].

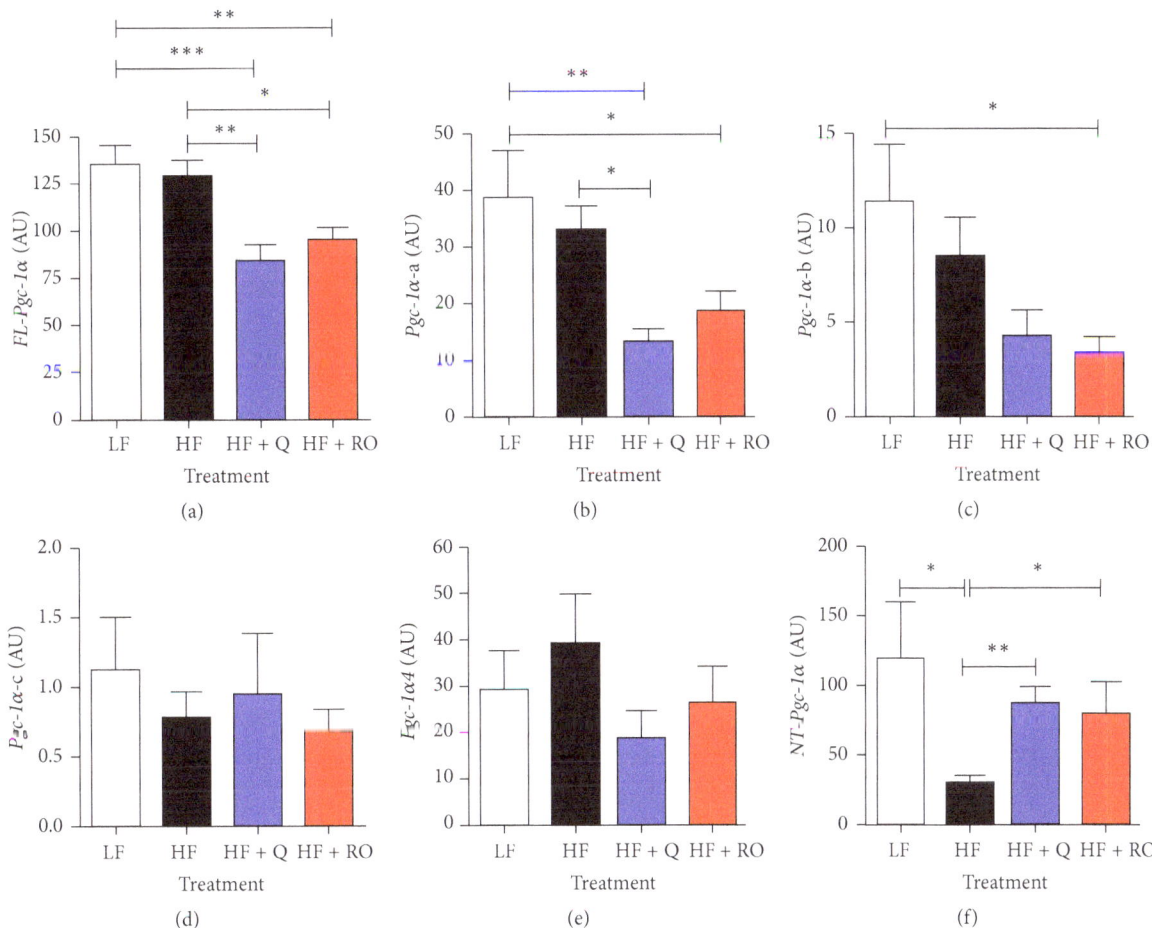

FIGURE 3: Expressions of (a) *FL-Pgc-1α*, (b) *Pgc-1α-a*, (c) *Pgc-1α-b*, (d) *Pgc-1α-c*, (e) *Pgc-1α4*, and total *NT-Pgc-1α* isoforms were measured by qRT-PCR in skeletal muscle samples of mice fed a low fat (LF), high fat (HF), high fat plus quercetin (HF + Q), or high fat plus red onion extract (HF + RO) diet for 9 wks. Values are shown as means ± SEM in arbitrary units (AU). ∗ denotes significant difference with $P < 0.05$, ∗∗$P < 0.01$, and ∗∗∗$P < 0.001$.

Environmental inputs, such as diet and exercise, alter *Pgc-1α* expression to determine skeletal muscle mitochondrial adaptations [1, 2, 4, 14]. Dietary supplementation with the flavonoid Q and/or the botanical extract from red onions prevents HFD-induced obesity and insulin resistance by increasing skeletal muscle *Pgc-1α* expression and mitochondrial function and number [7, 31, 32]. Due to their effects on *Pgc-1α* and mitochondrial adaptations and the ability of *Pgc-1α* to be epigenetically regulated, it is possible that the effects of Q and ROE occur through an epigenetic mechanism involving DNA methylation. Here, we show that 9 wks of HFD feeding, which causes increases in adiposity and insulin resistance in C57BL/6J mice [32], leads to hypermethylation at the −260 nt of the *Pgc-1α* promoter. Both Q and ROE attenuate HFD-induced obesity and insulin resistance while preventing HFD-induced hypermethylation of the −260 nt in *Pgc-1α*. Although we have previously found that 50 ug/day of Q supplementation upregulates skeletal muscle *Pgc-1α* in association with increased mitochondrial function in the form of more complete beta oxidation of fatty acids [7] and the mice in the present study showed an ~50% increase in skeletal

muscle mitochondrial number [32], in the present study we observed no difference in *Pgc-1α* expression (measured as the total *Pgc-1α* expression) between HF and HF + Q or HF + RO.

Importantly, the effects of dietary Q supplementation on skeletal muscle *Pgc-1α* expression and mitochondrial adaptations occur in a dose- and time-dependent manner [7, 31]. Our previous study showed an increase in *Pgc-1α* at 8 wks of supplementation [7] and, in the present study, *Pgc-1α* was measured after 9 wks of supplementation. Despite the lack of increase in total *Pgc-1α*, we continued to observe Q- and ROE-induced increases in energy expenditure and mitochondrial number [32], which may partially be the result of prior *Pgc-1α* upregulation at 8 wks. However, mitochondrial turnover occurs rapidly, ranging from ~1 to 17 days in a tissue-specific manner, and this turnover rate can be increased by dietary interventions, such as caloric restriction [35, 36]. Thus, one would expect that if the effects of Q and ROE are no longer beneficial after 9 wks due to the lack of change in total *Pgc-1α* expression, the continuous impetus of the HFD would lead to similar skeletal muscle physiologies in HF, HF + Q, and HF + RO groups; yet at

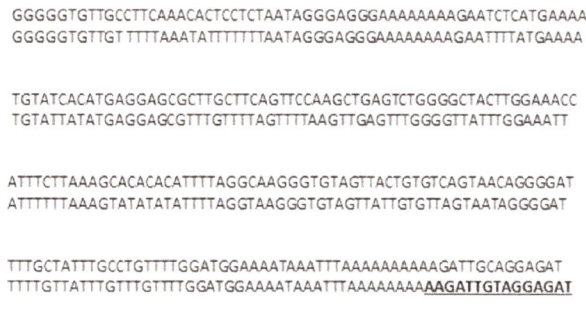

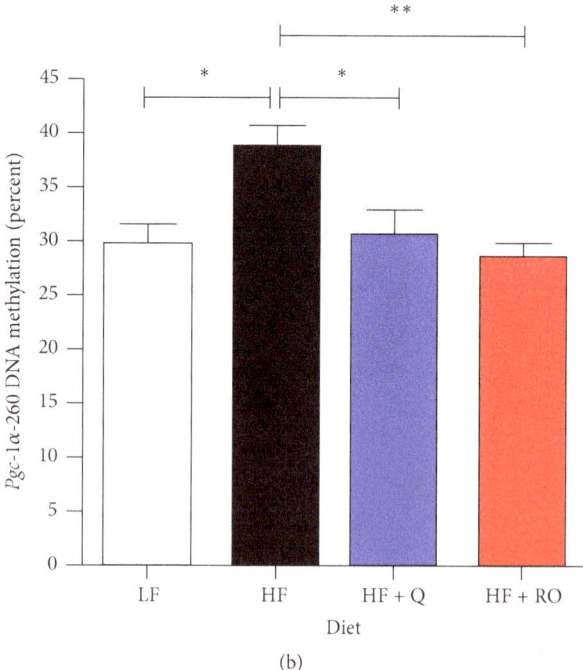

(a)   (b)

Figure 4: Bisulfite sequencing of the *Pgc-1α* promoter was used to determine DNA methylation levels at the −260 nt. The original (top line) and bisulfite converted (corresponding bottom line) sequences are shown in (a). The bold and underlined region within the bisulfite converted sequence indicates where the pyrosequencing primer is located. The red highlighted, bold, and underlined region is the regulatory −260 nt that undergoes DNA methylation. The percent of DNA methylation present at the −260 nt in skeletal muscle is shown as the mean ± SEM for low fat (LF), high fat (HF), high fat plus quercetin (HF + Q), and high fat plus red onion extract (HF + RO) animals after 9 wks of feeding the respective diets. ∗ denotes significant difference with $P < 0.05$ and ∗∗$P < 0.01$.

9 wks, we still observed increased mitochondrial number [32] and decreased *Pgc-1α* methylation in HF + Q and HF + RO. Thus, it appears that although total *Pgc-1α* remains unchanged, other mechanisms may compensate for this loss of *Pgc-1α* upregulation to perpetuate beneficial mitochondrial adaptations in HF + Q and HF + RO.

Interestingly, DNA methylation has been shown to drive mRNA splicing and *Pgc-1α* has several known isoforms that result from alternative splicing and alternate promoter start sites [17–19, 21, 26]. These isoforms have unique and complementary or overlapping functions, specific to each variant [17, 18, 21, 25]. Thus, it is possible that the effects of Q and ROE may be due to epigenetic regulation of mRNA splicing and subsequent alterations in *Pgc-1α* splice variant expression. Indeed, we show here that Q and ROE decreased expression of *FL-Pgc-1α* and isoform a, without changing isoforms b, c, or 4. Additionally, Q but not ROE decreased *Pgc-1α* isoform B in comparison to LF but HF. Here, none of the treatments had an effect on *Pgc-1α* isoforms 4 and c. The only isoform shown to decrease after 9 wks of HFD feeding was *NT-Pgc-1α*; and, both Q and ROE were able to prevent this HFD-induced decrease. These results are consistent with changes in DNA methylation status at the −260 nt, with HF increasing in methylation but HF + Q and HF + RO showing similar levels of methylation as LF. Thus at 9 wks of feeding, it is possible that the beneficial effects of Q and ROE on mitochondrial number

and function are mediated via upregulation of *NT-Pgc-1α* and that isoform expression is dependent on epigenetic regulation of *Pgc-1α*. Indeed, *NT-Pgc-1α* has known complementary and overlapping functions to *FL-Pgc-1α* and may compensate for loss of *FL-Pgc-1α* or other isoforms [17, 25]; and it has recently been shown that *Pgc-1α* isoform expression is epigenetically regulated by histone methylation in response to exercise, with expression of *Pgc-1α-b* and of *Pgc-1α-c* but not of *Pgc-1α-a* being upregulated in conjunction with increased histone methylation in the promoter of exon 1b compared to exon 1a [16].

Here, we measured the percentage of −260 nt DNA methylation, a methylation site known to regulate *Pgc-1α* expression and skeletal muscle mitochondrial adaptations which is located within the proximal promoter upstream of exon 1a. Given that Q and ROE decreased *Pgc-1α* isoforms *Pgc-1α-a* and *Pgc-1α-b* without changing *Pgc-1α-c*, and *Pgc-1α-a* includes exon 1a, *Pgc-1α-b* includes exon 1b, and *Pgc-1α-c* includes exon 1b′, it appears that −260 nt methylation does not play a role in regulating 5′ splicing or transcription initiation within *Pgc-1α* proximal versus alternative, distal promoters. This is consistent with the recent publication by Lochmann et al. 2015, who similarly showed that *Pgc-1α* methylation was not related to *Pgc-1α* isoform a, b, or c expression [16]. Interestingly, total *Pgc-1α* expression was also not associated with DNA methylation at the −260 nt.

However, it is unclear in previous publications what isoforms of *Pgc-1α* were measured and correlated with −260 nt DNA methylation. It is possible that previous reports use primers that measure isoforms which are differentially spliced at the 3′ prime end; as in the present study, although we did not observe associations between −260 nt methylation and 5′ splicing or specific promoter initiation, we did see alterations in isoform expression based on splicing at the 3′ region in association with DNA methylation levels at the −260 nt. Notably, *FL-Pgc-1α* decreased in HF + Q and HF + RO and total *NT-Pgc-1α* increased. Although alternative splicing that produces these isoforms occurs at exons 6 and 7 and the intronic region between these exons [17] and DNA methylation occurs within the promoter region, promoter structure is known to be important for alternative splicing [26]. Promoter methylation regulates splicing through a complex process involving epigenetic modifications and promoter occupation of transcriptional activators [26]. DNA methylation not only alters transcription factor binding, but also directly regulates alternative splicing by recruiting RNA-binding proteins that can be transferred to the mRNA to alter the splicing pattern [26]. Although the present study is limited by measuring only the −260 nt methylation status, others have shown that methylation at the −260 nt occurs when the entire *Pgc-1α* promoter is hypermethylated [6]. Thus, hyper- and hypomethylation of the −260 nt may serve as a surrogate measure to indicate methylation status across the entire promoter or gene, whose methylation may play a role in determining alternative splicing and isoform expression.

In conclusion, Q and ROE show similar effects in preventing *Pgc-1α*−260 nt methylation induced by HFD feeding, upregulating total *NT-Pgc-1α* splice variant expression in skeletal muscle. Thus, the perpetuating beneficial effects of Q and ROE on body weight, body composition, energy expenditure, insulin sensitivity, and skeletal muscle mitochondrial number and function in mice after 9 wks of supplementation [32] may be mediated via upregulation of total *NT-Pgc-1α*. There is a further need to study the functions and epigenetic regulation of total *NT-Pgc-1α* and other isoforms of *Pgc-1α* to determine their specific roles in regulating skeletal muscle adaptations and contribute to a lean, insulin sensitive state.

5. Conclusions

HFD causes *Pgc-1α* hypermethylation at the −260 nt in the *Pgc-1α* proximal promoter in conjunction with alterations in *Pgc-1α* splice variant expression in skeletal muscle. Q and ROE similarly prevent HFD-induced hypermethylation of *Pgc-1α* and increase *NT-Pgc-1α* expression in skeletal muscle. Q- and ROE-induced upregulation of *NT-Pgc-1α* may occur through an epigenetic mechanism and may be sufficient to increase skeletal muscle mitochondrial number and complete beta oxidation of fatty acids, contributing to attenuation of obesity and insulin resistance.

Competing Interests

The authors declare no competing interests.

Authors' Contributions

Prasad P. Devarshi and Aarin D. Jones contributed equally to this work. Aarin D. Jones performed experiments, analyzed data, and edited the manuscript. Prasad P. Devarshi analyzed data and wrote and edited the manuscript. Erin M. Taylor and Barbara Stefanska performed experiments and edited the manuscript. Tara M. Henagan conceptualized, designed, and performed experiments, analyzed data, wrote and edited the manuscript, and provided funding.

Acknowledgments

This work was funded by Indiana CTSI Core Pilot Funding UL1TR001108 and NIH NCCAM 5P50-AT002776-09 grants.

References

[1] D. Knutti and A. Kralli, "PGC-1, a versatile coactivator," *Trends in Endocrinology & Metabolism*, vol. 12, no. 8, pp. 360–365, 2001.

[2] H. Liang and W. F. Ward, "PGC-1α: a key regulator of energy metabolism," *Advances in Physiology Education*, vol. 30, no. 4, pp. 145–151, 2006.

[3] J. Lin, H. Wu, P. T. Tarr et al., "Transcriptional co-activator PGC-1α drives the formation of slow-twitch muscle fibres," *Nature*, vol. 418, pp. 797–801, 2002.

[4] Z. Wu, P. Puigserver, U. Andersson et al., "Mechanisms controlling mitochondrial biogenesis and respiration through the thermogenic coactivator PGC-1," *Cell*, vol. 98, no. 1, pp. 115–124, 1999.

[5] R. Barrès, J. Yan, B. Egan et al., "Acute exercise remodels promoter methylation in human skeletal muscle," *Cell Metabolism*, vol. 15, no. 3, pp. 405–411, 2012.

[6] R. Barrès, M. E. Osler, J. Yan et al., "Non-CpG methylation of the PGC-1α promoter through DNMT3B controls mitochondrial density," *Cell Metabolism*, vol. 10, no. 3, pp. 189–198, 2009.

[7] T. M. Henagan, N. R. Lenard, T. W. Gettys, and L. K. Stewart, "Dietary quercetin supplementation in mice increases skeletal muscle PGC1α expression, improves mitochondrial function and attenuates insulin resistance in a time-specific manner," *PLoS ONE*, vol. 9, no. 2, Article ID e89365, 2014.

[8] I. Pagel-Langenickel, J. Bao, L. Pang, and M. N. Sack, "The role of mitochondria in the pathophysiology of skeletal muscle insulin resistance," *Endocrine Reviews*, vol. 31, no. 1, pp. 25–51, 2010.

[9] M.-E. Patti and S. Corvera, "The role of mitochondria in the pathogenesis of type 2 diabetes," *Endocrine Reviews*, vol. 31, no. 3, pp. 364–395, 2010.

[10] J.-A. Kim, Y. Wei, and J. R. Sowers, "Role of mitochondrial dysfunction in insulin resistance," *Circulation Research*, vol. 102, no. 4, pp. 401–414, 2008.

[11] J. C. Bournat and C. W. Brown, "Mitochondrial dysfunction in obesity," *Current Opinion in Endocrinology, Diabetes and Obesity*, vol. 17, no. 5, pp. 446–452, 2010.

[12] L. M. Sparks, H. Xie, R. A. Koza et al., "A high-fat diet coordinately downregulates genes required for mitochondrial oxidative phosphorylation in skeletal muscle," *Diabetes*, vol. 54, no. 7, pp. 1926–1933, 2005.

[13] T. M. Henagan, B. Stefanska, Z. Fang et al., "Sodium butyrate epigenetically modulates high-fat diet-induced skeletal muscle mitochondrial adaptation, obesity and insulin resistance

through nucleosome positioning," *British Journal of Pharmacology*, vol. 172, no. 11, pp. 2782–2798, 2015.

[14] P. J. Fernandez-Marcos and J. Auwerx, "Regulation of PGC-1α, a nodal regulator of mitochondrial biogenesis," *American Journal of Clinical Nutrition*, vol. 93, no. 4, pp. 884S–890S, 2011.

[15] T. M. Henagan, L. K. Stewart, L. A. Forney, L. M. Sparks, N. Johannsen, and T. S. Church, "PGC1 -1 nucleosome position and splice variant expression and cardiovascular disease risk in overweight and obese individuals," *PPAR Research*, vol. 2014, Article ID 895734, 7 pages, 2014.

[16] T. L. Lochmann, R. R. Thomas, J. P. Bennett Jr., and S. M. Taylor, "Epigenetic modifications of the PGC-1α promoter during exercise induced expression in mice," *PLoS ONE*, vol. 10, no. 6, Article ID e0129647, 2015.

[17] Y. Zhang, P. Huypens, A. W. Adamson et al., "Alternative mRNA splicing produces a novel biologically active short isoform of PGC-1α," *Journal of Biological Chemistry*, vol. 284, no. 47, pp. 32813–32826, 2009.

[18] S. Miura, Y. Kai, Y. Kamei, and O. Ezaki, "Isoform-specific increases in murine skeletal muscle peroxisome proliferator-activated receptor-γ coactivator-1α (PGC-1α) mRNA in response to β2-adrenergic receptor activation and exercise," *Endocrinology*, vol. 149, no. 9, pp. 4527–4533, 2008.

[19] X. Wen, J. Wu, J. S. Chang et al., "Effect of exercise intensity on isoform-specific expressions of NT-PGC-1α mRNA in mouse skeletal muscle," *BioMed Research International*, vol. 2014, Article ID 402175, 11 pages, 2014.

[20] D. V. Popov, E. A. Lysenko, I. V. Kuzmin, O. L. Vinogradova, and A. I. Grigoriev, "Regulation of PGC-1α isoform expression in skeletal muscles," *Acta Naturae*, vol. 7, no. 1, pp. 48–59, 2015.

[21] J. L. Ruas, J. P. White, R. R. Rao et al., "A PGC-1α isoform induced by resistance training regulates skeletal muscle hypertrophy," *Cell*, vol. 151, no. 6, pp. 1319–1331, 2012.

[22] M. Ydfors, H. Fischer, H. Mascher, E. Blomstrand, J. Norrbom, and T. Gustafsson, "The truncated splice variants, *NT–PGC–1α* and *PGC–1α4*, increase with both endurance and resistance exercise in human skeletal muscle," *Physiological Reports*, vol. 1, Article ID e00140, 2013.

[23] V. Martínez-Redondo, A. T. Pettersson, and J. L. Ruas, "The hitchhiker's guide to PGC-1α isoform structure and biological functions," *Diabetologia*, vol. 58, no. 9, pp. 1969–1977, 2015.

[24] M. Tadaishi, S. Miura, Y. Kai, Y. Kano, Y. Oishi, and O. Ezaki, "Skeletal muscle-specific expression of PGC-1α-b, an exercise-responsive isoform, increases exercise capacity and peak oxygen uptake," *PLoS ONE*, vol. 6, no. 12, Article ID e28290, 2011.

[25] H.-J. Jun, Y. Joshi, Y. Patil, R. C. Noland, and J. S. Chang, "NT-PGC-1α activation attenuates high-fat diet-induced obesity by enhancing brown fat thermogenesis and adipose tissue oxidative metabolism," *Diabetes*, vol. 63, no. 11, pp. 3615–3625, 2014.

[26] A. R. Kornblihtt, M. De La Mata, J. P. Fededa, M. J. Muñoz, and G. Nogués, "Multiple links between transcription and splicing," *RNA*, vol. 10, no. 10, pp. 1489–1498, 2004.

[27] J. M. Davis, E. A. Murphy, M. D. Carmichael, and B. Davis, "Quercetin increases brain and muscle mitochondrial biogenesis and exercise tolerance," *American Journal of Physiology—Regulatory Integrative and Comparative Physiology*, vol. 296, no. 4, pp. R1071–R1077, 2009.

[28] C. Carrasco-Pozo, M. L. Mizgier, H. Speisky, and M. Gotteland, "Differential protective effects of quercetin, resveratrol, rutin and epigallocatechin gallate against mitochondrial dysfunction induced by indomethacin in Caco-2 cells," *Chemico-Biological Interactions*, vol. 195, no. 3, pp. 199–205, 2012.

[29] N. Rayamajhi, S.-K. Kim, H. Go et al., "Quercetin induces mitochondrial biogenesis through activation of HO-1 in HEPG2 cells," *Oxidative Medicine and Cellular Longevity*, vol. 2013, Article ID 154279, 10 pages, 2013.

[30] L. Rivera, R. Morón, M. Sánchez, A. Zarzuelo, and M. Galisteo, "Quercetin ameliorates metabolic syndrome and improves the inflammatory status in obese Zucker rats," *Obesity*, vol. 16, no. 9, pp. 2081–2087, 2008.

[31] L. K. Stewart, J. L. Soileau, D. Ribnicky et al., "Quercetin transiently increases energy expenditure but persistently decreases circulating markers of inflammation in C57BL/6J mice fed a high-fat diet," *Metabolism: Clinical and Experimental*, vol. 57, supplement 1, pp. S39–S46, 2008.

[32] T. M. Henagan, W. T. Cefalu, D. M. Ribnicky et al., "In vivo effects of dietary quercetin and quercetin-rich red onion extract on skeletal muscle mitochondria, metabolism, and insulin sensitivity," *Genes & Nutrition*, vol. 10, article 2, 2015.

[33] K. Højlund, M. Mogensen, K. Sahlin, and H. Beck-Nielsen, "Mitochondrial dysfunction in type 2 diabetes and obesity," *Endocrinology and Metabolism Clinics of North America*, vol. 37, no. 3, pp. 713–731, 2008.

[34] T. R. Koves, J. R. Ussher, R. C. Noland et al., "Mitochondrial overload and incomplete fatty acid oxidation contribute to skeletal muscle insulin resistance," *Cell Metabolism*, vol. 7, no. 1, pp. 45–56, 2008.

[35] S. Miwa, C. Lawless, and T. Von Zglinicki, "Mitochondrial turnover in liver is fast in.vivo and is accelerated by dietary restriction: application of a simple dynamic model," *Aging Cell*, vol. 7, no. 6, pp. 920–923, 2008.

[36] R. A. Menzies and P. H. Gold, "The turnover of mitochondria in a variety of tissues of young adult and aged rats," *Journal of Biological Chemistry*, vol. 246, no. 8, pp. 2425–2429, 1971.

7

PPARγ in Bacterial Infections: A Friend or Foe?

Aravind T. Reddy,[1,2] Sowmya P. Lakshmi,[1,2] and Raju C. Reddy[1,2]

[1]Department of Medicine, Division of Pulmonary, Allergy and Critical Care Medicine,
 University of Pittsburgh School of Medicine, Pittsburgh, PA 15213, USA
[2]Veterans Affairs Pittsburgh Healthcare System, Pittsburgh, PA 15240, USA

Correspondence should be addressed to Raju C. Reddy; reddyrc@upmc.edu

Academic Editor: Paul D. Drew

Peroxisome proliferator-activated receptor γ (PPARγ) is now recognized as an important modulator of leukocyte inflammatory responses and function. Its immunoregulatory function has been studied in a variety of contexts, including bacterial infections of the lungs and central nervous system, sepsis, and conditions such as chronic granulomatous disease. Although it is generally believed that PPARγ activation is beneficial for the host during bacterial infections via its anti-inflammatory and antibacterial properties, PPARγ agonists have also been shown to dampen the host immune response and in some cases exacerbate infection by promoting leukocyte apoptosis and interfering with leukocyte migration and infiltration. In this review we discuss the role of PPARγ and its activation during bacterial infections, with focus on the potential of PPARγ agonists and perhaps antagonists as novel therapeutic modalities. We conclude that adjustment in the dosage and timing of PPARγ agonist administration, based on the competence of host antimicrobial defenses and the extent of inflammatory response and tissue injury, is critical for achieving the essential balance between pro- and anti-inflammatory effects on the immune system.

1. Introduction

The family of transcription factors designated peroxisome proliferator-activated receptors (PPARs) has long been studied for its role in regulation of lipid and glucose metabolism [1, 2]. More recently, PPARs' role in immunoregulation has been recognized and is the subject of intense investigation [1, 2]. PPARs are expressed by a variety of cells of the immune system including monocytes, macrophages, B and T lymphocytes, natural killer cells, dendritic cells, neutrophils, eosinophils, and mast cells [1]. In this review, we discuss the role of PPARγ specifically in bacterial infections.

PPARs belong to the nuclear hormone receptor superfamily that regulates a multitude of genes [2]. There are three PPARs encoded by separate genes: PPARα, PPARβ/δ, and PPARγ [3]. The three PPARs differ in their structure, function, and tissue distribution [4]. PPARγ has received significant attention as a key regulator of adipocyte differentiation as well as glucose and lipid homeostasis [2, 4]. PPARγ can be transcribed from three distinct mRNAs, γ1, γ2, and γ3, based on sites of transcription initiation and splicing [4–6]. However, there are only two protein isoforms, PPARγ1 and PPARγ2, as translation of γ1 and γ3 mRNAs results in indistinguishable proteins [6]. PPARγ1 is the predominant isoform [5]. Whereas expression of PPARγ2 and PPARγ3 mRNAs is restricted [6], PPARγ1 mRNA is expressed fairly ubiquitously [4].

A variety of ligands, natural and synthetic, are capable of stimulating PPARγ activity. Natural PPARγ ligands include saturated and unsaturated fatty acids, eicosanoid derivatives such as 15-deoxy-$\Delta^{12,14}$-prostaglandin J_2 (15d-PGJ$_2$), and nitrated fatty acids such as nitrated linoleic and oleic acids [4, 7]. Synthetic PPARγ agonists are represented by thiazolidinediones (TZDs) such as pioglitazone, rosiglitazone, troglitazone, and ciglitazone. In addition, some nonsteroidal anti-inflammatory drugs such as indomethacin, fenoprofen, and ibuprofen can activate PPARγ, although their binding affinity is lower than that of TZDs. In the absence of these agonists,

PPARγ remains inactive, bound to a series of corepressors. Upon ligand activation, these corepressors are displaced, allowing PPARγ to heterodimerize with retinoid X receptors and initiate transcriptional control by binding to specific peroxisome proliferator response elements in the promoter regions of target genes [4]. PPARγ agonists may have other activities, though. For example, pioglitazone has been shown to alter mitochondrial function in a PPARγ-independent manner [8] and nitrated fatty acids are electrophiles that alkylate and may inactivate target proteins [9, 10]. These off-target effects may be either helpful or harmful, depending on the context. Additionally, PPARγ agonists are known to upregulate the receptor's expression, which may render the effects of repeated dosing greater than would be anticipated from single-dose results [11, 12].

Recognition that PPARγ is expressed by a variety of immune cells stimulated interest in its immunoregulatory function, especially its anti-inflammatory role [13]. Involvement of PPARγ in several leukocyte functions supports its prominent role in immunoregulation [13, 14]. Protein and mRNA expression and activity of PPARγ are altered during many inflammatory conditions, and such alterations appear to be a significant factor in the pathogenesis of some diseases [15].

We are surrounded by a variety of microbial species and are constantly interacting with them throughout our lives. Some of these microorganisms are commensal or even beneficial, while others are pathogens that can cause significant morbidity and mortality. The innate immune system, characterized by secretion of proinflammatory cytokines and antimicrobial molecules and recruitment of phagocytes, is a major mediator of resistance to infection by pathogenic bacteria. Compromised or dysregulated immunity can allow development of major illnesses requiring therapeutic intervention, yet in some cases inflammatory responses themselves can become life-threatening. Although many infectious diseases can be controlled by antibacterial drugs, antimicrobial resistance poses a significant threat to our healthcare system worldwide, compromising therapy, complicating treatment, increasing mortality, and resulting in substantial financial costs [16]. Drugs with novel mechanisms of action are therefore urgently needed. Recent advances in our understanding of PPARγ's role in immunity, infection, and inflammation, as discussed below, offer the opportunity for intervention with a novel approach to bacterial infections. Appropriate antimicrobial therapy will continue to be the standard of care, but adjunctive use of PPARγ agonists or antagonists may reduce the required antibiotic dosages and improve outcomes.

Human disease is complex, however, and effects on one cell type may be beneficial while those on another may tend to exacerbate the disease. Outcomes may also depend crucially on the exact nature of the disease—not only pathogen but also the state of disease development and potential comorbidities. Nevertheless, despite these complexities and resulting uncertainties, evidence supports the desirability of further investigation of PPARγ ligands as potential adjunctive therapy in many infectious diseases.

2. PPARγ: A Friend

The positive effect of PPARγ (and/or its ligands) in bacterial infections, especially its anti-inflammatory effects via inhibition of proinflammatory molecules such as IL-6, TNF-α, IL-1β, and IL-12, has been well documented. In the *ex vivo* study by Aronoff et al., troglitazone, rosiglitazone, and 15d-PGJ$_2$ increased the Fcγ receptor-mediated phagocytosis of *Klebsiella pneumoniae* as well as that of IgG-opsonized nonphysiological targets by primary lung macrophages abundantly expressing PPARγ [17]. This effect appears to be mediated through PPARγ, demonstrating the role of PPARγ in pathogen clearance during bacterial infections. This phagocytic role of PPARγ is in line with other studies showing that PPARγ activation increases expression of CD36 cell surface receptors and uptake of apoptotic neutrophils by macrophages, a process critical for resolution of inflammation [18, 19]. Likewise, Stegenga et al. reported that the PPARγ ligand ciglitazone alleviates *Streptococcus pneumoniae*-induced lung inflammation in mice by suppressing bacterial outgrowth and proinflammatory cytokine secretion, thereby improving survival of the infected animals [20]. Interestingly, however, contrary to previous findings [17], Stegenga et al. observed no ciglitazone-induced increase in *in vitro* phagocytosis or killing ability of alveolar macrophages in response to *S. pneumoniae* infection [20]. This discrepancy may reflect differences in agonists and pathogens used as well as the cell types employed in their studies. Nevertheless, these studies highlight the role of PPARγ activation in reducing inflammation and improving pathogen clearance.

Anti-inflammatory effects of PPARγ activation are not confined to bacterial infections of the lungs. In a study using a mouse model of central nervous system infection by *Staphylococcus aureus*, which is associated with brain abscesses in humans, ciglitazone reduced the expression of proinflammatory mediators as well as iNOS and inhibited microglia/macrophage activation. The authors of the study noted that ciglitazone's ability to suppress proinflammatory mediator secretion is only partial, a significant observation as complete absence of proinflammatory responses would result in persistence of bacteria in the brain parenchyma and therefore would be detrimental to survival of the infected animals. Another key finding in this study was that ciglitazone is capable not only of preventing microglial activation when administered prophylactically but also of dampening the activity of microglia that have already been stimulated by on-going bacterial infections. This is clinically relevant and important because typically patients seeking treatment for brain abscess would already exhibit inflammatory central nervous system responses. In addition to attenuation of microglial response, ciglitazone-treated animals show reduced bacterial burdens, probably due to the enhanced microglial phagocytic ability that was observed. Moreover, ciglitazone accelerates brain abscess encapsulation, as evidenced by the increased deposition and compact organization of fibronectin as well as the early emergence of α-smooth muscle actin-expressing myofibroblasts associated with development of the capsule, which could prevent further dissemination of the pathogens [21]. Altogether, these observations provide evidence that

PPARγ activation by synthetic agonists is an attractive therapeutic intervention for brain abscesses since it is capable of achieving a balance between effective clearance of pathogen and minimal damage to the brain tissue.

PPARγ's anti-inflammatory function is also prominent in chronic granulomatous disease (CGD), an inherited disorder in which phagocytes' defective ability to kill certain infectious pathogens results in chronic and recurrent infections and inflammation. In a mouse model of CGD, macrophages demonstrate reduced PPARγ expression and activation and impaired efferocytosis of apoptotic neutrophils during zymosan-induced acute inflammation [22]. Monocytes from human CGD patients similarly show defective efferocytosis [23]. Furthermore, neutrophils and monocytes/macrophages from these CGD mice as well as monocytes from human CGD patients exhibit defects in PPARγ-dependent production of mitochondrial reactive oxygen species (ROS) that contribute to bacterial killing [24]. These defects can be largely restored by PPARγ activation with pioglitazone, given prophylactically or during preexisting inflammation [22–24], providing further evidence for the antibacterial effect of PPARγ activation. Importantly, the authors showed that pioglitazone is capable of enhancing CGD phagocytes' ability to clear pathogens such as *S. aureus* and *Burkholderia cepacia*, restoring host defense against these pathogens [24]. Furthermore, the PPARγ agonist pioglitazone produced marked clinical improvement in a 5-month-old boy with CGD and multiple severe infections [25]. Significantly improved ROS production was associated with reductions in pathogen burden and improvements in overall clinical condition that allowed curative hematopoietic stem cell transplantation. Although this reflects an unusual setting, these direct clinical results support the ability of PPARγ agonists to upregulate pathogen killing and clearance.

Infections by a variety of bacteria can result in sepsis, in which blood-borne toxins lead to an exaggerated and dysregulated inflammatory response that frequently results in tissue injury [26]. In severe sepsis, potentially lethal septic shock and multiple organ failure become strong possibilities [27]. PPARγ signaling has shown a protective effect in multiple models of sepsis. In the mouse model of lipopolysaccharide- (LPS-) induced sepsis involving pulmonary inflammation and injury, endothelial cell PPARγ (ePPARγ) deficiency intensifies the tissue injury with increased pulmonary edema and capillary permeability, elevated ROS and cytokine/chemokine production, infiltration of neutrophils to the lungs, and expression of inflammation-associated adhesion molecules such as ICAM-1 and PECAM-1. This exacerbation of inflammatory responses in ePPARγ-deficient mice is due to enhanced toll-like receptor-4 (TLR4) expression in the lung tissues and upregulation of TLR4 downstream signaling including the NF-κB pathway [26]. TLR4 signaling has been shown to play a key role in modulating inflammation/sepsis [28, 29]. In addition to the effects of PPARγ agonists reported by others, Reddy et al. observed that physiologically relevant concentrations of 10-nitro-oleic acid reduce LPS-induced transcription of many inflammatory markers and inhibit neutrophil transmigration *in vitro* [26].

The protective effect of PPARγ activation is also demonstrated in mouse and rat models of polymicrobial sepsis using cecal ligation and puncture (CLP) [27, 30]. Zingarelli et al. found that rats subjected to CLP exhibit reduced PPARγ expression in the lungs and thoracic aortas, increased circulating neutrophils accompanied by reduction in lymphocytes, and increased accumulation of neutrophils in multiple vital organs. Elevated levels of mediators of sepsis-associated vascular dysfunction and hypotension were also detected. These cellular and molecular changes were shown to reflect upregulation of the proinflammatory transcription factors NF-κB and AP-1. 15d-PGI$_2$ and ciglitazone prolong the animals' survival, reversing the sepsis-associated proinflammatory events and improving arterial blood pressure [27]. Likewise, in mice experiencing polymicrobial sepsis, pioglitazone reduces bacterial burden at the site of infection (the peritoneum) and in the blood and alleviates edema and capillary congestion at target tissues such as the lungs by reducing neutrophil infiltration and cytokine accumulation. Survival rate of septic mice consequently improves. The authors found that PPARγ activation exerts its protective effect against bacterial sepsis via an IL-10-dependent reduction in expression of MyD88, a critical downstream component of the TLR pathway [30].

Remarkably, several of these studies [20, 21, 30] report that PPARγ agonists exhibit both anti-inflammatory and antibacterial properties, two seemingly contradictory effects. Mechanisms underlying this unique characteristic of PPARγ agonists are currently unclear. It is possible that these two properties are the results of two distinct activities of the drugs. Alternatively, limited inflammatory response may simply reflect improved pathogen clearance and thus reduced inflammatory stimulus [31]. Further research is needed to address this question.

Regardless, in bacterial infections where optimal pathogen clearance and prevention of excessive inflammation are equally critical for the health and survival of patients, PPARγ agonists offer new therapeutic strategies. This may be particularly true for lung infections due to effects on resident alveolar macrophages. PPARγ activation reduces the ability of inflammation to stimulate alveolar macrophage switching from an anti-inflammatory to a proinflammatory state yet simultaneously increases macrophage phagocytosis of both opsonized and unopsonized particles [32]. Differentiation of monocytes into alveolar macrophages is associated with appearance of PPARγ, and macrophage-specific PPARγ knockout is associated with mild steady-state inflammation in lungs but not elsewhere [33]. Additionally, absence of macrophage PPARγ led to reduced bacterial clearance and increased mortality following *S. pneumoniae* infection.

Lastly, adding a new layer to PPARγ's involvement in bacterial infections is the study by Kelly et al. Here, the authors showed that *Bacteroides thetaiotaomicron*, a commensal bacterium prevalent in the human gut microflora, blocks the dysfunctional acute inflammatory response to infection by pathogenic *Salmonella enterica* by inducing binding of PPARγ to the NF-κB RelA subunit and their joint nuclear export and cytosolic localization, thereby inhibiting the consequent transcription of proinflammatory IL-8. Intestinal structure is mostly preserved in rats infected with both bacteria, compared to the animals exposed to *S. enterica* alone, providing evidence for the attenuation of inflammation. Importantly, this anti-inflammatory function of *B. thetaiotaomicron* is dependent on PPARγ, as RNAi-mediated reduction in PPARγ expression abolishes the inhibitory effect on IL-8 [34]. Thus, not only host defense but also bacteria themselves can engage PPARγ for its anti-inflammatory functions during pathogenic bacterial infections.

3. PPARγ: A Foe

Whereas the above studies present clear evidence of the protective role of PPARγ and/or its agonists in bacterial infections, other research shows that PPARγ expression/activation is harmful for the host, in at least two distinct fashions.

PPARγ activation triggers apoptosis in a variety of leukocytes, which can dampen the host immune response during bacterial infections. Pioglitazone has been shown to induce caspase-3- and caspase-9-dependent apoptosis in macrophage-like cells derived from a human monocyte cell line. This effect is reversed by a functionally selective PPARγ antagonist, GW9662, supporting its PPARγ dependence [35]. Likewise, rosiglitazone, troglitazone, and ciglitazone induce and GW9662 and another PPARγ antagonist, BADGE, block apoptosis of human leukemia cells in a caspase-3-dependent manner [36]. PPARγ activation with 15d-PGJ₂, troglitazone, or ciglitazone is likewise antiproliferative and proapoptotic in multiple mouse B lymphoma cell lines representing different stages of maturation and in human B lymphocytes and B lymphoma cells [37, 38]. Tautenhahn et al. observed that ciglitazone treatment causes apoptosis in phytohemagglutinin-stimulated T lymphocytes [39].

Apoptosis is thought to contribute to the lymphopenia seen in septic patients [40]. Indeed, T cell depletion leads to immunosuppression or immunoparalysis that underlies persistent infection and/or predisposes patients with sepsis to secondary infections and increased mortality [41]. The proapoptotic role of PPARγ activation established by the studies previously mentioned potentially implicates the receptor in these effects. Soller et al. demonstrated that ciglitazone-mediated PPARγ activation significantly increases apoptosis of human septic T lymphocytes, which is blocked by the PPARγ antagonist SR-202. Intriguingly, sera from human septic patients seem to contain molecule(s) capable of specifically activating PPARγ and inducing PPARγ-dependent apoptosis of human T lymphocyte cells, although the exact identity of such molecules has yet to be determined. The authors therefore concluded that PPARγ activation contributes to the lymphopenia observed during sepsis [40]. Schmidt et al. presented similar findings using the mouse CLP polymicrobial sepsis model as well as LPS-induced endotoxemia. They found that PPARγ expression triggers T lymphocyte apoptosis and is associated with poor survival of mice experiencing endotoxemia or peritonitis whereas mice whose T lymphocytes lack PPARγ or those treated with GW9662 show significantly fewer apoptotic T lymphocytes, reduced organ damage, and improved survival [41].

PPARγ can also negatively affect hosts' response to bacterial infections by other mechanisms. PPARγ activation can downregulate neutrophil migration, rolling, and adhesion, key processes during their chemotactic response to invading pathogens [42, 43]. This inhibition may reflect PPARγ-dependent reduction in neutrophils' ability to adhere to fibrinogen and to polymerize actin [42] and/or suppression of ICAM-1 expression [43] and contributes to the host's failure to contain infections. 15d-PGJ₂-induced PPARγ activation also exacerbates pulmonary edema and tissue injury associated with LPS-induced endotoxemia by locally elevating chemokine and IL-1β expression and increasing the number of mucin-producing cells [44]. Other studies, however, have found that 15d-PGJ₂ treatment improves survival in mouse [45] and rat [46] endotoxemia. Dose, timing, and species do not provide obvious explanations for the discrepant results.

Philipson et al. showed that abrogation of PPARγ expression, by T lymphocyte specific conditional knockout or GW9662, enhances inflammatory and effector responses in the early stage of enteroaggregative *Escherichia coli* infection and improves bacterial clearance by increasing infiltration of leukocytes, including T lymphocytes, dendritic cells, and macrophages [47], implying a deleterious effect of PPARγ activation/expression on host defense. These results must be interpreted with caution, however, since prolonged *E. coli* infection was seen only in mice on a protein-deficient diet. Mice on a normal diet clear the infection within 14 days without regard to PPARγ deficiency. Despite this caveat, however, this group of studies suggests that PPARγ may adversely affect the host's ability to combat bacterial infections.

Interestingly, some bacteria seem capable of modulating PPARγ to assist their pathogenesis by manipulating its function in lipid metabolism: mycobacteria, such as those associated with tuberculosis and leprosy, use the hosts' lipids for intracellular survival and replication [1]. *Mycobacterium bovis* bacillus Calmette-Guérin (BCG) infection induces PPARγ expression and its nuclear localization in human monocytes and enhances lipid body formation in the activated macrophages. The PPARγ agonist BRL49653 (rosiglitazone) also increases and the antagonist GW9662 blocks this lipid body biogenesis, confirming its PPARγ dependence. Furthermore, the enhanced ability of macrophages to kill *Mycobacterium bovis* BCG in response to GW9662 treatment and failure of a nonpathogenic bacterium to induce PPARγ expression strongly indicate that *Mycobacterium bovis* BCG specifically employs PPARγ signaling for its pathogenesis [48]. Findings that lipid droplets within *Mycobacterium bovis* BCG-activated macrophages and *Mycobacterium leprae*-infected Schwann cells and macrophages are major production sites of eicosanoids, a class of PPARγ agonists, further reinforce PPARγ's supportive role in survival and replication of mycobacteria [49–51].

The negative effect of PPARγ activation during bacterial infections is supported by a systematic review and meta-analysis of 13 long-term randomized controlled trials of TZDs that involved 17,627 participants (8,163 receiving TZDs and 9,464 receiving control drugs) [52]. The analysis revealed that long-term (1–5.5 years) use of TZDs, compared to control drugs, significantly increases the risk of participants acquiring pneumonia or lower respiratory tract infection, some of which result in hospitalization, disability, or death [52]. It is important to note, however, that the effect was small even with prolonged treatment and that diabetic individuals, the subject population, are at increased risk of infection. Nevertheless, these results suggest caution in using TZDs in patients who may be particularly susceptible to infection.

4. Conclusions

In contrast to the use of antimicrobial drugs that directly target the problem's source, bacteria, treating infections with immunomodulatory agents such as PPARγ ligands is more complex. The innate immune responses to invading pathogens can be divided broadly into an initial hyperinflammatory stage, termed the systemic inflammatory response syndrome, and a subsequent immunosuppressive stage called the compensatory anti-inflammatory response syndrome [53]. Thus, immunomodulatory drugs must achieve a fine balance between pro- and anti-inflammatory effects on the immune system, dampening excessive systemic inflammatory responses to prevent severe tissue damage and other complications without significantly affecting the essential ability of the host immune system to clear the infection.

We have here reviewed research investigating the effects of PPARγ activation or inhibition during bacterial infections. These studies clearly show that PPARγ is a double-edged sword, possessing both pro- and anti-inflammatory effects and exerting beneficial as well as harmful effects upon host defenses against pathogenic bacteria. While differences in the type of pathogens, disease models, and PPARγ agonists/antagonists used in the research can explain many of the variations in results reported by different research groups, timing, the point during the host immune response at which drugs are administered, likely plays a large part in determining which PPARγ agonist/antagonist effect predominates. For instance, blocking the anti-inflammatory cytokine IL-10, which is associated with reduced secretion of proinflammatory mediators, at an early stage of sepsis is detrimental to the host, whereas IL-10 suppression later in sepsis is linked with longer survival of the affected animals. Similarly, established sepsis may respond to immune-stimulating strategies but not to therapeutic interventions designed to suppress proinflammatory mediators secreted early during sepsis. In addition, in human patients, the effect of a PPARγ agonist or antagonist would likely differ with the immune status of each individual—the exact pathophysiologic nature of immune imbalance—as well as other factors such as age, comorbidities, and genetic background [53]. Patients suffering damage and symptoms due to exaggerated immune response would benefit from the anti-inflammatory effect of PPARγ ligands, while those experiencing immunoparalysis-induced symptoms would require the immune-enhancing effect of PPARγ antagonists to alleviate damage and symptoms [54]. Thus, it is imperative to aim for a carefully defined balance between immune stimulation and immunosuppression in each patient. Close assessment of the competence of host antimicrobial defenses and the extent of inflammation and tissue injury, including measurement of mediators of the immune response, and adjustment in the dosage and timing of PPARγ agonist/antagonist administration would be valuable for achieving the most desired outcome [55, 56].

Disclosure

The contents in this article do not represent the views of the US Department of Veterans Affairs or the US government.

Competing Interests

The authors declare that they have no conflicts of interests.

Acknowledgments

This work was supported by a Merit Review award from the US Department of Veterans Affairs and National Institutes of Health Grants HL093196 and AI125338 (to Raju C. Reddy).

References

[1] P. E. Almeida, A. B. Carneiro, A. R. Silva, and P. T. Bozza, "PPARγ expression and function in mycobacterial infection: roles in lipid metabolism, immunity, and bacterial killing," *PPAR Research*, vol. 2012, Article ID 383829, 7 pages, 2012.

[2] R. B. Clark, "The role of PPARs in inflammation and immunity," *Journal of Leukocyte Biology*, vol. 71, no. 3, pp. 388–400, 2002.

[3] B. P. Kota, T. H.-W. Huang, and B. D. Roufogalis, "An overview on biological mechanisms of PPARs," *Pharmacological Research*, vol. 51, no. 2, pp. 85–94, 2005.

[4] J. Berger and D. E. Moller, "The mechanisms of action of PPARs," *Annual Review of Medicine*, vol. 53, no. 1, pp. 409–435, 2002.

[5] L. Fajas, D. Auboeuf, E. Raspé et al., "The organization, promoter analysis, and expression of the human PPARγ gene," *The Journal of Biological Chemistry*, vol. 272, no. 30, pp. 18779–18789, 1997.

[6] L. Fajas, J.-C. Fruchart, and J. Auwerx, "PPARγ3 mRNA: a distinct PPARγ mRNA subtype transcribed from an independent promoter," *FEBS Letters*, vol. 438, no. 1-2, pp. 55–60, 1998.

[7] Y. Li, J. Zhang, F. J. Schopfer et al., "Molecular recognition of nitrated fatty acids by PPARγ," *Nature Structural & Molecular Biology*, vol. 15, no. 8, pp. 865–867, 2008.

[8] D. L. Feinstein, A. Spagnolo, C. Akar et al., "Receptor-independent actions of PPAR thiazolidinedione agonists: is mitochondrial function the key?" *Biochemical Pharmacology*, vol. 70, no. 2, pp. 177–188, 2005.

[9] L. M. S. Baker, P. R. S. Baker, F. Golin-Bisello et al., "Nitro-fatty acid reaction with glutathione and cysteine. Kinetic analysis of thiol alkylation by a Michael addition reaction," *The Journal of Biological Chemistry*, vol. 282, no. 42, pp. 31085–31093, 2007.

[10] A. T. Reddy, S. P. Lakshmi, R. R. Muchumarri, and R. C. Reddy, "Nitrated fatty acids reverse cigarette smoke-induced alveolar macrophage activation and inhibit protease activity via electrophilic S-alkylation," *PLoS ONE*, vol. 11, no. 4, Article ID e0153336, 2016.

[11] U. Panchapakesan, C. A. Pollock, and X. M. Chen, "The effect of high glucose and PPAR-γ agonists on PPAR-γ expression and

function in HK-2 cells," *American Journal of Physiology-Renal Physiology*, vol. 287, no. 3, pp. F528–F534, 2004.

[12] S. P. Lakshmi, A. T. Reddy, Y. Zhang et al., "Down-regulated peroxisome proliferator-activated receptor γ (PPARγ) in lung epithelial cells promotes a PPARγ agonist-reversible proinflammatory phenotype in chronic obstructive pulmonary disease (COPD)," *The Journal of Biological Chemistry*, vol. 289, no. 10, pp. 6383–6393, 2014.

[13] M. V. Schmidt, B. Brüne, and A. Von Knethen, "The nuclear hormone receptor PPARγ as a therapeutic target in major diseases," *TheScientificWorldJOURNAL*, vol. 10, pp. 2181–2197, 2010.

[14] A. Croasdell, P. F. Duffney, N. Kim, S. H. Lacy, P. J. Sime, and R. P. Phipps, "PPARγ and the innate immune system mediate the resolution of inflammation," *PPAR Research*, vol. 2015, Article ID 549691, 20 pages, 2015.

[15] J. M. Kaplan and B. Zingarelli, "Novel therapeutic agents in pediatric sepsis: peroxisome proliferator receptor γ (PPAR γ) agonists," *The Open Inflammation Journal*, vol. 4, no. 1, pp. 120–124, 2011.

[16] F. C. Tenover, "Mechanisms of antimicrobial resistance in bacteria," *The American Journal of Medicine*, vol. 119, no. 6, pp. S3–S10, 2006.

[17] D. M. Aronoff, C. H. Serezani, J. K. Carstens et al., "Stimulatory effects of peroxisome proliferator-activated receptor-γ on Fcγ receptor-mediated phagocytosis by alveolar macrophages," *PPAR Research*, vol. 2007, Article ID 52546, 8 pages, 2007.

[18] K. Asada, S. Sasaki, T. Suda, K. Chida, and H. Nakamura, "Antiinflammatory roles of peroxisome proliferator-activated receptor γ in human alveolar macrophages," *American Journal of Respiratory and Critical Care Medicine*, vol. 169, no. 2, pp. 195–200, 2004.

[19] A. T. Reddy, S. P. Lakshmi, S. Dornadula, S. Pinni, D. R. Rampa, and R. C. Reddy, "The nitrated fatty acid 10-nitro-oleate attenuates allergic airway disease," *The Journal of Immunology*, vol. 191, no. 5, pp. 2053–2063, 2013.

[20] M. E. Stegenga, S. Florquin, A. F. de Vos, and T. van der Poll, "The thiazolidinedione ciglitazone reduces bacterial outgrowth and early inflammation during *Streptococcus pneumoniae* pneumonia in mice," *Critical Care Medicine*, vol. 37, no. 2, pp. 614–618, 2009.

[21] T. Kielian, M. M. Syed, S. Liu et al., "The synthetic peroxisome proliferator-activated receptor-γ agonist ciglitazone attenuates neuroinflammation and accelerates encapsulation in bacterial brain abscesses," *The Journal of Immunology*, vol. 180, no. 7, pp. 5004–5016, 2008.

[22] R. Fernandez-Boyanapalli, S. C. Frasch, D. W. H. Riches, R. W. Vandivier, P. M. Henson, and D. L. Bratton, "PPARγ activation normalizes resolution of acute sterile inflammation in murine chronic granulomatous disease," *Blood*, vol. 116, no. 22, pp. 4512–4522, 2010.

[23] R. F. Fernandez-Boyanapalli, E. L. Falcone, C. S. Zerbe et al., "Impaired efferocytosis in human chronic granulomatous disease is reversed by pioglitazone treatment," *Journal of Allergy and Clinical Immunology*, vol. 136, no. 5, pp. 1399.e3–1401.e3, 2015.

[24] R. F. Fernandez-Boyanapalli, S. C. Frasch, S. M. Thomas et al., "Pioglitazone restores phagocyte mitochondrial oxidants and bactericidal capacity in chronic granulomatous disease," *Journal of Allergy and Clinical Immunology*, vol. 135, no. 2, pp. 517–527.e12, 2015.

[25] M. Migliavacca, A. Assanelli, F. Ferrua et al., "Pioglitazone as a novel therapeutic approach in chronic granulomatous disease," *The Journal of Allergy and Clinical Immunology*, vol. 137, no. 6, pp. 1913–1915.e2, 2016.

[26] A. T. Reddy, S. P. Lakshmi, J. M. Kleinhenz, R. L. Sutliff, C. M. Hart, and R. C. Reddy, "Endothelial cell peroxisome proliferator-activated receptor γ reduces endotoxemic pulmonary inflammation and injury," *The Journal of Immunology*, vol. 189, no. 11, pp. 5411–5420, 2012.

[27] B. Zingarelli, M. Sheehan, P. W. Hake, M. O'Connor, A. Denenberg, and J. A. Cook, "Peroxisome proliferator activator receptor-γ ligands, 15-deoxy-Δ12,14-prostaglandin J2 and ciglitazone, reduce systemic inflammation in polymicrobial sepsis by modulation of signal transduction pathways," *The Journal of Immunology*, vol. 171, no. 12, pp. 6827–6837, 2003.

[28] S. Ogawa, J. Lozach, C. Benner et al., "Molecular determinants of crosstalk between nuclear receptors and toll-like receptors," *Cell*, vol. 122, no. 5, pp. 707–721, 2005.

[29] B. M. Necela, W. Su, and E. A. Thompson, "Toll-like receptor 4 mediates cross-talk between peroxisome proliferator-activated receptor γ and nuclear factor-κB in macrophages," *Immunology*, vol. 125, no. 3, pp. 344–358, 2008.

[30] A. E. Ferreira, F. Sisti, F. Sônego et al., "PPAR-γ/IL-10 axis inhibits MyD88 expression and ameliorates murine polymicrobial sepsis," *The Journal of Immunology*, vol. 192, no. 5, pp. 2357–2365, 2014.

[31] H. S. Warren, "Peroxisome proliferator-activated receptor-gamma agonists, control of bacterial outgrowth, and inflammation," *Critical Care Medicine*, vol. 37, no. 2, pp. 773–774, 2009.

[32] R. C. Reddy, "Immunomodulatory role of PPAR-gamma in alveolar macrophages," *Journal of Investigative Medicine*, vol. 56, no. 2, pp. 522–527, 2008.

[33] E. L. Gautier, A. Chow, R. Spanbroek et al., "Systemic analysis of PPARγ in mouse macrophage populations reveals marked diversity in expression with critical roles in resolution of inflammation and airway immunity," *The Journal of Immunology*, vol. 189, no. 5, pp. 2614–2624, 2012.

[34] D. Kelly, J. I. Campbell, T. P. King et al., "Commensal anaerobic gut bacteria attenuate inflammation by regulating nuclear-cytoplasmic shutting of PPAR-γ and RelA," *Nature Immunology*, vol. 5, no. 1, pp. 104–112, 2004.

[35] A. M. Bodles, V. Varma, A. Yao-Borengasser et al., "Pioglitazone induces apoptosis of macrophages in human adipose tissue," *Journal of Lipid Research*, vol. 47, no. 9, pp. 2080–2088, 2006.

[36] Y.-C. Chen, S.-C. Shen, and S.-H. Tsai, "Prostaglandin D$_2$ and J$_2$ induce apoptosis in human leukemia cells via activation of the caspase 3 cascade and production of reactive oxygen species," *Biochimica et Biophysica Acta (BBA)—Molecular Cell Research*, vol. 1743, no. 3, pp. 291–304, 2005.

[37] J. Padilla, K. Kaur, H. J. Cao, T. J. Smith, and R. P. Phipps, "Peroxisome proliferator activator receptor-γ agonists and 15-deoxy-Δ12,14-PGJ2 induce apoptosis in normal and malignant B-lineage cells," *The Journal of Immunology*, vol. 165, no. 12, pp. 6941–6948, 2000.

[38] J. Padilla, E. Leung, and R. P. Phipps, "Human B lymphocytes and B lymphomas express PPAR-γ and are killed by PPAR-γ agonists," *Clinical Immunology*, vol. 103, no. 1, pp. 22–33, 2002.

[39] A. Tautenhahn, B. Brüne, and A. von Knethen, "Activation-induced PPARγ expression sensitizes primary human T cells toward apoptosis," *Journal of Leukocyte Biology*, vol. 73, no. 5, pp. 665–672, 2003.

[40] M. Soller, A. Tautenhahn, B. Brüne et al., "Peroxisome proliferator-activated receptor γ contributes to T lymphocyte apoptosis during sepsis," *Journal of Leukocyte Biology*, vol. 79, no. 1, pp. 235–243, 2006.

[41] M. V. Schmidt, P. Paulus, A.-M. Kuhn et al., "Peroxisome proliferator-activated receptor γ-induced T cell apoptosis reduces survival during polymicrobial sepsis," *American Journal of Respiratory and Critical Care Medicine*, vol. 184, no. 1, pp. 64–74, 2011.

[42] R. C. Reddy, V. R. Narala, V. G. Keshamouni, J. E. Milam, M. W. Newstead, and T. J. Standiford, "Sepsis-induced inhibition of neutrophil chemotaxis is mediated by activation of peroxisome proliferator-activated receptor-γ," *Blood*, vol. 112, no. 10, pp. 4250–4258, 2008.

[43] M. H. Napimoga, S. M. Vieira, D. Dal-Secco et al., "Peroxisome proliferator-activated receptor-γ ligand, 15-deoxy-Δ12,14-prostaglandin J2, reduces neutrophil migration via a nitric oxide pathway," *The Journal of Immunology*, vol. 180, no. 1, pp. 609–617, 2008.

[44] K.-I. Inoue, H. Takano, R. Yanagisawa et al., "Effect of 15-deoxy-$\Delta^{12,14}$-prostaglandin J_2 on acute lung injury induced by lipopolysaccharide in mice," *European Journal of Pharmacology*, vol. 481, no. 2-3, pp. 261–269, 2003.

[45] J. M. Kaplan, J. A. Cook, P. W. Hake, M. O'Connor, T. J. Burroughs, and B. Zingarelli, "15-Deoxy-$\Delta^{12,14}$-prostaglandin J_2 (15D-PGJ$_2$), a peroxisome proliferator activated receptor γ ligand, reduces tissue leukosequestration and mortality in endotoxic shock," *Shock*, vol. 24, no. 1, pp. 59–65, 2005.

[46] D. Liu, Z. Geng, W. Zhu, H. Wang, Y. Chen, and J. Liang, "15-deoxy-Delta(1)(2, (1)(4)-prostaglandin J(2) ameliorates endotoxin-induced acute lung injury in rats," *Chinese Medical Journal*, vol. 127, no. 5, pp. 815–820, 2014.

[47] C. W. Philipson, J. Bassaganya-Riera, M. Viladomiu et al., "The role of peroxisome proliferator-activated receptor γ in immune responses to enteroaggregative escherichia coli infection," *PLoS ONE*, vol. 8, no. 2, Article ID e57812, 2013.

[48] P. E. Almeida, A. R. Silva, C. M. Maya-Monteiro et al., "Mycobacterium bovis bacillus Calmette-Guérin infection induces TLR2-dependent peroxisome proliferator-activated receptor γ expression and activation: functions in inflammation, lipid metabolism, and pathogenesis," *The Journal of Immunology*, vol. 183, no. 2, pp. 1337–1345, 2009.

[49] H. D'Avila, R. C. N. Melo, G. G. Parreira, E. Werneck-Barroso, H. C. Castro-Faria-Neto, and P. T. Bozza, "*Mycobacterium bovis* bacillus Calmette-Guérin induces TLR2-mediated formation of lipid bodies: intracellular domains for eicosanoid synthesis in vivo," *The Journal of Immunology*, vol. 176, no. 5, pp. 3087–3097, 2006.

[50] K. A. Mattos, H. D'Avila, L. S. Rodrigues et al., "Lipid droplet formation in leprosy: toll-like receptor-regulated organelles involved in eicosanoid formation and Mycobacterium leprae pathogenesis," *Journal of Leukocyte Biology*, vol. 87, no. 3, pp. 371–384, 2010.

[51] K. A. Mattos, V. G. C. Oliveira, H. D'Avila et al., "TLR6-driven lipid droplets in *Mycobacterium leprae*-infected Schwann cells: immunoinflammatory platforms associated with bacterial persistence," *The Journal of Immunology*, vol. 187, no. 5, pp. 2548–2558, 2011.

[52] S. Singh, Y. K. Loke, and C. D. Furberg, "Long-term use of thiazolidinediones and the associated risk of pneumonia or lower respiratory tract infection: systematic review and meta-analysis," *Thorax*, vol. 66, no. 5, pp. 383–388, 2011.

[53] E. Christaki, P. Anyfanti, and S. M. Opal, "Immunomodulatory therapy for sepsis: an update," *Expert Review of Anti-Infective Therapy*, vol. 9, no. 11, pp. 1013–1033, 2011.

[54] L.-A. Pirofski and A. Casadevall, "Immunomodulators as an antimicrobial tool," *Current Opinion in Microbiology*, vol. 9, no. 5, pp. 489–495, 2006.

[55] H. D. Volk, P. Reinke, and W. D. Döcke, "Clinical aspects: from systemic inflammation to 'immunoparalysis'," *Chemical Immunology*, vol. 74, pp. 162–177, 2000.

[56] S. C. A. Meijvis, E. M. W. van de Garde, G. T. Rijkers, and W. J. W. Bos, "Treatment with anti-inflammatory drugs in community-acquired pneumonia," *Journal of Internal Medicine*, vol. 272, no. 1, pp. 25–35, 2012.

8

Peroxisome Proliferator-Activated Receptor Modulation during Metabolic Diseases and Cancers: Master and Minions

Salvatore Giovanni Vitale,[1] Antonio Simone Laganà,[1] Angela Nigro,[2]
Valentina Lucia La Rosa,[3] Paola Rossetti,[2] Agnese Maria Chiara Rapisarda,[4]
Sandro La Vignera,[5] Rosita Angela Condorelli,[5] Francesco Corrado,[1]
Massimo Buscema,[2] and Rosario D'Anna[1]

[1]Unit of Gynecology and Obstetrics, Department of Human Pathology in Adulthood and Childhood "G. Barresi",
University of Messina, Messina, Italy
[2]Unit of Diabetology and Endocrino-Metabolic Diseases, Hospital for Emergency Cannizzaro, Catania, Italy
[3]Unit of Psychodiagnostics and Clinical Psychology, University of Catania, Catania, Italy
[4]Department of General Surgery and Medical Surgical Specialties, University of Catania, Catania, Italy
[5]Department of Clinical and Experimental Medicine-CRAMD (Research Centre of Motor Activity and
Metabolic Rehabilitation in Diabetes), University of Catania, Catania, Italy

Correspondence should be addressed to Salvatore Giovanni Vitale; vitalesalvatore@hotmail.com

Academic Editor: Daniele Fanale

The prevalence of obesity and metabolic diseases (such as type 2 diabetes mellitus, dyslipidaemia, and cardiovascular diseases) has increased in the last decade, in both industrialized and developing countries. This also coincided with our observation of a similar increase in the prevalence of cancers. The aetiology of these diseases is very complex and involves genetic, nutritional, and environmental factors. Much evidence indicates the central role undertaken by peroxisome proliferator-activated receptors (PPARs) in the development of these disorders. Due to the fact that their ligands could become crucial in future target-therapies, PPARs have therefore become the focal point of much research. Based on this evidence, this narrative review was written with the purpose of outlining the effects of PPARs, their actions, and their prospective uses in metabolic diseases and cancers.

1. Introduction

The prevalence of obesity and metabolic diseases (for example, type 2 diabetes mellitus (T2DM), dyslipidaemia, and cardiovascular diseases) has increased in the last decade, in both industrialized and developing countries. At the same time, we have observed similar increase in the prevalence of cancers. The aetiology of these disorders is very complex and involves genetic, nutritional, and environmental factors. There is much evidence that peroxisome proliferator-activated receptors (PPARs) play a significant part in the progression of these diseases [1, 2].

Peroxisome proliferator-activated receptors (PPARs) are a group of ligand-activated nuclear hormone receptors (NRs), existing within the steroid receptor superfamily, which includes the receptors for thyroid hormones, retinoids, 1,25-dihydroxyvitamin D_3, and steroid hormones [3]. After binding with their agonists (natural or synthetic) in cytoplasm, PPARs heterodimerize with the retinoid acid receptor (RNR or NR2B) and translocate to the nucleus, subsequently binding to specific DNA regions termed peroxisome proliferator response elements (PPREs). Here they activate the transcription of numerous genes that play a role in mechanisms associated with glucose and lipid metabolism, body energy production, inflammation, cell cycle arrest, apoptosis, and DNA damage response [4, 5].

Currently, we know of three different types of PPARs (PPARα, PPARβ/δ, and PPARγ), which present many different features, such as tissue distribution, ligand specificities, and effects. The principal differences among PPARs are due to their structure; despite the DNA-binding domains being 80% identical, the ligand-binding domains are different. The biological effects of PPARs depend on their different ligand and the presence of several proteins that operate as coactivators or corepressors and whose presence may alter the expression of genes [6]. About this point, recent evidence suggests that the E6-associated protein (E6-AP) is an E3 ubiquitin ligase that affects the activity of other NRs: in particular, E6-AP is able to inhibit the ligand-independent transcriptional activity of PPARα and PPARβ, with marginal effects on PPARγ, and decreased basal mRNA levels of PPARα target genes [7]. Similarly, Murine Double Minute 2 (MDM2), an E3 ubiquitin ligase, was identified as a PPARα-interacting protein that regulates the transcriptional activity of PPARα and PPARβ/δ, but not PPARγ [8].

2. PPARα Role in Metabolic Diseases

PPARα is expressed in large amounts in the liver, skeletal muscles, heart, intestinal mucosa, and brown adipose tissue, where it undertakes an important role in fatty acid metabolism, as well as glucose and lipid metabolism [9]. PPARα activation induces the expression of genes involved in lipid and lipoprotein metabolism (apolipoprotein genes A1, A2, and A5), in fatty acid oxidation (acyl-coenzyme A oxidase and carnitine palmitoyltransferases I and II), in the desaturation of fatty acyl-CoA (delta-6-desaturase), in High Density Lipoprotein (HDL) metabolism (Phospholipid Transfer Protein), and in ketone synthesis (3-Hydroxy-3-Methylglutaryl-CoA Synthase 2) [10]. Activated PPARα also stimulates the expression of the fibroblast growth factor gene 21 (FGF21) and the angiopoietin-like protein gene 4 (ANGPLT4). In response to PPARα activation, production of FGF21 in the liver begins, activating white adipose tissue lipolysis in order to provide nonadipose tissue with fatty acids as well as controlling ketogenesis in the liver with the purpose of procuring energy from fatty acids [11]. In partial agreement with these data, it was found that increased FGF21 expression was observed in the livers of PPARβ/δ-null mice and in mouse primary hepatocytes when this receptor was knocked down by small interfering RNA (siRNA) and that this increase was associated with enhanced protein levels in the heme-regulated eukaryotic translation initiation factor 2α (eIF2α) kinase (HRI) [12]. Recent studies indicate that the physiological fluctuations in lipoproteins lipase (LPL) activity are mediated by ANGPLT4 as well as the decrease in adipose LPL activity observed during intervals of fasting [13]. The natural and pharmacological ligands for PPARα are, respectively, omega-3 fatty acids resulting from diet (such as linolenic, α-linolenic, γ-linolenic, and arachidonic acids) and fibrate, normally used as potent hypolipidemic agents [14]. In the liver, PPARα plays the role of lipid sensor, normally undergoing activation due to fatty acids and resulting in the increased burning of energy, the reduction of fat storage, and the prevention of steatosis; conversely, when PPARα sensing is not efficient or when fatty acid concentration is decreased (for genetic, toxic, or metabolic causes), this causes a reduction in energy burning and the resulting lipotoxicity promotes hepatic steatosis and steatohepatitis [15].

These data were confirmed when liver and whole-body fatty acid homeostasis impairment was recently demonstrated in a hepatocyte-specific PPARα knockout mouse model. Results included hepatic lipid accumulation (nonalcoholic fatty liver disease, NAFLD) and hypercholesterolemia during ageing [16]. In addition, mice conditionally expressing human PPARδ demonstrated pronounced weight loss and promoted hepatic steatosis when treated with GW501516 (PPARδ-agonist) when compared to wild type mice [17]. Fibrates are weak PPARα ligands; they reduce triglyceride (30–50%) and very low-density lipoprotein (VLDL) levels through an increased rate of lipid uptake, lipoprotein lipase mediated lipolysis, and β- oxidation; in addition, fibrates also induce a modest increase in HDL cholesterol levels (5–20%), secondary to the transcriptional induction of apolipoprotein A-I/A-II synthesis found in the liver [18]. In this way, they decrease the systemic availability of fatty acids as well as fatty acid uptake in muscles [19], consequently leading to fibrates reducing arteriosclerosis progression and cardiovascular events. They also increase insulin sensitization and reduce plasma glucose levels.

PPARα activation by omega-3 fatty acids results in an anti-inflammatory effect, caused in all probability by the inhibition of their own oxidation due to the activation of the nuclear factor kappa-light-chain-enhancers of activated B cells (NF-κB). PPARα also plays a key role in the mediation of the anti-inflammatory actions of palmitoylethanolamide, the natural amide of palmitic acid, and ethanolamide [20]. Recently, a PPARα agonist (K-877) displaying high levels of potency and selectivity demonstrated optimal effects on atherogenic dyslipidemia [21]. In addition, a recent study indicated that statins, which are normally employed as cholesterol-lowering drugs, induce an increase in neurotrophin expression in the brain, as a result of their binding to a specific PPARα domain independent of the mevalonate pathway. In a mouse model with Alzheimer's disease, the use of Simvastatin led to an increase in neutrophin expression, as well as an improvement in memory and learning [22].

3. The Role of PPARβ/δ in Metabolic Diseases

PPARβ/δ is expressed ubiquitously, particularly in tissue which is metabolically active, such as the liver, skeletal and cardiac muscle, adipose tissue, and macrophages. Its involvement in the oxidation of fatty acids is crucial, and it improves lipid and cholesterol profiles. It plays a central role in the oxidation of fatty acids as well as improving lipid and cholesterol profiles, which reduces adiposity and prevents the development of obesity [23, 24]. It also regulates glucose blood levels. In several animal studies, PPARβ/δ acted as regulator of fat consumption; the deficiency of this receptor leads to obesity, while the activation of PPARβ/δ conversely results in resistance to this condition [25]. In the heart, in the presence of high-level dietary fat, PPARβ/δ lowers lipid accumulation and increases glucose metabolism and consequently seems to be useful in diabetic cardiomyopathy, as it protects the heart against ischemia-reperfusion injury [26]. For all these reasons, PPARβ/δ agonists (GW501516, GW0742, and L-165041) could become a potential target in the treatment of metabolic disorders. However, adverse effects, particularly for PPARγ agonists, are also observed with the use of investigational PPAR agonists and even some approved drugs [27].

Recently, it was found that GW501516 significantly increased fatty acid oxidation and reduced the triglyceride amount in VLDL-loaded foam cells, suggesting a key role of PPARβ/δ in modulating macrophage lipid overload [28]. Intriguingly, PPAR-δ agonist GW501516 decreases uptake of VLDL and expression of VLDL receptor at mRNA and protein levels through the regulation of miRNA-100 in Human Umbilical Vein Endothelial Cells [29]. Confirming the human findings, clear data from mouse model showed that PPARβ/δ-deficient mice fed with fructose exacerbated glucose intolerance and this led to macrophage infiltration, inflammation, enhanced mRNA and protein levels of CD36, and activation of the c-Jun N-terminal kinase pathway in white adipose tissue; fascinatingly, these effects were partially prevented by the PPARβ/δ activator GW501516 [30]. In addition, topical application of polymer-encapsulated GW501516 was found to have therapeutic wound healing activity, through stimulation of glutathione peroxidase 1 (GPx1) and catalase expression in fibroblasts: indeed, GPx1 and catalase are known to scavenge excessive H_2O_2 accumulation in diabetic wound beds, preventing H_2O_2-induced extracellular matrix modification and facilitating keratinocyte migration [31]. Furthermore, PPARδ plays pivotal roles in wound healing by promoting fibroblast-to-myofibroblast differentiation via transforming growth factor (TGF)-β/Smad3 signalling: according to recent findings [32], GW501516-activated PPARδ increases the migration and contractile properties of human dermal fibroblasts and upregulates the expression of myofibroblast markers such as collagen I and fibronectin, with a concomitant reduction in expression of the epithelial marker E-cadherin.

Regarding GW0742, it was recently demonstrated that it can reverse the lung tissue damage induced by elastase in emphysema-model mice and improves respiratory function in mouse model: in particular, GW0742 increases the in vivo expression of surfactant proteins A and D, which are known alveolar type II epithelial cell markers, reduces the average distance between alveolar walls in the lungs, and improves tissue elastance, as well as the ratio of the forced expiratory volume in the first 0.05 s to the forced vital capacity [33]. In addition, recent evidence suggests that GW0742 administration to mice fed in high-fat diet prevented the gain of body weight, heart and kidney hypertrophy, and fat accumulation: namely, it prevents the increase of in plasma levels of fasting glucose, glucose tolerance test, homeostatic model assessment of insulin resistance, and triglyceride; from the molecular point of view, it increases both protein kinase B (Akt) and endothelial nitric oxide synthase phosphorylation and inhibits the increase in caveolin-1/endothelial nitric oxide synthase interaction, ethidium fluorescence, nicotinamide adenine dinucleotide phosphate (NADPH) oxidase 1, Toll-like receptor 4, tumor necrosis factor-α, and interleukin-6 expression, and IκBα phosphorylation [34].

Regarding the PPARβ agonist L-165041, it was demonstrated that it induces vascular endothelial growth factor

(VEGF) (121), VEGF(165), and VEGF(189) expression in HPV (Human Papillomavirus) positive HeLa cells: considering the intrinsic connection between HPV-related cancer of uterine cervix and VEGF levels, it is possible that PPARβ-mediated pathway may play a key role in the development of this type of cancer [35]. Confirming these data, L-165041 was found to inhibit VEGF-stimulated angiogenesis by suppressing the cell cycle progression independently of PPARδ: in particular, it reduces the number of endothelial cells in the S phase and the expression levels of cell cycle regulatory proteins such as cyclin A, cyclin E, cyclin-dependent kinase (CDK) 2, and CDK4 [36]. Furthermore, a recent in vitro study found that L-165041 significantly inhibits high glucose-induced interleukin-6 and TNF-α production, receptor for advanced glycation end products expression, and NF-κB translocation in human embryonic kidney 293 (HEK) cells; in addition, it increases superoxide dismutase expression and attenuates apoptosis in HEK and mesangial cells [37].

4. PPARα/δ Role in Metabolic Diseases

The dual PPARα/δ agonist (GFT-505-Elafibranor) seems to have potentially beneficial effects in the treatment of NAFLD. In 2013, Staels et al. [38] showed in a mouse model that GFT505 protects liver from steatosis, inflammation, and fibrosis. This agonist also improves liver markers, decreases hepatic lipid accumulation, and inhibits proinflammatory (IL-1, TNFα) and profibrotic (transforming growth factor beta, tissue inhibitor of metalloproteinase 2, collagen type I, alpha 1, and collagen type I, alpha 2) gene expression with a PPARα dependent and independent mechanism [38]. In partial agreement with these data, it was recently found that Biliverdin reductase A protects against hepatic steatosis by inhibiting glycogen synthase kinase 3β (GSK3β) by enhancing serine 9 phosphorylation, which inhibits its activity: in particular, GSK3β phosphorylates serine 73 of the PPARα, which in turn increased ubiquitination and protein turnover, as well as decreasing activity [39].

In phase 2a trials (duration 8 weeks) involving twenty-two obese males with dyslipidemia, prediabetes, or T2DM, GFT505 reduced fasting plasma triglycerides, low-density lipoprotein (LDL) cholesterol, and liver enzyme concentrations improving peripheral insulin sensitivity and hepatic insulin sensitivity [40]. The liver-specific action of GFT505 was suggested by the fact that neither PPARα nor PPARδ target genes were induced in skeletal muscle. Recently, it was demonstrated that Elafibranor was capable of improving the histological features of severe and moderate nonalcoholic steatohepatitis (NASH) and presents a favorable safety profile [41].

5. PPARγ Role in Metabolic Diseases

PPARγ was the first to be cloned and studied in depth, due to its being the target of a class of antidiabetic drugs called thiazolidinediones (TZD). Currently, we know of three isoforms of PPARγ: PPARγ_1 and PPARγ_3, which are expressed in the liver, intestine, and spleen; PPARγ_2 is present only in white and brown adipose tissue. Activated PPARγ induces the expression of many genes, essential for adipogenesis, energy balance, insulin sensitivity, lipid and glucose metabolism, and inflammation [42]. In adipocytes, PPARγ is necessary in order for adipose tissue to develop. PPARγ₂ is a potent transcription activator and is triggered as a response to nutrient intake and obesity [43]. Indeed, mice deprived of PPARγ₂ (obese POKO mice) presented higher levels of fat accumulation in adipocytes in comparison with normally obese mice fed an identical diet [44]. According to these data, PPARγ₂ is essential for preventing lipotoxicity by promoting the expansion of adipose tissue and an increased lipid-buffering capacity in liver, muscle, and pancreatic beta cells. A proliferative response of β-cells to insulin resistance is also promoted by PPARγ [45]. In adipocytes, activated PPARγ causes a both balanced and adequate adipocytokine secretion (adiponectin and leptin), which regulates the behavior of insulin when introduced to peripheral tissues (such as the liver, skeletal muscle). As a consequence, PPARγ leads to improved insulin sensitivity in the entire body, additionally protecting the nonadipose tissue against excessive lipid levels [46]. Activated PPARγ induces the expression of genes that regulate the release, transport, and storage of fatty acid, such as the gene of LPL and fatty acid transporter CD36 [44]. PPARγ is also found in endothelial cells and vascular smooth muscle cells, where it seems to be an important factor in inflammation and atherosclerosis [47]. Polyunsaturated fatty acids are the natural ligand of PPARγ; they increase glucose uptake and insulin sensitivity, but they do not have many effects on adipocytes differentiation [48]. As already mentioned, TZDs (pioglitazone, rosiglitazone) are synthetic agonists of PPARγ and are widely used for the treatment of type 2 diabetes. TZDs are also described as insulin sensitizing, as they indirectly induce a higher insulin-stimulated glucose uptake in adipocytes, hepatocytes, and skeletal muscle; they also reduce free fatty acids levels and increase lipid storage in adipocytes. In the liver, TZDs decrease fasting plasma glucose levels through the increase of insulin sensitivity and the inhibition of gluconeogenesis [34]. In the muscles, TZDs reduces postprandial glucose levels [49]. A typical effect of TZDs is weight gain, due (at least in part) to fat being redistributed from visceral depot to subcutaneous depot [49].

In diabetic patients, the two principal types of TZDs (rosiglitazone e pioglitazone) have different effects on cardiovascular outcomes. According to the data of a PROactive study, pioglitazone reduced 16% of cardiovascular complications compared to a placebo [50]. Conversely, rosiglitazone was linked with a significantly increased death rate due to cardiovascular causes; consequently, in 2010 the European Medicines Agency withdrew the usage of this molecule [51]. These existing differences between pio- and rosiglitazone are most likely due to their differing effects on lipid levels; in fact, pioglitazone leads to an increased level of HDL cholesterol whilst lowering levels of triglycerides and fasting fatty acids. Rosiglitazone increases total and HDL cholesterol but also LDL cholesterol, which is negatively associated with cardiovascular diseases [52].

Recently, a new synthetic antidiabetic drug (SR1664) was proposed: when compared to TZDs, it does not induce weight gain. SR1664, with respect to the classic agonist of PPARγ,

blocks only the phosphorylation of serine 273 by CDK5. In a recent study, CDK5 deficient mice (CDK5 KO) demonstrated a paradoxical augmentation of PPARγ phosphorylation at serine 273 by a protein kinase (extracellular signal-regulated kinase, ERK), normally suppressed by CDK5 [53], suggesting a key role in the modulation of the abovementioned pathways. Finally, as extensively summarized elsewhere [54, 55], it was showed that natural PPARγ ligands have different binding modalities to the receptor with respect to the full TZD agonists and can activate also PPARα (as it occurs for genistein, biochanin A, sargaquinoic acid, sargahydroquinoic acid, resveratrol, and amorphastilbol) or the PPARγ-dimer partner retinoid X receptor (RXR; as it occurs for the neolignans, magnolol, and honokiol).

6. PPARα and Tumorigenesis

To date, many studies have analysed the role played by PPARs in the complex mechanism of tumorigenesis. Not all data are clear and PPARs seem to possess both positive and negative effects, depending on the type of tumor. In particular, it leads to negatively regulated colonic inflammation and proliferation. In an animal model of IL-10 −/− mice, the inhibition of colitis was mediated by fenofibrate, increasing the PPARα expression of lymphocytes, macrophages, and colonic epithelial cells and resulting in proinflammatory cytokine production, such as interleukin-17, interferon-γ, and chemokine (C-C motif) ligand 20 (CCL20), being inhibited [56]. In partial agreement with these results in the mouse model, it was recently found that activation of PPARα through fenofibrate suppressed migration of oral cancer cells: in particular, differential protein profiling demonstrated that expressions of genes related to mitochondrial energy metabolism were either upregulated (Atp5g3, Cyc1, Ndufa5, Ndufa10, and Sdhd) or downregulated (Cox5b, Ndufa1, Ndufb7, and Uqcrh), conforming the key role of PPARα activation and response in mitochondrial energy metabolism [57]. In addition, recent data suggests that the selective activation of PPARα by palmitoylethanolamide inhibits colitis-associated angiogenesis, decreasing VEGF release and new vessels formation, via the phosphatidylinositol 3-kinase/Akt/mammalian-target-of-rapamycin (mTOR) signalling pathway [58].

In breast cancer, the data are still not clear. In some studies, PPARα inhibits breast cancer progression, promoting apoptosis of cancer cells through NFκB signalling. Recently, it was demonstrated that clofibrate presents a high chemosensitivity towards breast cancer cells, in all likelihood through the inhibition of NF-κB and ERK1/2 activation, which lowers cyclin D1, cyclin A, and cyclin E and induces proapoptotic P21 levels [59]. In contrast, in other studies PPARα promoted breast cancer progression by releasing leukotriene B4 that activates PPARα in B cells, inducing the differentiation of B cells and metastasis [60].

Despite the fact that PPARα clearly acts in a tumor-dependent fashion [61], recent evidence suggests that its overexpression enhances cancer cell chemotherapy sensitivity, whereas silenced PPARα decreased this event. In this regard, it is possible that it induces cell apoptosis by destructing

B-cell lymphoma 2 (Bcl2): as summarized elsewhere [62], PPARα serves as an E3 ubiquitin ligase to govern Bcl2 protein stability; PPARα binds to BH3 domain of Bcl2 and, subsequently, transfers K48-linked polyubiquitin to lysine-22 site of Bcl2 resulting in its ubiquitination and proteasome-dependent degradation. Confirming these results, it was found that ectopic expression of PPARα in hepatocarcinoma cells significantly suppressed cell proliferation and induced apoptosis by inhibition of NF-κB promoter activity, diminution of phosphor-p65, phosphor-p50, and BCL2 levels, and enhancing IkBα protein [63].

7. PPARγ and Tumorigenesis

PPARγ or dual PPAR α/γ agonists, in rodent carcinogenicity studies, were frequently associated with the development of hemangioma or hemangiosarcoma, fibrosarcoma, bladder, and hepatic tumors [64], suggesting that these types of cancer are drug specific [65].

Recently, a hypothetical mechanism was proposed that could clarify the induction of liposarcoma by differing PPAR agonists: in this model, the first stage of tumor development is initiation, during which DNA damage ensues independent of PPAR activation. The second step, promotion, relies on PPAR and is defined by tumor cell recruitment, proliferation, and differentiation [44]. A multitude of in vitro and in vivo studies have demonstrated much evidence for the antitumor effects of natural and synthetic PPARγ, since it seems to be upregulated in several human cancer lines. Indeed, recent data suggest that PPARγ ligands have an antitumorigenic effect in prostate cancer as a result of antiproliferative and prodifferentiation effects [66]. It would appear that TZDs possess protective effects in the development of pancreatic ductal adenocarcinoma, through improvement in insulin sensitivity and inflammation [67]. Interestingly, it was recently found that PPARβ/δ plays a role in regulating pancreatic cancer cell invasion through regulation of genes via ligand-dependent release of B-cell lymphoma-6 and that activation of the receptor may provide an alternative therapeutic method for controlling migration and metastasis [68].

Despite the fact that data are still elusive, recent evidence from human follicular thyroid carcinoma seems to underlie a key role for paired box gene 8 (PAX8)/PPARγ fusion protein in enhancing in vivo angiogenesis through VEGF expression [69]. PPARγ has positive effects on breast cell cancer: it downregulates the expression of the C-X-C chemokine receptor type 4 (CXCR-4) gene, which is crucial in the growth and progression of cancer, as well as in the development of metastasis. This mechanism seems to be PPARγ dependent, because it could be reversed by GW9662, that is, a PPARγ antagonist [70]. In partial agreement with these results, it was recently found that γ-tocopherol-rich tocopherol decreased tumor volume and multiplicity in estrogen-induced breast cancer female rats, increasing the expression of PPARγ and its downstream genes, phosphatase and tensin homolog (PTEN), and p27 [71]. In addition, it was found that in vivo PPARγ expression in mammary stromal adipocytes attenuates breast tumorigenesis through breast cancer 1 (BRCA1) upregulation and decreased leptin

secretion, and that 7,12-dimethylbenz[a]anthracene (DMBA) plus Rosiglitazone is able to reduce average mammary tumor volumes by 50% [72]. Conversely, heterozygous or homozygous intestinal-specific PPARγ deficiency enhanced small intestine and colon tumorigenesis in Apc(Min/+) mice [73]. Last but not least, robust data from myeloid-specific bitransgenic mouse model allow us to hypothesize that anti-inflammatory PPARγ in myeloid-lineage cells plays a key role in controlling proinflammatory cytokine synthesis, myeloid-derived suppressor cell expansion, immunosuppression, and the development of cancer [74]. Finally, recent evidence suggests that PPARγ is able to induce apoptosis in lung cancer, although it can be inhibited by NR0B1, an orphan nuclear receptor whose knockdown reduces tumorigenic and antiapoptotic potential [75].

8. PPARδ and Tumorigenesis

The role of PPARδ in carcinogenesis is uncertain and seems to be context-dependent. In particular, PPARδ, through its anti-inflammatory effects, seems to prevent cancer before its development; conversely, after the development of cancer, the activation of PPARδ promotes angiogenesis and cancer growth [76]. Clinical data suggest a strong association between PPARδ and aggressive cancer; in particular, inverse correlation of PPARδ expression with survival in gastrointestinal cancer has been noted [77]. In addition, PPARδ is required for chronic colonic inflammation and colitis-associated carcinogenesis: specifically, the cyclooxygenase (COX)-2-derived prostaglandin E2 (PGE2) signalling mediates crosstalk between tumor epithelial cells and macrophages to promote chronic inflammation and colitis-associated tumor genesis [78]. In agreement with what reported in the previous chapters, high-fat diet is associated with increased colorectal cancer incidence, probably because many of its effects on stem and progenitor cell compartment are driven by a robust PPAR-δ program and contribute to the early steps of intestinal tumorigenesis [79]. In addition, recent evidence suggests that high-fat diet modifies the PPARγ pathway leading to disruption of microbial and physiological ecosystem in murine small intestine [80].

Recently, the expression of PPARδ in breast cancer has been negatively linked with patient survival. In 2016, Wang et al. [81] showed that PPARδ upregulation increases the expression of catalase and Akt in breast cancer cells and in this way cells are able to survive in harsh conditions (including in the presence of chemotherapies), promoting progression and metastasis. Not surprisingly, both the proinflammatory PGE2 and the BRCA1 tumor-suppressor gene were found to regulate aromatase expression [82] and, furthermore, pioglitazone is able to inhibit aromatase expression by inhibition of PGE2 signalling and upregulation of BRCA [83]. Finally, recent evidence suggests that PPARδ modulates the migration and invasion of melanoma cells by upregulating Snail expression: in an elegant in vitro study, it was found that activation of PPARδ by GW501516 significantly increased the migration and invasion of highly metastatic A375SM cells, but not that of low metastatic A375P cells, by upregulating Snail expression [84]. Despite the promising results, further studies are necessary in order to clarify the role of PPAR pathway modulation during cancer, also taking into account their paramount importance in regulating pro- and anti-inflammatory activities [85, 86] as well as possible interaction with the immune system [87–89] and other metabolic determinants [90–93].

9. Conclusion

The fact that a link between PPAR signalling, metabolism, and cancer exists currently represents one of the most active research fields in the literature. As discussed in this review, PPARs have many important functions. PPARs could be considered the crossroads of obesity, diabetes, inflammation, and cancer. These molecules are extremely interesting and are capable of treating numerous metabolic and nonmetabolic diseases. Currently, not all the effects of PPARs are known or fully explained, especially those related to tumorigenesis. Further research is necessary to identify a high-affinity and high-specificity agonist in order to counteract the abovementioned diseases.

Competing Interests

The authors declare that there is no conflict of interests regarding the publication of this paper.

References

[1] G. S. Harmon, M. T. Lam, and C. K. Glass, "PPARs and lipid ligands in inflammation and metabolism," *Chemical Reviews*, vol. 111, no. 10, pp. 6321–6340, 2011.

[2] J.-C. Fruchart, "Peroxisome proliferator-activated receptor-alpha (PPARα): at the crossroads of obesity, diabetes and cardiovascular disease," *Atherosclerosis*, vol. 205, no. 1, pp. 1–8, 2009.

[3] J. Berger and D. E. Moller, "The Mechanisms of Action of PPARs," *Annual Review of Medicine*, vol. 53, no. 1, pp. 409–435, 2002.

[4] S. Kersten, B. Desvergne, and W. Wahli, "Roles of PPARS in health and disease," *Nature*, vol. 405, no. 6785, pp. 421–424, 2000.

[5] B. Desvergne and W. Wahli, "Peroxisome proliferator-activated receptors: nuclear control of metabolism," *Endocrine Reviews*, vol. 20, no. 5, pp. 649–688, 1999.

[6] T. M. Willson, P. J. Brown, D. D. Sternbach, and B. R. Henke, "The PPARs: from orphan receptors to drug discovery," *Journal of Medicinal Chemistry*, vol. 43, no. 4, pp. 527–550, 2000.

[7] L. Gopinathan, D. B. Hannon, R. W. Smith III, J. M. Peters, and J. P. Vanden Heuvel, "Regulation of peroxisome proliferator-activated receptors by E6-associated protein," *PPAR Research*, Article ID 746935, 2008.

[8] L. Gopinathan, D. B. Hannon, J. M. Peters, and J. P. Vanden Heuvel, "Regulation of peroxisome proliferator-activated receptor-α by MDM2," *Toxicological Sciences*, vol. 108, no. 1, pp. 48–58, 2009.

[9] J. K. Reddy and M. S. Rao, "Lipid metabolism and liver inflammation. II. Fatty liver disease and fatty acid oxidation," *American Journal of Physiology—Gastrointestinal and Liver Physiology*, vol. 290, no. 5, pp. G852–G858, 2006.

[10] A. Shah, D. J. Rader, and J. S. Millar, "The effect of PPAR-α agonism on apolipoprotein metabolism in humans," *Atherosclerosis*, vol. 210, no. 1, pp. 35–40, 2010.

[11] T. Inagaki, P. Dutchak, G. Zhao et al., "Endocrine regulation of the fasting response by PPARα-mediated induction of fibroblast growth factor 21," *Cell Metabolism*, vol. 5, no. 6, pp. 415–425, 2007.

[12] M. Zarei, E. Barroso, R. Leiva et al., "Heme-regulated eIF2α kinase modulates hepatic FGF21 and is activated by PPARβ/δ deficiency," *Diabetes*, vol. 65, no. 10, pp. 3185–3199, 2016.

[13] W. Dijk and S. Kersten, "Regulation of lipoprotein lipase by Angptl4," *Trends in Endocrinology and Metabolism*, vol. 25, no. 3, pp. 146–155, 2014.

[14] S. Neschen, K. Morino, J. Dong et al., "n-3 fatty acids preserve insulin sensitivity in vivo in a peroxisome proliferator-activated receptor-α-dependent manner," *Diabetes*, vol. 56, no. 4, pp. 1034–1041, 2007.

[15] A. Montagner, A. Polizzi, E. Fouché et al., "Liver PPARα is crucial for whole-body fatty acid homeostasis and is protective against NAFLD," *Gut*, vol. 65, no. 7, pp. 1202–1214, 2016.

[16] E. Ip, G. C. Farrell, G. Robertson, P. Hall, R. Kirsch, and I. Leclercq, "Central role of PPARα-dependent hepatic lipid turnover in dietary steatohepatitis in mice," *Hepatology*, vol. 38, no. 1, pp. 123–132, 2003.

[17] W. G. Garbacz, J. T. J. Huang, L. G. Higgins, W. Wahli, and C. N. A. Palmer, "PPARα is required for PPARδ action in regulation of body weight and hepatic steatosis in mice," *PPAR Research*, vol. 2015, Article ID 927057, 15 pages, 2015.

[18] B. Staels, J. Dallongeville, J. Auwerx, K. Schoonjans, E. Leitersdorf, and J.-C. Fruchart, "Mechanism of action of fibrates on lipid and lipoprotein metabolism," *Circulation*, vol. 98, no. 19, pp. 2088–2093, 1998.

[19] M. P. Mosti, M. Ericsson, R. G. Erben, C. Schüler, U. Syversen, and A. K. Stunes, "The PPARα agonist fenofibrate improves the musculoskeletal effects of exercise in ovariectomized rats," *Endocrinology*, vol. 157, no. 10, pp. 3924–3934, 2016.

[20] J. Lo Verme, J. Fu, G. Astarita et al., "The nuclear receptor peroxisome proliferator-activated receptor-α mediates the anti-inflammatory actions of palmitoylethanolamide," *Molecular Pharmacology*, vol. 67, no. 1, pp. 15–19, 2005.

[21] Z.-M. Liu, M. Hu, P. Chan, and B. Tomlinson, "Early investigational drugs targeting PPAR-α for the treatment of metabolic disease," *Expert Opinion on Investigational Drugs*, vol. 24, no. 5, pp. 611–621, 2015.

[22] A. Roy, M. Jana, M. Kundu et al., "HMG-CoA reductase inhibitors bind to PPARα to upregulate neurotrophin expression in the brain and improve memory in mice," *Cell Metabolism*, vol. 22, no. 2, pp. 253–265, 2015.

[23] Y. Wang, C. Lee, S. Tiep et al., "Peroxisome-proliferator-activated receptor δ activates fat metabolism to prevent obesity," *Cell*, vol. 113, no. 2, pp. 159–170, 2003.

[24] J. Berger, M. D. Leibowitz, T. W. Doebber et al., "Novel peroxisome proliferator-activated receptor (PPAR) γ and PPARδ ligands produce distinct biological effects," *The Journal of Biological Chemistry*, vol. 274, no. 10, pp. 6718–6725, 1999.

[25] R. A. Ngala, C. J. Stocker, A. G. Roy et al., "A new, highly selective murine peroxisome proliferator-activated receptor δ agonist increases responsiveness to thermogenic stimuli and glucose uptake in skeletal muscle in obese mice," *Diabetes, Obesity and Metabolism*, vol. 13, no. 5, pp. 455–464, 2011.

[26] B. Yu, C. Chang, H. Ou, K. Cheng, and J. Cheng, "Decrease of peroxisome proliferator-activated receptor delta expression in cardiomyopathy of streptozotocin-induced diabetic rats," *Cardiovascular Research*, vol. 80, no. 1, pp. 78–87, 2008.

[27] F. A. Monsalve, R. D. Pyarasani, F. Delgado-Lopez, and R. Moore-Carrasco, "Peroxisome proliferator-activated receptor targets for the treatment of metabolic diseases," *Mediators of Inflammation*, vol. 2013, Article ID 549627, 18 pages, 2013.

[28] M. Kemmerer, F. Finkernagel, M. F. Cavalcante et al., "AMP-activated protein kinase interacts with the peroxisome proliferator-activated receptor delta to induce genes affecting fatty acid oxidation in human macrophages," *PLoS ONE*, vol. 10, no. 6, Article ID e0130893, 2015.

[29] X. Fang, L. Fang, A. Liu, X. Wang, B. Zhao, and N. Wang, "Activation of PPAR-δ induces microRNA-100 and decreases the uptake of very low-density lipoprotein in endothelial cells," *British Journal of Pharmacology*, vol. 172, no. 15, pp. 3728–3736, 2015.

[30] E. Barroso, R. Rodríguez-Rodríguez, M. R. Chacón et al., "PPARβ/δ ameliorates fructose-induced insulin resistance in adipocytes by preventing Nrf2 activation," *Biochimica et Biophysica Acta*, vol. 1852, no. 5, pp. 1049–1058, 2015.

[31] X. Wang, M. K. Sng, S. Foo et al., "Early controlled release of peroxisome proliferator-activated receptor β/δ agonist GW501516 improves diabetic wound healing through redox modulation of wound microenvironment," *Journal of Controlled Release*, vol. 197, pp. 138–147, 2015.

[32] S. A. Ham, J. S. Hwang, T. Yoo et al., "Ligand-activated PPARδ upregulates α-smooth muscle actin expression in human dermal fibroblasts: a potential role for PPARδ in wound healing," *Journal of Dermatological Science*, vol. 80, no. 3, pp. 186–195, 2015.

[33] C. Ozawa, M. Horiguchi, T. Akita et al., "Pulmonary administration of GW0742, a high-affinity peroxisome proliferator-activated receptor agonist, repairs collapsed alveoli in an elastase-induced mouse model of emphysema," *Biological & Pharmaceutical Bulletin*, vol. 39, no. 5, pp. 778–785, 2016.

[34] M. Toral, M. Gómez-Guzmán, R. Jiménez et al., "Chronic peroxisome proliferator-activated receptorβ/δ agonist GW0742 prevents hypertension, vascular inflammatory and oxidative status, and endothelial dysfunction in diet-induced obesity," *Journal of Hypertension*, vol. 33, no. 9, pp. 1831–1844, 2015.

[35] E. Roche, I. Lascombe, H. Bittard, C. Mougin, and S. Fauconnet, "The PPARβ agonist L-165041 promotes VEGF mRNA stabilization in HPV18-harboring HeLa cells through a receptor-independent mechanism," *Cellular Signalling*, vol. 26, no. 2, pp. 433–443, 2014.

[36] J.-H. Park, K.-S. Lee, H.-J. Lim, H. Kim, H.-J. Kwak, and H.-Y. Park, "The PPARδ ligand L-165041 inhibits vegf-induced angiogenesis, but the antiangiogenic effect is not related to PPARδ," *Journal of Cellular Biochemistry*, vol. 113, no. 6, pp. 1947–1954, 2012.

[37] Y.-J. Liang, J.-H. Jian, C.-Y. Chen, C.-Y. Hsu, C.-Y. Shih, and J.-G. Leu, "L-165,041, troglitazone and their combination treatment to attenuate high glucose-induced receptor for advanced glycation end products (RAGE) expression," *European Journal of Pharmacology*, vol. 715, no. 1–3, pp. 33–38, 2013.

[38] B. Staels, A. Rubenstrunk, B. Noel et al., "Hepatoprotective effects of the dual peroxisome proliferator-activated receptor alpha/delta agonist, GFT505, in rodent models of nonalcoholic fatty liver disease/nonalcoholic steatohepatitis," *Hepatology*, vol. 58, no. 6, pp. 1941–1952, 2013.

[39] T. D. Hinds, K. A. Burns, P. A. Hosick et al., "Biliverdin reductase A attenuates hepatic steatosis by inhibition of glycogen synthase kinase (GSK) 3β phosphorylation of serine 73 of peroxisome proliferator-activated receptor (PPAR) α," *The Journal of Biological Chemistry*, vol. 291, no. 48, pp. 25179–25191, 2016.

[40] B. Cariou, R. Hanf, S. Lambert-Porcheron et al., "Dual peroxisome proliferator- activated receptor α/δ agonist GFT505 improves hepatic and peripheral insulin sensitivity in abdominally obese subjects," *Diabetes Care*, vol. 36, no. 10, pp. 2923–2930, 2013.

[41] V. Ratziu, S. A. Harrison, S. Francque et al., "Elafibranor, an agonist of the peroxisome proliferator-activated receptor-α and -δ, induces resolution of nonalcoholic steatohepatitis without fibrosis worsening," *Gastroenterology*, vol. 150, no. 5, pp. 1147–1159.e5, 2016.

[42] C. Janani and B. Ranjitha Kumari, "PPAR gamma gene—a review," *Diabetes & Metabolic Syndrome: Clinical Research & Reviews*, vol. 9, no. 1, pp. 46–50, 2015.

[43] J. N. Feige, L. Gelman, L. Michalik, B. Desvergne, and W. Wahli, "From molecular action to physiological outputs: peroxisome proliferator-activated receptors are nuclear receptors at the crossroads of key cellular functions," *Progress in Lipid Research*, vol. 45, no. 2, pp. 120–159, 2006.

[44] G. Medina-Gomez, S. L. Gray, L. Yetukuri et al., "PPAR gamma 2 prevents lipotoxicity by controlling adipose tissue expandability and peripheral lipid metabolism," *PLoS Genetics*, vol. 3, no. 4, pp. 634–647, 2007.

[45] G. Medina-Gomez, S. Gray, and A. Vidal-Puig, "Adipogenesis and lipotoxicity: role of peroxisome proliferator-activated receptor γ (PPARγ) and PPARγcoactivator-1 (PGC1)," *Public Health Nutrition*, vol. 10, no. 10 A, pp. 1132–1137, 2007.

[46] U. Kintscher and R. E. Law, "PPARγ-mediated insulin sensitization: the importance of fat versus muscle," *American Journal of Physiology—Endocrinology and Metabolism*, vol. 288, no. 2, pp. E287–E291, 2005.

[47] N. Marx, T. Bourcier, G. K. Sukhova, P. Libby, and J. Plutzky, "PPARγ activation in human endothelial cells increases plasminogen activator inhibitor type-1 expression: PPARγ as a potential mediator in vascular disease," *Arteriosclerosis, Thrombosis, and Vascular Biology*, vol. 19, no. 3, pp. 546–551, 1999.

[48] M. Heim, J. Johnson, F. Boess et al., "Phytanic acid, a natural peroxisome proliferator-activated receptor (PPAR) agonist, regulates glucose metabolism in rat primary hepatocytes," *The FASEB Journal*, vol. 16, no. 7, pp. 718–720, 2002.

[49] A. Krishnaswami, S. Ravi-Kumar, and J. M. Lewis, "Thiazolidinediones: a 2010 perspective," *The Permanente Journal*, vol. 14, pp. 64–72, 2010.

[50] J. Dormandy, M. Bhattacharya, and A.-R. Van Troostenburg De Bruyn, "Safety and tolerability of pioglitazone in high-risk patients with type 2 diabetes: an overview of data from PROactive," *Drug Safety*, vol. 32, no. 3, pp. 187–202, 2009.

[51] S. E. Nissen and K. Wolski, "Effect of rosiglitazone on the risk of myocardial infarction and death from cardiovascular causes," *The New England Journal of Medicine*, vol. 356, no. 24, pp. 2457–2471, 2007.

[52] M. A. Deeg and M. H. Tan, "Pioglitazone versus rosiglitazone: effects on lipids, lipoproteins, and apolipoproteins in head-to-head randomized clinical studies," *PPAR Research*, vol. 2008, Article ID 520465, 6 pages, 2008.

[53] J. H. Choi, A. S. Banks, T. M. Kamenecka et al., "Antidiabetic actions of a non-agonist PPARγ ligand blocking Cdk5-mediated phosphorylation," *Nature*, vol. 477, no. 7365, pp. 477–481, 2011.

[54] X. Liu, O. Kunert, M. Blunder et al., "Polyyne hybrid compounds from notopterygium incisum with peroxisome proliferator-activated receptor gamma agonistic effects," *Journal of Natural Products*, vol. 77, no. 11, pp. 2513–2521, 2014.

[55] L. Wang, B. Waltenberger, E.-M. Pferschy-Wenzig et al., "Natural product agonists of peroxisome proliferator-activated receptor gamma (PPARγ): a review," *Biochemical Pharmacology*, vol. 92, no. 1, pp. 73–89, 2014.

[56] J. W. Lee, P. J. Bajwa, M. J. Carson et al., "Fenofibrate represses interleukin-17 and interferon-γ expression and improves colitis in interleukin-10–deficient mice," *Gastroenterology*, vol. 133, no. 1, pp. 108–123, 2007.

[57] Y.-P. Huang and N. W. Chang, "PPARα modulates gene expression profiles of mitochondrial energy metabolism in oral tumorigenesis," *BioMedicine*, vol. 6, no. 1, article 3, 2016.

[58] G. Sarnelli, A. D'Alessandro, T. Iuvone et al., "Palmitoylethanolamide modulates inflammation-associated Vascular Endothelial Growth Factor (VEGF) signaling via the akt/mtor pathway in a selective Peroxisome Proliferator-Activated Receptor Alpha (PPAR-α)-dependent manner," *PLoS One*, vol. 11, no. 5, Article ID e0156198, 2016.

[59] K. Chandran, S. Goswami, and N. Sharma-Walia, "Implications of a peroxisome proliferator-activated receptor alpha (PPARα) ligand clofibrate in breast cancer," *Oncotarget*, vol. 7, no. 13, pp. 15577–15599, 2015.

[60] K. Wejksza, C. Lee-Chang, M. Bodogai et al., "Cancer-produced metabolites of 5-lipoxygenase induce tumor-evoked regulatory B cells via peroxisome proliferator-activated receptor α," *The Journal of Immunology*, vol. 190, no. 6, pp. 2575–2584, 2013.

[61] J. Gao, S. Yuan, J. Jin, J. Shi, and Y. Hou, "PPARα regulates tumor progression, foe or friend?" *European Journal of Pharmacology*, vol. 765, pp. 560–564, 2015.

[62] J. Gao, Q. Liu, Y. Xu et al., "PPARα induces cell apoptosis by destructing Bcl2," *Oncotarget*, vol. 6, no. 42, pp. 44635–44642, 2015.

[63] N. Zhang, E. S. H. Chu, J. Zhang et al., "Peroxisome proliferator activated receptor alpha inhibits hepatocarcinogenesis through mediating NF-κB signaling pathway," *Oncotarget*, vol. 5, no. 18, pp. 8330–8340, 2014.

[64] T. Aoki, "Current status of carcinogenicity assessment of peroxisome proliferator-activated receptor agonists by the US FDA and a mode-of-action approach to the carcinogenic potential," *Journal of Toxicologic Pathology*, vol. 20, no. 4, pp. 197–202, 2008.

[65] I. M. Pruimboom-Brees, O. Francone, J. C. Pettersen et al., "The development of subcutaneous sarcomas in rodents exposed to peroxisome proliferators agonists: hypothetical mechanisms of action and de-risking attitude," *Toxicologic Pathology*, vol. 40, no. 5, pp. 810–818, 2012.

[66] H. K. Park, H. K. Kim, H.-G. Kim et al., "Expression of peroxisome proliferator activated receptor gamma in prostatic adenocarcinoma," *Journal of Korean Medical Science*, vol. 30, no. 5, pp. 533–541, 2015.

[67] S. Polvani, M. Tarocchi, S. Tempesti, L. Bencini, and A. Galli, "Peroxisome proliferator activated receptors at the crossroad of obesity, diabetes, and pancreatic cancer," *World Journal of Gastroenterology*, vol. 22, no. 8, pp. 2441–2459, 2016.

[68] J. D. Coleman, J. T. Thompson, R. W. Smith III, B. Prokopczyk, and J. P. Vanden Heuvel, "Role of peroxisome proliferator-activated receptor β/δ and B-cell lymphoma-6 in regulation of genes involved in metastasis and migration in pancreatic cancer cells," *PPAR Research*, vol. 2013, Article ID 121956, 11 pages, 2013.

[69] H. V. Reddi, P. Madde, L. A. Marlow et al., "Expression of the PAX8/PPARγ fusion protein is associated with decreased neovascularization in vivo: impact on tumorigenesis and disease prognosis," *Genes and Cancer*, vol. 1, no. 5, pp. 480–492, 2010.

[70] D. Rovito, G. Gionfriddo, I. Barone et al., "Ligand-activated PPARγ downregulates CXCR4 gene expression through a novel identified PPAR response element and inhibits breast cancer progression," *Oncotarget*, 2016.

[71] S. Das Gupta, S. Sae-Tan, J. Wahler et al., "Dietary γ-tocopherol-rich mixture inhibits estrogen-induced mammary tumorigenesis by modulating estrogen metabolism, antioxidant response, and PPARγ," *Cancer Prevention Research*, vol. 8, no. 9, pp. 807–816, 2015.

[72] G. Skelhorne-gross, A. L. Reid, A. J. Apostoli et al., "Stromal adipocyte PPARγ protects against breast tumorigenesis," *Carcinogenesis*, vol. 33, no. 7, pp. 1412–1420, 2012.

[73] C. A. McAlpine, Y. Barak, I. Matise, and R. T. Cormier, "Intestinal-specific PPARγ deficiency enhances tumorigenesis in ApcMin/+ mice," *International Journal of Cancer*, vol. 119, no. 10, pp. 2339–2346, 2006.

[74] L. Wu, C. Yan, M. Czader et al., "Inhibition of PPARγ in myeloid-lineage cells induces systemic inflammation, immunosuppression, and tumorigencsis," *Blood*, vol. 119, no. 1, pp. 115–126, 2012.

[75] Y. Susaki, M. Inoue, M. Minami et al., "Inhibitory effect of PPARγ on NR0B1 in tumorigenesis of lung adenocarcinoma," *International Journal of Oncology*, vol. 41, no. 4, pp. 1278–1284, 2012.

[76] J. M. Peters, F. J. Gonzalez, and R. Müller, "Establishing the Role of PPARβ/δ in Carcinogenesis," *Trends in Endocrinology and Metabolism*, vol. 26, no. 11, pp. 595–607, 2015.

[77] A. Abdollahi, C. Schwager, J. Kleeff et al., "Transcriptional network governing the angiogenic switch in human pancreatic cancer," *Proceedings of the National Academy of Sciences of the United States of America*, vol. 104, no. 31, pp. 12890–12895, 2007.

[78] D. Wang and R. N. DuBois, "PPARδ and PGE2 signaling pathways communicate and connect inflammation to colorectal cancer," *Inflammation and Cell Signaling*, vol. 1, no. 4, 2014.

[79] S. Beyaz and Ö. H. Yilmaz, "Molecular pathways: dietary regulation of stemness and tumor initiation by the PPAR-δ pathway," *Clinical Cancer Research*, vol. 22, no. 23, pp. 5636–5641, 2016.

[80] J. Tomas, C. Mulet, A. Saffarian et al., "High-fat diet modifies the PPAR-γ pathway leading to disruption of microbial and physiological ecosystem in murine small intestine," *Proceedings of the National Academy of Sciences*, vol. 113, no. 40, pp. E5934–E5943, 2016.

[81] X. Wang, G. Wang, Y. Shi et al., "PPAR-delta promotes survival of breast cancer cells in harsh metabolic conditions," *Oncogenesis*, vol. 5, no. 6, article e232, 2016.

[82] O. Margalit, D. Wang, and R. N. DuBois, "PPARγ agonists target aromatase via both PGE2 and BRCA1," *Cancer Prevention Research*, vol. 5, no. 10, pp. 1169–1172, 2012.

[83] K. Subbaramaiah, L. R. Howe, X. K. Zhou et al., "Pioglitazone, a PPARγ agonist, suppresses CYP19 transcription: evidence for involvement of 15-hydroxyprostaglandin dehydrogenase and BRCA1," *Cancer Prevention Research*, vol. 5, no. 10, pp. 1183–1194, 2012.

[84] S. A. Ham, T. Yoo, J. S. Hwang et al., "Ligand-activated PPARδ modulates the migration and invasion of melanoma cells by regulating Snail expression," *American Journal of Cancer Research*, vol. 4, no. 6, pp. 674–682, 2014.

[85] A. Laganà, S. Vitale, A. Nigro et al., "Pleiotropic actions of Peroxisome Proliferator-Activated Receptors (PPARs) in dysregulated metabolic homeostasis, inflammation and cancer: current evidence and future perspectives," *International Journal of Molecular Sciences*, vol. 17, no. 7, article no. 999, 2016.

[86] M. Terrasi, V. Bazan, S. Caruso et al., "Effects of PPARγ agonists on the expression of leptin and vascular endothelial growth factor in breast cancer cells," *Journal of Cellular Physiology*, vol. 228, no. 6, pp. 1368–1374, 2013.

[87] V. Vetvicka, A. S. Laganà, F. M. Salmeri et al., "Regulation of apoptotic pathways during endometriosis: from the molecular basis to the future perspectives," *Archives of Gynecology and Obstetrics*, vol. 294, no. 5, pp. 897–904, 2016.

[88] A. S. Laganà, O. Triolo, F. M. Salmeri et al., "Natural Killer T cell subsets in eutopic and ectopic endometrium: a fresh look to a busy corner," *Archives of Gynecology and Obstetrics*, pp. 1–9, 2016.

[89] V. Sofo, M. Götte, A. S. Laganà et al., "Correlation between dioxin and endometriosis: an epigenetic route to unravel the pathogenesis of the disease," *Archives of Gynecology and Obstetrics*, vol. 292, no. 5, pp. 973–986, 2015.

[90] S. G. Vitale, P. Rossetti, F. Corrado et al., "How to achieve high-quality oocytes? The key role of myo-inositol and melatonin," *International Journal of Endocrinology*, vol. 2016, Article ID 4987436, 9 pages, 2016.

[91] A. Cianci, N. Colacurci, A. M. Paoletti et al., "Soy isoflavones, inulin, calcium, and vitamin D3 in post-menopausal hot flushes: An Observational Study," *Clinical and experimental obstetrics & gynecology*, vol. 42, no. 6, pp. 743–745, 2015.

[92] F. Colonese, A. S. Laganà, E. Colonese et al., "The pleiotropic effects of vitamin D in gynaecological and obstetric diseases: an overview on a hot topic," *BioMed Research International*, vol. 2015, Article ID 986281, 11 pages, 2015.

[93] C. Paul, A. S. Laganà, P. Maniglio, O. Triolo, and D. M. Brady, "Inositol's and other nutraceuticals' synergistic actions counteract insulin resistance in polycystic ovarian syndrome and metabolic syndrome: state-of-the-art and future perspectives," *Gynecological Endocrinology*, vol. 32, no. 6, pp. 431–438, 2016.

9

Fluid Retention Caused by Rosiglitazone is Related to Increases in AQP2 and αENaC Membrane Expression

Jinghua Xu, Mingyue Pan, Xiaoli Wang, Lishi Xu, Lanfang Li, and Cheng Xu

Department of Physiology, School of Life Science and Biopharmaceutics, Shenyang Pharmaceutical University, 103 Wenhua Road, Shenyang 110016, China

Correspondence should be addressed to Cheng Xu; 2443759092@qq.com

Academic Editor: Swasti Tiwari

Peroxisome proliferator activated receptor-γ (PPARγ) is a ligand-activated transcription factor of the nuclear hormone receptor superfamily. The decreased phosphorylation of PPARγ due to rosiglitazone (ROS) is the main reason for the increased insulin sensitivity caused by this antidiabetic drug. However, there is no clear evidence whether the nuclear translocation of p-PPARγ stimulated by ROS is related to fluid retention. It is also unclear whether the translocation of p-PPARγ is associated with the change of aquaporin-2 (AQP2) and epithelial sodium channel α subunit (αENaC) in membranes, cytoplasm, and nucleus. Our experiments indicate that ROS significantly downregulates nuclear p-PPARγ and increases membrane AQP2 and αENaC; however, SR1664 (a nonagonist PPARγ ligand) reduces p-PPARγ and has no effect on AQP2 and αENaC. Therefore, we conclude that in vitro the fluid retention caused by ROS is associated with the increases in membrane αENaC and AQP2 but has little relevance to the phosphorylation of PPARγ.

1. Introduction

Rosiglitazone (ROS), a classic clinical oral antidiabetic drug, is a PPARγ agonist; studies have shown that the decreased phosphorylation of PPARγ due to ROS is the main reason for the increase in insulin sensitivity caused by this drug [1]. However, long-term clinical observations have revealed that ROS has the side effect of fluid retention, which leads to heart failure [2, 3]. SR1664, a novel compound developed by the Scripps Institute in the United States and other institutions, is a PPARγ ligand that activates PPARγ to suppress PPARγ Ser^{273} phosphorylation, leading to enhanced insulin sensitivity, thereby playing a role in treating type 2 diabetes [4]. However, in vivo experiments showed that SR1664 can increase insulin sensitivity and does not cause fluid retention [5].

Substantial research showed that fluid retention is closely related to AQP2 and αENaC proteins [6, 7], and in vitro experiments indicated that the expression of AQP2 and αENaC is upregulated after PPARγ agonist treatment [8, 9]. Nevertheless, the mechanism of ROS on membrane, cytoplasmic, and nuclear AQP2 and αENaC has yet to be clarified.

In this study, we investigated the effects of ROS, SR1664, and TNFα (increased phosphorylation of PPARγ) on p-PPARγ, AQP2, and αENaC in HEK293 and mIMCD-3 cells, being then coincubated with PPARγ antagonist GW9662; results showed that the effects disappeared. So we concluded that in vitro the decrease of PPARγ phosphorylation has little relationship with fluid retention, and the fluid retention induced by ROS is mainly related to the increase of membranes AQP2 and αENaC.

2. Materials and Methods

2.1. Chemicals and Reagents. Reagents were purchased from the following sources: rosiglitazone and GW9662 (Sigma, St Louis, MO); RPMI-1640 medium (GIBCO, Invitrogen) and fetal bovine serum (FBS; Shenyang Huibai Biotechnology Co., Ltd.); 3-(4,5-dimethylthiazol-2-yl)-2,5-diphenyl tetrazolium (MTT; Biosharp); and ECL Western Blotting Detection Reagent (Bio-Rad, Hercules, CA, USA). Antibodies were selected using polyclonal antibody, PPARγ (Santa Cruz, CA, USA), p-PPARγ (Proteintech, CA, USA), αENaC (Santa Cruz, USA), AQP2 (Santa Cruz, USA), and β-tubulin (Santa

Cruz, USA); FITC Alexa 488-conjugated goat anti-rabbit secondary antibodies were from Santa Cruz Biotechnology (USA); and horseradish peroxidase-conjugated anti-rabbit secondary antibodies were from Proteintech (USA).

2.2. Cell Culture and Administration.

Mouse kidney inner medullary collecting duct (mIMCD) cells (Shanghai Bogu Biological Technology Co., Ltd.) and human embryo kidney (HEK293) cells (ATCC, Manassas, VA, USA) were routinely cultured in RPMI-1640 medium supplemented with 10% FBS and antibiotics (Serva & AMRESCO), in a humidified chamber containing 5% CO_2 at 37°C. Combined administration regimen is as follows: when the cells reached 80%–90% confluence, GW9662 (5 μM) was incubated for 6 h before the addition of ROS (1, 10 μM) or SR1664 (1, 10 μM). After 24 h, cells were collected for extraction of total, cytoplasmic, nucleus, or membrane protein, respectively.

2.3. Cell Viability Experiment.

For the MTT assay, cells were seeded at 6×10^3 cells per well onto 96-well culture plates and allowed to grow for 24 h after treatment with various concentrations of ROS, SR1664, GW9662, TNFα, or ROS and SR1664 combined with GW9662. After removing the medium, MTT solution (5 mg/ml in PBS) was added and incubated for 4 h and the resulting formazan was solubilized with DMSO (150 μl). The absorption was measured at 490 nm in a multifunctional enzyme marking instrument.

2.4. Preparation of Protein Samples

2.4.1. Preparation of Total Protein.

RIPA lysis buffer was added to the cell precipitations and resuspended. After 30 min of lysis at 4°C, the lysates were centrifuged at 12,000 g for 20 min, and the obtained supernatant was used as the total protein.

2.4.2. Preparation of Cytoplasm and Nuclear Proteins.

The reagents were dissolved at room temperature and put on the ice immediately. Then, 200 μl cytoplasmic protein extraction reagent A (to which 1 mM PMSF had been added a few minutes previously) was added to 20-μl cell precipitations. Five seconds' vortex was performed to ensure adequate resuspension, followed by incubation on ice for 10–15 min. Then, 10 μM cytoplasmic protein extraction reagent B was added. Vortexing was again performed for 5 s, followed by incubation on ice for 1 min. Centrifugation was then performed at 12,000 g and 4°C for 5 min, and the obtained supernatant was used as cytoplasmic protein. Then, 50 μl of PMSF-added nucleoprotein extraction reagent was added to the nuclear pellet, followed by vortexing for 15–30 s, to ensure complete suspension and dispersal. Then, after incubation on ice, vortexing for 30 s was performed every 1-2 minutes for 30 min. This was followed by vortexing at 12,000 g at 4°C for 10 min, from which the obtained supernatant was used to represent nuclear protein. The nuclear and cytoplasmic extracts were then analyzed for protein content using BCA assay.

2.4.3. Preparation of Membrane Proteins.

The cellular membrane fraction was prepared in accordance with the manufacturer's instructions. 1 ml membrane protein extraction reagent A with PMSF was added to 2–5 billion cells, for gentle and complete suspension, followed by incubation on ice for 10–15 min. Next, centrifuging was applied at 700 g for 10 min at 4°C. The supernatant obtained from this procedure was then centrifuged at 14,000 g for 30 min at 4°C to precipitate membrane fragments, with the obtained supernatant being used to represent cytoplasmic protein. The precipitate was also centrifuged at 14,000 g for 10 s at 4°C and exhausted the supernatant completely. Then, after the addition of 200 μl of membrane protein extraction reagent B, vortexing was performed for 5 s for resuspension, followed by incubation on ice for 5–10 min. The previous steps were then repeated 1-2 times to extract the membrane protein completely. Subsequently, centrifugation was performed at 14,000 g for 5 min at 4°C, with the obtained supernatant being used as the membrane protein. The membrane extracts were then analyzed for protein content using BCA assay.

2.5. Western Blot Analysis.

Cells were first washed with cold PBS three times and lysed in RIPA buffer. The BCA protein assay was used to determine the protein concentrations of the samples. Equal amounts (25 ug) of cellular proteins were loaded into each well and separated by 10% SDS-PAGE after denaturation with 5x loading buffer and then transferred onto PVDF membranes, incubated in 5% nonfat dry milk for 2 h on shaker at room temperature and then incubated with PPARγ (1 : 500), p-PPARγ (1 : 500), AQP2 (1 : 800), and αENaC (1 : 800) antibodies, respectively; β-tublin (1 : 1000) was used as internal control. Finally, blots were also incubated with secondary antibody (1 : 5000) and visualized using enhanced ECL luminous fluid.

2.6. Immunocytochemistry.

Cells in the logarithmic growth phase were collected and, following adjustment of cell suspension density to 1×10^5 cells/ml after digestion, the cells were inoculated on coverslips with concentrations of drugs diluted with culture medium, cultured at 37°C for 24 h, and blocked for 30 min without light at room temperature [4% paraformaldehyde (PFA), 0.2% Triton X-100, and 5% BSA]. Overnight incubation with primary antibodies (diluted with 1% BSA) was performed at 4°C followed by 30 min of incubation with secondary antibodies (diluted with 1% BSA). Washing with PBS was then performed three times for 10 min after each step, along with exposure to 100 ng/ml Hoechst 33258 dye for 10 min, then washing again with PBS for 5 min three times. Finally, confocal microscopy was performed using a 60x oil objective on a Nikon C2-si laser-scanning confocal microscope, and images were manipulated using Photoshop software.

2.7. Data Analysis.

All experiments were repeated at least three times independently, and data are expressed as mean $\pm$ s.e.m. Statistical analysis was performed using SPSS 17.0 by one-way analysis of variance (ANOVA). The LSD test was used to compare differences in the means between groups; if

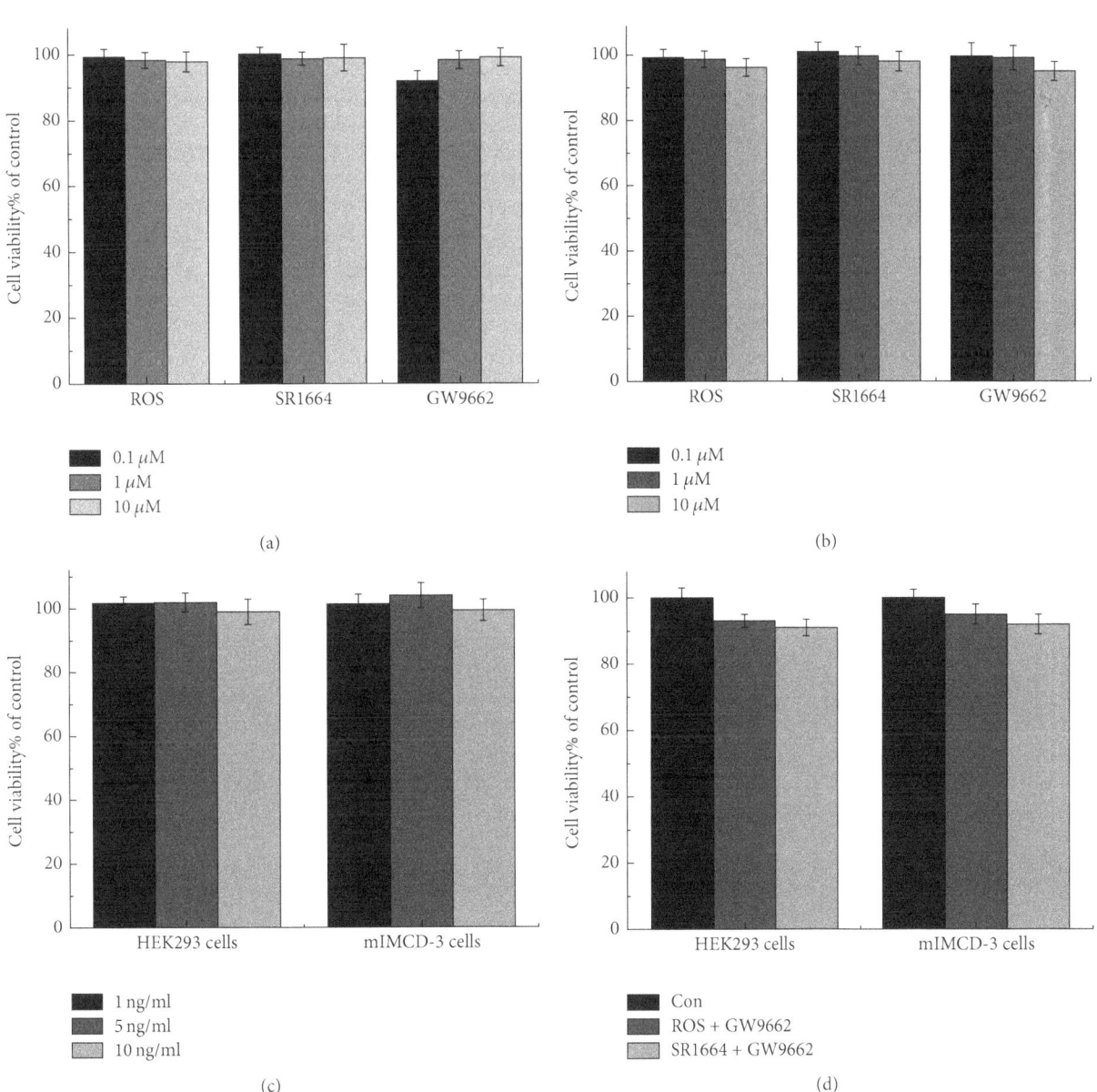

FIGURE 1: In vitro experiments on the cytotoxic effects of ROS, GW9662, SR1664, and TNFα in HEK293 and mIMCD-3 cells. (a) The effects of ROS, SR1664, and GW9662 (0.1, 1, and 10 μM) in HEK293 cells. (b) The effects of ROS, SR1664, and GW9662 (0.1, 1, and 10 μM) in mIMCD-3 cells. (c) The effects of TNFα (1, 5, and 10 ng/ml) in HEK293 and mIMCD-3 cells. (d) Coincubation with ROS (10 μM) and GW9662 (5 μM) and SR1664 (10 μM) and GW9662 (5 μM). The results show that the concentrations that we used in the experiments have no significant cytotoxic effects. Results are shown as mean ± s.e.m., $n = 3$.

the variance is different, Dunnett's t-test was used. A value of $P < 0.05$ was considered to represent a significant difference, while $P < 0.01$ was considered to present a very significant difference.

3. Results

3.1. Cell Viability Analysis. First, to consider the cytotoxic effects of ROS, SR1664, GW9662, and TNFα, 3-(4,5-dimethylthiazol-2-yl)-2,5-diphenyltetrazolium bromide (MTT) experiments were used to determine the doses of these drugs and combination therapies. The administration

of ROS, SR1664, and GW9662 at 0.1, 1, and 10 μM (Figures 1(a) and 1(b)) and TNFα at 1, 5, and 10 ng/ml (Figure 1(c)) to HEK293 cells and mIMCD-3 cells showed no significant effects on cell viability. The administration of these agents in combination (Figure 1(d) also had no such effects.

3.2. Immunofluorescence Assay. Activation of nuclear receptor promotes the translocation of transcription factors from the cytoplasm to the nucleus to improve the transcriptional activity of transcription factor response element binding (CREB) protein. Therefore, a cell immunofluorescence experiment was used to detect the changes in the distribution of

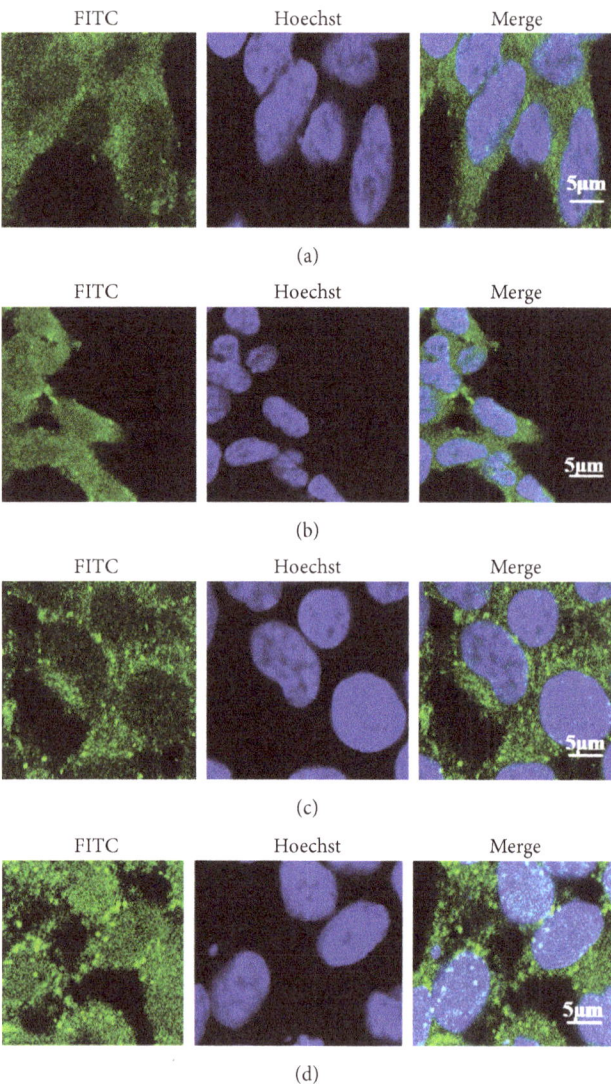

FIGURE 2: Altered localization of PPARγ in response to rosiglitazone. (a, c) Control in HEK293 and mIMCD-3 cells, respectively. PPARγ immunoreactivity following 24 h of culture without rosiglitazone; (b, d) PPARγ immunoreactivity following 24 h of culture with rosiglitazone (10 μM). Column 2 demonstrates nuclear staining (Hoechst; blue); column 3 illustrates PPARγ immunoreactivity (localized using Alexa 488; green). Column 1 features overlay images. PPARγ is redistributed to the nucleus in response to elevated rosiglitazone at 10 μM.

nuclear receptor PPARγ after the administration of agonists, which was based on the binding of a green fluorescence in the cytoplasm and nucleus; Hoechst stains the nucleus and indicates the localization of PPARγ in cells. The results are shown in Figure 2, indicating that, after ROS administration, green fluorescence in the cell nucleus increased compared with that in the blank group. Data analysis suggested that there was no significant difference in this activity in the cytoplasm, but it increased markedly in the nucleus.

3.3. Effects of ROS on PPARγ, p-PPARγ, AQP2, and αENaC in HEK293 Cells.
To investigate the effects of ROS on PPARγ,

p-PPARγ, AQP2, and αENaC at different locations, total, nuclear, membrane, and cytoplasmic proteins were extracted. The data show that ROS at 10 μM can significantly increase nuclear PPARγ (N-PPARγ) (Figure 3(a)) but downregulated total p-PPARγ (T-p-PPARγ) and nuclear p-PPARγ (N-p-PPARγ) and had no influence on cytoplasmic p-PPARγ (C-p-PPARγ) (Figure 3(b)). As for AQP2, membrane (M-AQP2) and cytoplasmic (C-AQP2) proteins levels were increased (Figure 3(c)), while, for αENaC, the findings show that just membrane (M-αENaC) translocation increased (Figure 3(d)). After coincubation with GW9662, the effects of ROS on PPARγ, p-PPARγ, AQP2, and αENaC disappeared (Figures 3(e)–3(h)).

3.4. Effects of ROS on PPARγ, p-PPARγ, AQP2, and αENaC in mIMCD-3 Cells.
To validate the above findings in HEK293 cells, the same experiments were conducted in mIMCD-3 cells. The data indicate that ROS (10 μM) also critically increased nuclear PPARγ (Figure 4(a)), downregulated total and nuclear p-PPARγ in mIMCD-3 cells (Figure 4(b)), and increased the expression of AQP2 in cytoplasm and membrane (Figure 4(c)), as well as membrane expression of αENaC (Figure 4(d)). Upon coincubation with GW9662, these effects disappeared (Figure 4(e)–4(h)). The results are consistent with those in HEK293 cells.

3.5. Effects of SR1664 and TNFα on PPARγ, p-PPARγ, AQP2, and αENaC in mIMCD-3 Cells.
SR1664 is a new type of PPARγ ligand that blocks the cyclin-dependent kinase 5-(Cdk5-) mediated phosphorylation of PPARγ. Research has shown that it improves insulin sensitivity by lowering glucose and has no side effects, as is the case for ROS. To confirm these effects, we detected PPARγ, p-PPARγ, AQP2, and αENaC proteins in mIMCD-3 cells. The data suggest that SR1664 (10 μM) can dramatically limit the p-PPARγ (Figure 5(a)); upon coincubation with GW9662, the effects on p-PPARγ disappeared (Figure 5(b)). Nevertheless, the expression of AQP2 in the cytoplasm and membrane and the membrane expression of αENaC exhibited no significant difference (Figures 5(c) and 5(d)).

Obesity-linked insulin resistance is associated with inflammation in adipocytes. Among the different types of proinflammatory cytokines, TNFα is the first one identified to connect obesity, inflammation, and insulin resistance. Notably, TNFα at both 5 and 10 ng/ml can upregulate p-PPARγ (Figure 5(e)), while it had no effect on αENaC in membrane and AQP2 in the cytoplasm and membrane (Figures 5(f) and 5(g)).

4. Discussion

In this study, we determined the reason for the relationship between fluid retention caused by ROS and the expression of AQP2 and αENaC in HEK293 and mIMCD-3 cells. Immunofluorescence experiment reveals that the green fluorescence in the nucleus increased after ROS application compared with that in the control, illustrating that ROS can activate the transcriptional activity of transcription factors

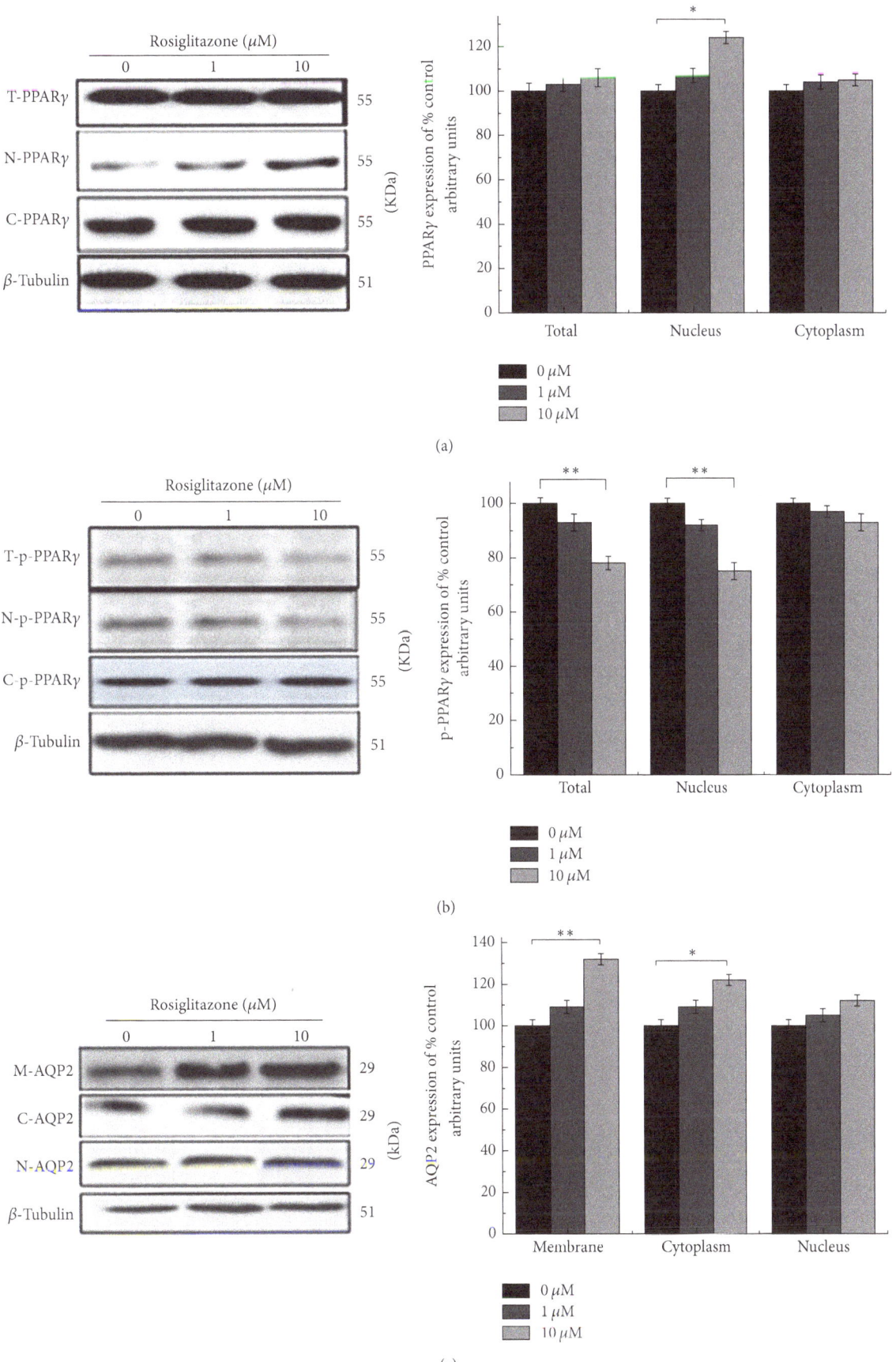

FIGURE 3: Continued.

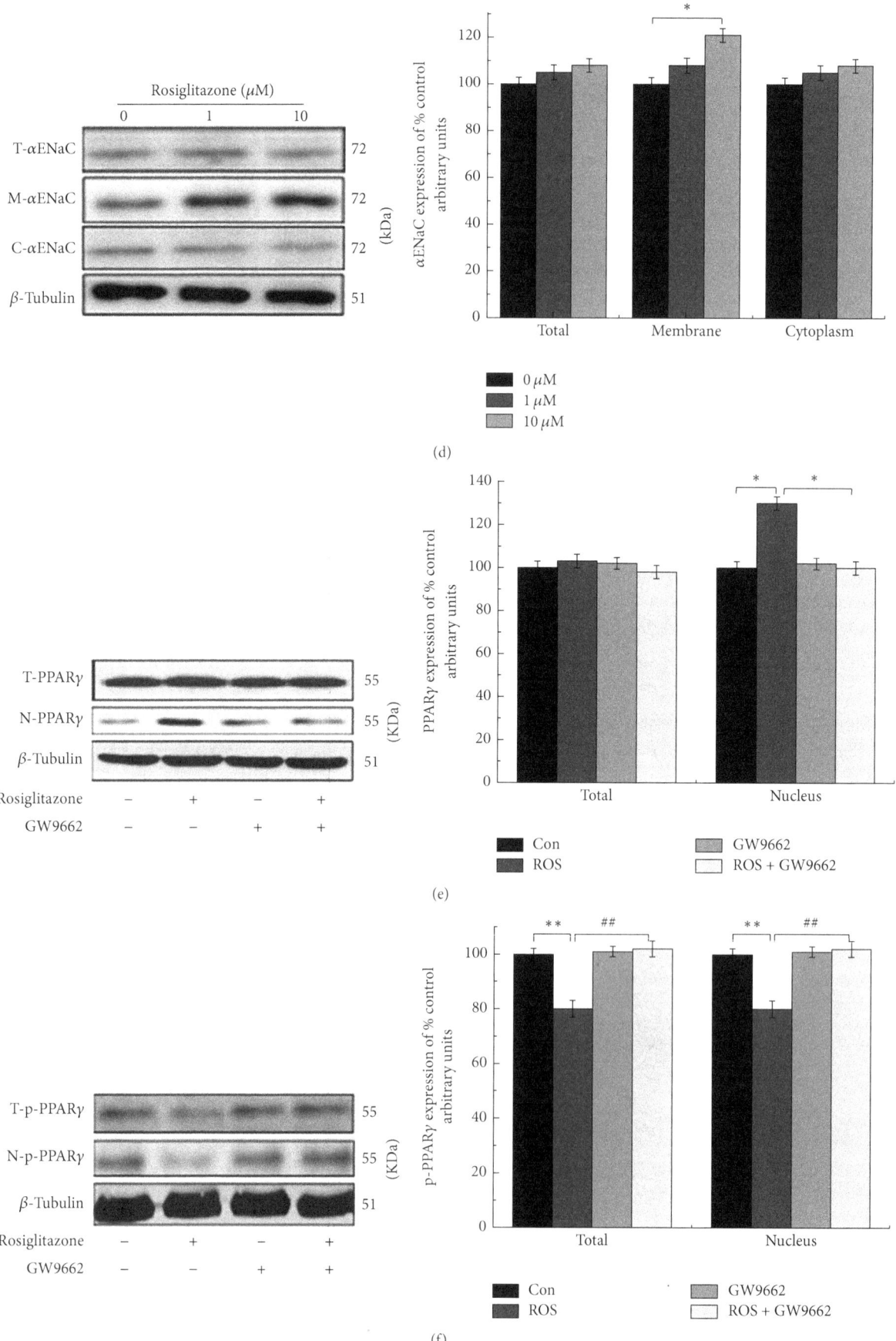

FIGURE 3: Continued.

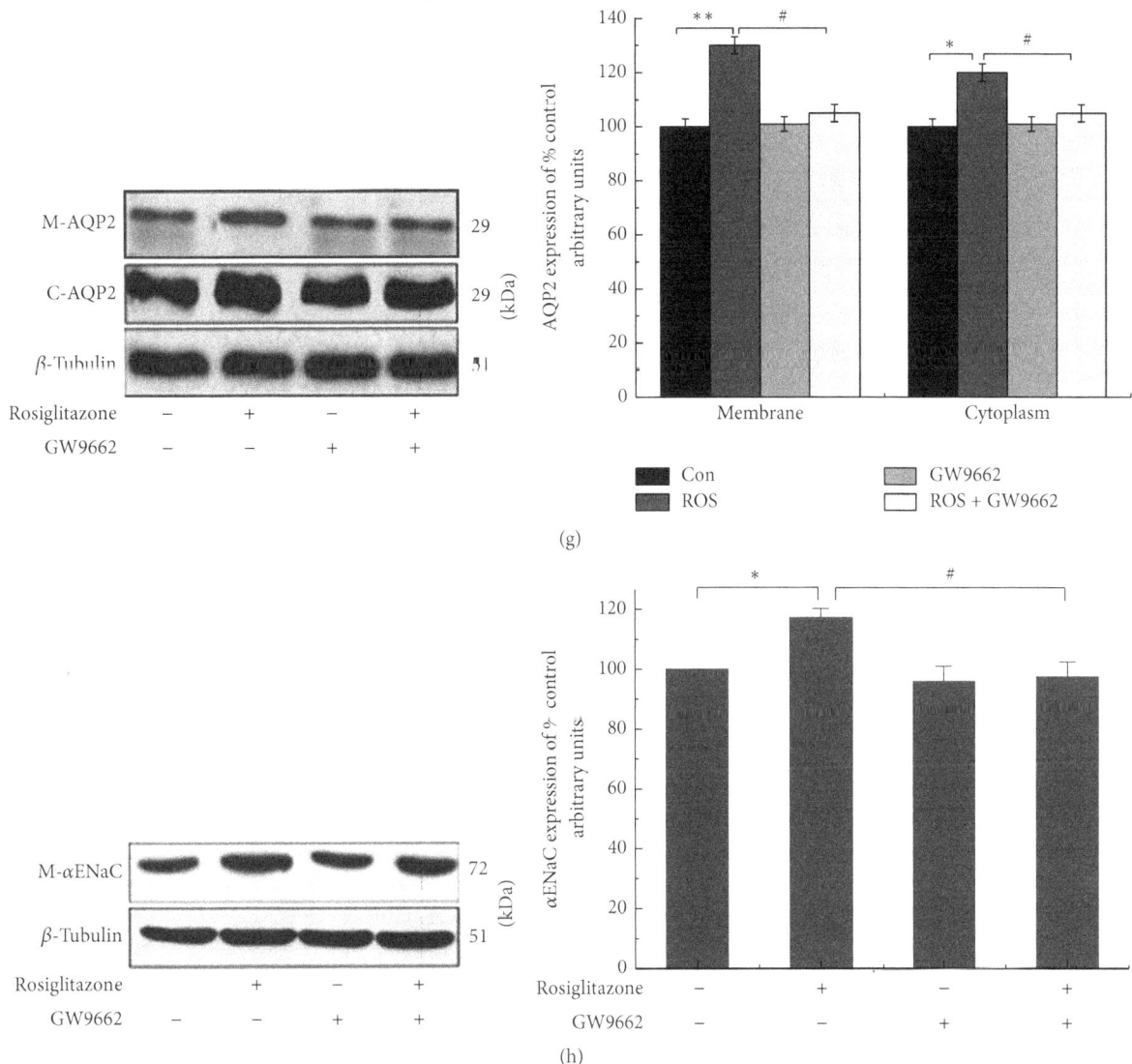

FIGURE 3: Effects of rosiglitazone and coincubation with GW9662 in HEK293 cells. (a–d) The effects of rosiglitazone on PPARγ, p-PPARγ, AQP2, and αENaC. (e–h) The changes of PPARγ, p-PPARγ, AQP2, and αENaC upon coincubation with GW9662 (10 μM ROS + 5 μM GW9662). The results show that rosiglitazone at 10 μM can significantly decrease total and nuclear p-PPARγ but critically upregulated nuclear PPARγ and AQP2 and αENaC membrane transposition. After coincubation with GW9662 (10 μM ROS + 5 μM GW9662), the effects of rosiglitazone on PPARγ, p-PPARγ, AQP2, and αENaC disappeared. The results are shown as mean ± s.e.m., $n = 3$. $^{*/\#} P < 0.05$. $^{**/\#\#} P < 0.01$. ∗ means compared to control; # means compared to rosiglitazone.

and promote their transfer from the cytoplasm to the nucleus. Next, we studied the effects of ROS on p-PPARγ at the protein level in HEK293 and mIMCD-3 cells. As shown in Figures 3(b) and 4(b), in both HEK293 and mIMCD-3 cells, ROS (10 μM) can critically inhibit PPARγ phosphorylation, in terms of both the total level and that in the nucleus; upon coincubation with GW9662, an antagonist of PPARγ, all of these effects disappeared. Taking these findings together, ROS activated PPARγ, leading to the reduction of p-PPARγ.

Against this background, to determine whether the reduction of p-PPARγ could lead to fluid retention, we examined the expression of AQP2 and αENaC proteins, which are related to body fluid homeostasis [10, 11]. The trafficking

mechanism of AQP2 was mainly induced by arginine vasopressin (AVP); when AVP increased, the cytoplasmic vesicles and lumen membrane fused, and AQP2 was transferred to the luminal membrane, increasing the permeability to water [12]. Based on these findings, an abnormal mechanism of AQP2 trafficking would affect the number of AQP2 molecules in the luminal membrane [13]. In diabetic model mice in vivo, after feeding on PPARγ agonist, PCR detection results showed that ADH had no significant changes, but AQP2 significantly increased [14]. Our results revealed that ROS (10 μM) can increase the expression of AQP2 in the cytoplasm and facilitate AQP2 vesicles fusing to the cell membrane; in addition, after coincubation with GW9662, these effects were all offset. These findings may be explained by ROS increasing

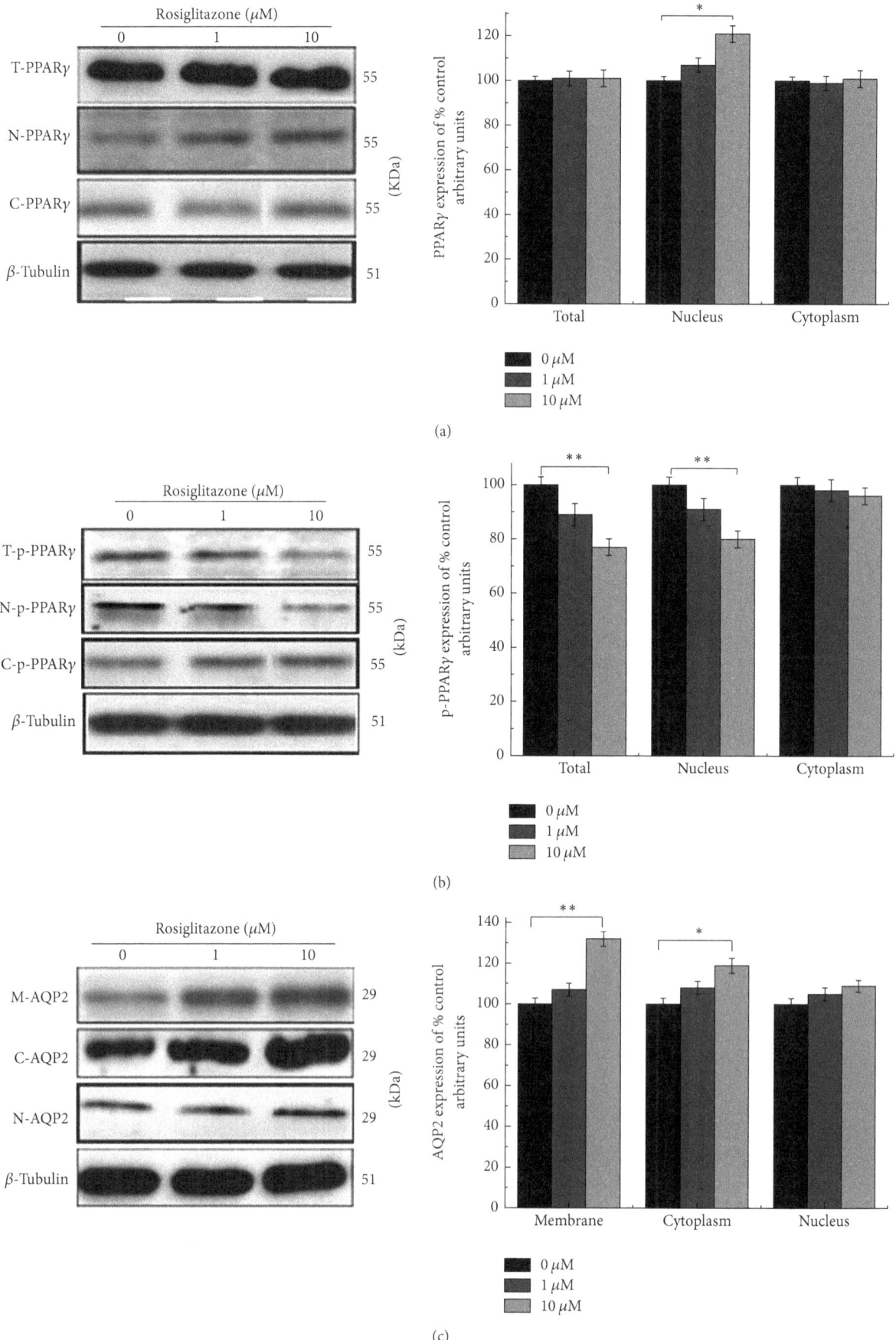

FIGURE 4: Continued.

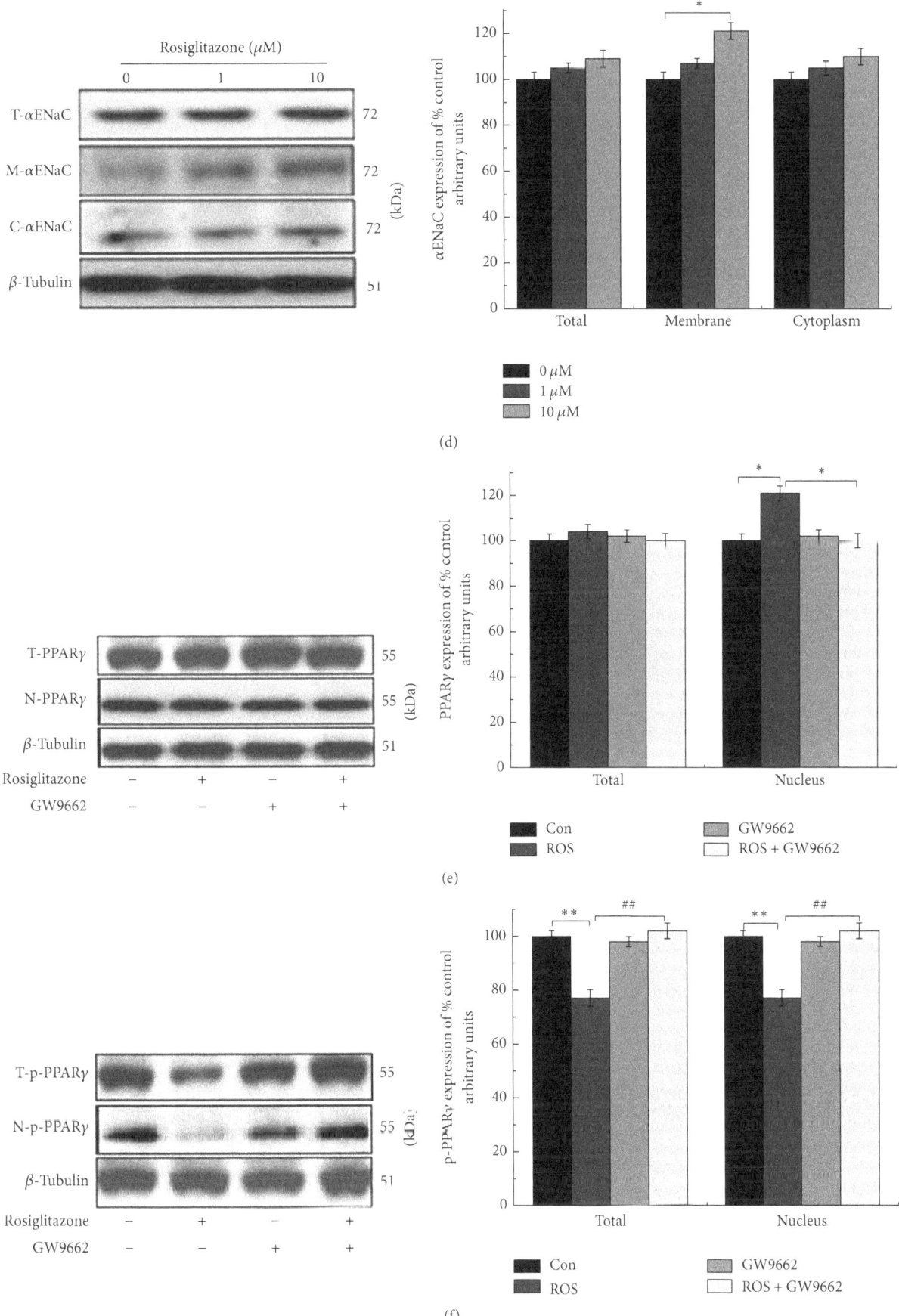

FIGURE 4: Continued.

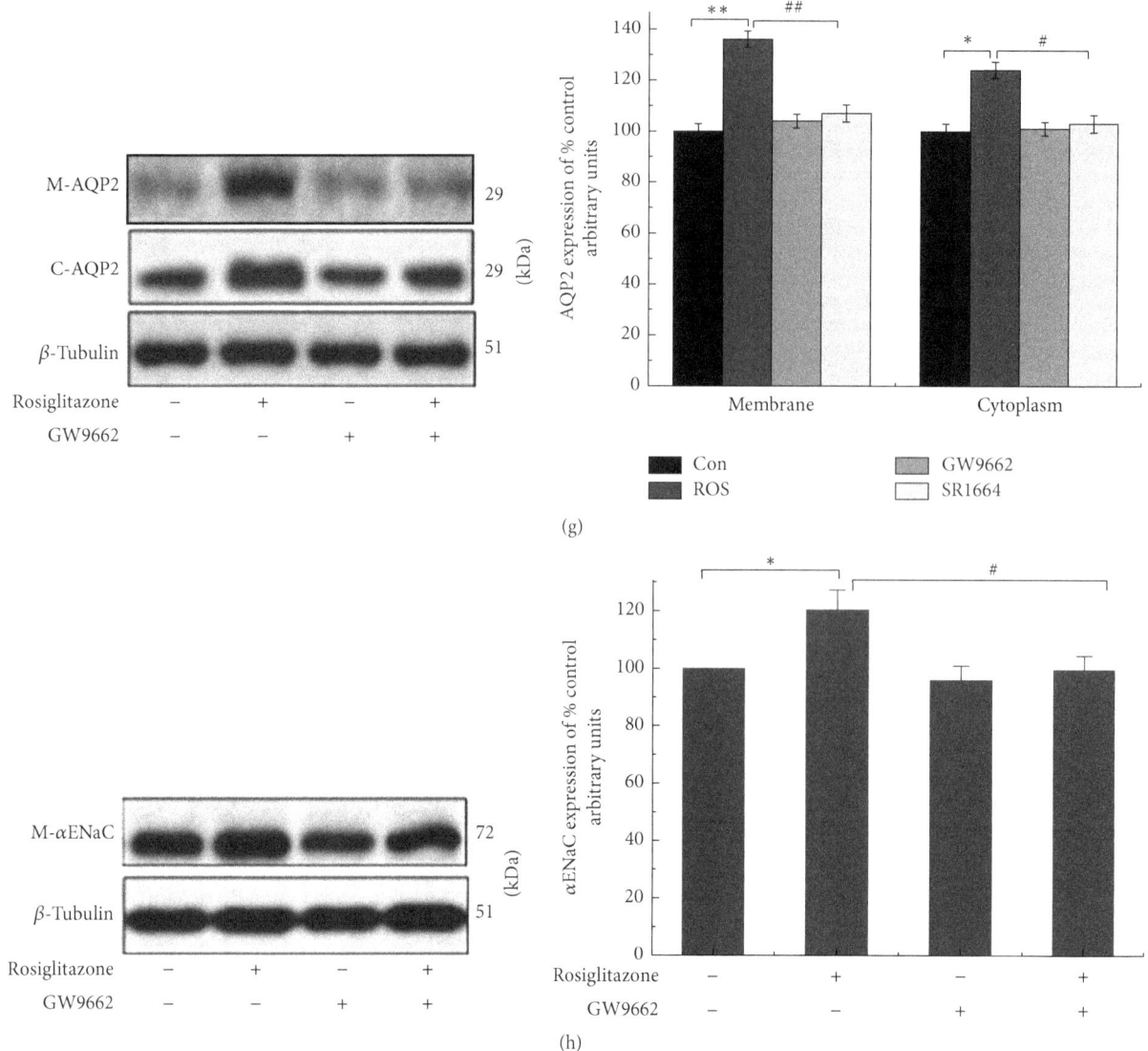

FIGURE 4: Effects of rosiglitazone and coincubation with GW9662 in mIMCD-3 cells. (a–d) The effects of rosiglitazone on PPARγ, p-PPARγ, AQP2, and αENaC. (e–h) The changes of PPARγ, p-PPARγ, AQP2, and αENaC upon coincubation with GW9662 (10 μM ROS + 5 μM GW9662). The results show that rosiglitazone at 10 μM can significantly decrease total and nuclear p-PPARγ but critically upregulated nuclear PPARγ and AQP2 and αENaC membrane transpositions. After coincubation with GW9662 (10 μM ROS + 5 μM GW9662), the effects of rosiglitazone on PPARγ, p-PPARγ, AQP2, and αENaC disappeared. The results are shown as mean ± s.e.m., $n = 3$. $^{*/\#}P < 0.05$. $^{**/\#\#}P < 0.01$. $*$ means compared to control; $\#$ means compared to rosiglitazone.

the expression of AQP2 in the collecting duct membrane and increasing water reabsorption, leading to fluid retention.

The regulation of renal sodium (Na^+) handling is a key determinant of the long-term control of extracellular fluid volume homeostasis. Na^+ reabsorption is mediated via the amiloride-sensitive epithelial sodium channel (ENaC), which exhibits high selectivity for sodium [15] and is a central requirement for Na^+ reabsorption across renal epithelia. ENaC expression and translocation to the plasma membrane are tightly regulated by a diverse array of hormonal [16, 17] and physical factors [18]. Our experiments show that ROS (10 μM) remarkably raised the membrane level of αENaC, and thus more and more Na^+ flowed into the lumen, which

accelerated water reabsorption and caused more serious fluid retention. After incubation with GW9662, this effect dissipated.

SR1664 is a novel PPARγ ligand (a nonagonist PPARγ ligand) that blocked the cyclin-dependent kinase 5 (CDK5)-mediated phosphorylation of PPARγ. In vivo experiments show that it can increase insulin sensitivity and does not cause fluid retention [5]. This study focused on the relationship between SR1664 and AQP2/αENaC proteins in vitro, indicating that SR1664 downregulated p-PPARγ, but did not cause any significant changes in AQP2 and αENaC in the membrane, demonstrating that SR1664 increased insulin sensitivity without affecting water and sodium channel protein expression.

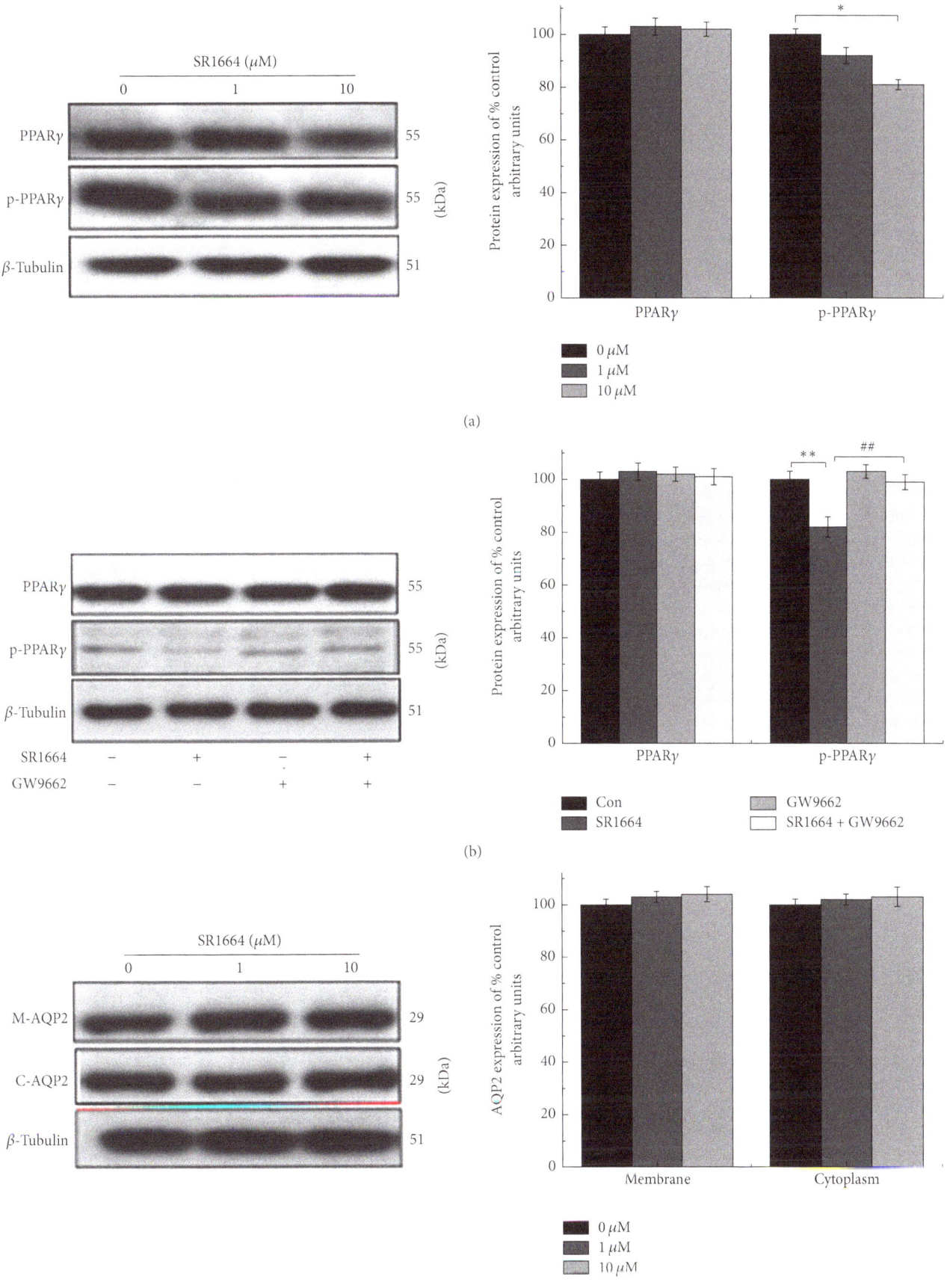

FIGURE 5: Continued.

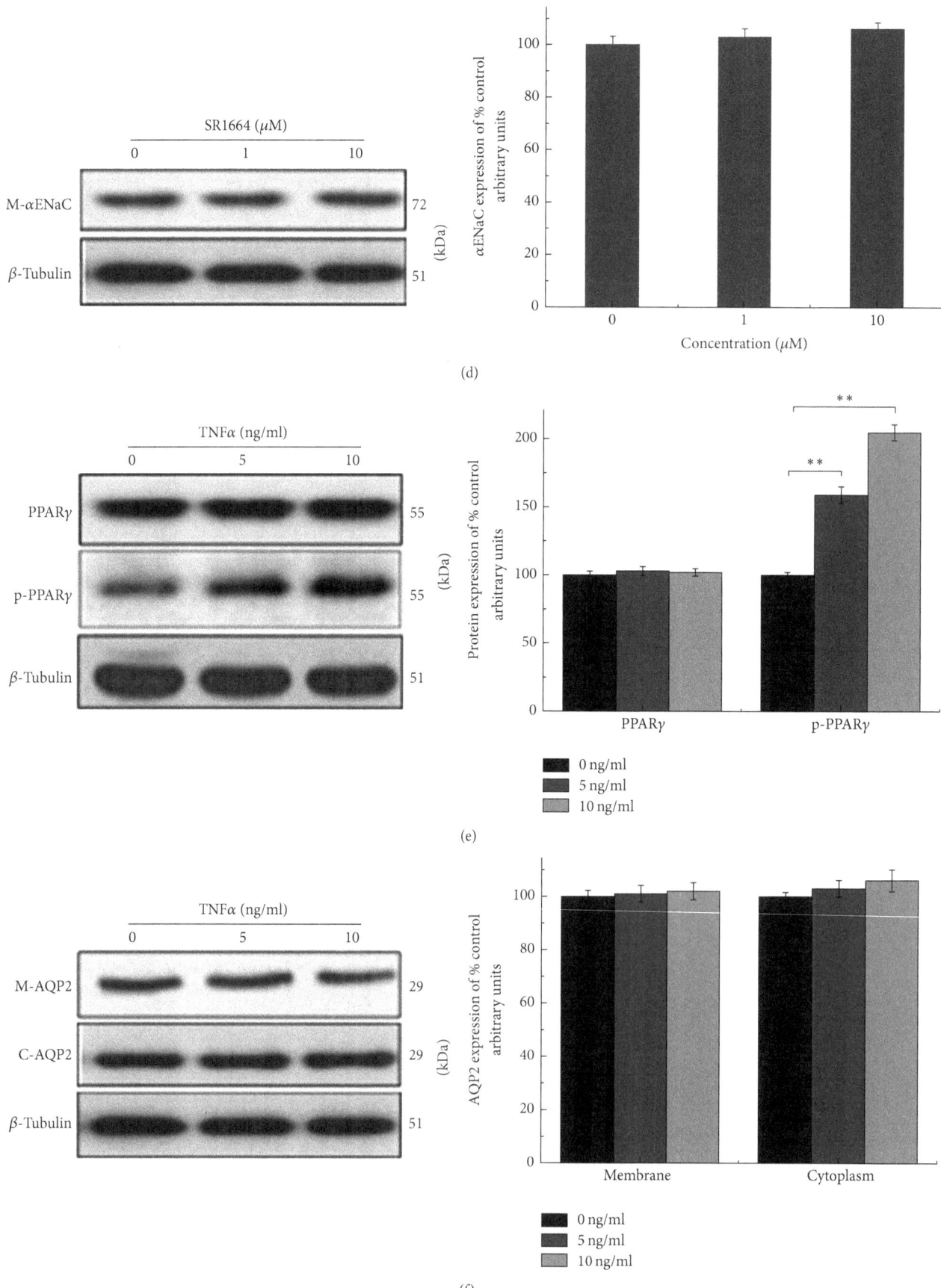

FIGURE 5: Continued.

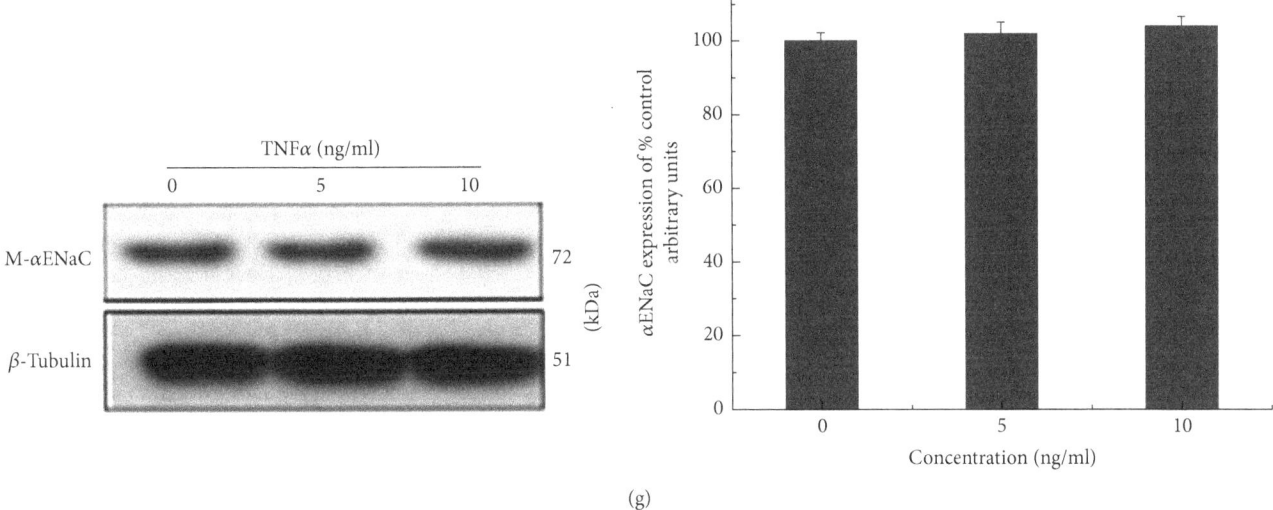

(g)

FIGURE 5: Effects of SR1664 and TNFα on PPARγ, p-PPARγ, AQP2, and αENaC in mIMCD-3 cells. (a, c, d) The effects of SR1664 on PPARγ, p-PPARγ, AQP2, and αENaC. (b) The changes of PPARγ and p-PPARγ upon coincubation with GW9662 (10 μM SR1664 + 5 μM GW9662). (e–g) The effects of TNFα on PPARγ, p-PPARγ, AQP2, and αENaC. The results show that SR1664 at 10 μM can significantly inhibit p-PPARγ; TNFα even 5 ng/ml can critically increase p-PPARγ, while there was no significant difference in the expression of AQP2 in cell membrane and cytoplasm and αENaC in membrane. After coincubation with GW9662 (10 μM SR1664 + 5 μM GW9662), the effect of SR1664 on p-PPARγ disappeared. The results are shown as mean ± s.e.m., $n = 3$. $^*P < 0.05$. $^{**}/^{##}P < 0.01$. ∗ means compared to control; # means compared to SR1664.

Activated PPARγ suppresses the expression of TNFα [19, 20], and TNFα increases the level of insulin antagonistic hormones by phosphorylating serine residue of the substrates of the insulin receptor, inhibiting tyrosine phosphorylation of this receptor, which in turn limits signal transmission [21]. Furthermore, both ROS and SR1664 are reported to eliminate p-PPARγ upregulated by TNFα [22]. Prompted by these findings, we also studied the correlation of phosphorylated PPARγ induced by TNFα with AQP2 and αENaC expression. As shown in Figure 5, TNFα at both 5 and 10 ng/ml can upregulate p-PPARγ, but the expression of AQP2 and αENaC in the cytoplasm and membrane was not changed by it.

In conclusion, in vitro the fluid retention induced by ROS is closely associated with two major aspects: the first includes the increase of cytoplasmic AQP2 and promotion of AQP2 vesicles to undergo membrane fusion, thereby increasing water reabsorption; the second involves ROS enhancing membrane αENaC expression, thus accelerating Na⁺ reabsorption, which further increases the absorption of water. In contrast, SR1664 and TNFα experiments reveal that whether activated PPARγ was up- or downregulated did not affect AQP2 and αENaC expression. From the former evidence, we deduced that in vitro there was little association between the fluid retention induced by ROS and the phosphorylation of PPARγ.

Conflicts of Interest

The authors declare that there are no competing or financial interests.

Authors' Contributions

Jinghua Xu and Mingyue Pan performed the molecular biology experiments and analyzed data, and Mingyue Pan wrote the manuscript. Xiaoli Wang designed the methodology. Lishi Xu and Lanfang Li prepared the figures and images. Cheng Xu guided the whole experiments. Jinghua Xu and Mingyue Pan contributed equally to the work.

Acknowledgments

The authors thank Liwen Beijing, Edanz Group China (http://www.liwenbianji.cn/ac), for editing the English text of a draft of this manuscript.

References

[1] T. Yamauchi, J. Kamon, H. Waki et al., "The mechanisms by which both heterozygous peroxisome proliferator-activated receptor γ (PPARγ) deficiency and PPARγ agonist improve insulin resistance," *The Journal of Biological Chemistry*, vol. 276, no. 44, pp. 41245–41254, 2001.

[2] S. Paredes, C. Matta-Coelho, A. M. Monteiro et al., "Cardiovascular safety of type 2 diabetes medications: Review of existing literature and clinical implications," *Hormones*, vol. 15, no. 2, pp. 170–185, 2016.

[3] E. R. Blasi, J. Heyen, M. Hemkens, A. McHarg, C. M. Ecelbarger, and S. Tiwari, "Effects of chronic PPAR-agonist treatment on cardiac structure and function, blood pressure, and kidney in healthy sprague-dawley rats," *PPAR Research*, vol. 2009, Article ID 237865, 13 pages, 2009.

[4] S.-S. Choi, E. S. Kim, M. Koh et al., "A novel non-agonist peroxisome proliferator-activated receptor γ (PPARγ) ligand UHC1 blocks PPARγ phosphorylation by cyclin-dependent kinase 5 (CDK5) and improves insulin sensitivity," *The Journal of Biological Chemistry*, vol. 289, no. 38, pp. 26618–26629, 2014.

[5] J. H. Choi, A. S. Banks, T. M. Kamenecka et al., "Antidiabetic actions of a non-agonist PPARγ ligand blocking Cdk5-mediated phosphorylation," *Nature*, vol. 477, no. 7365, pp. 477–481, 2011.

[6] H. Zhang, A. Zhang, D. E. Kohan, R. D. Nelson, F. J. Gonzalez, and T. Yang, "Collecting duct-specific deletion of peroxisome proliferator-activated receptor gamma blocks thiazolidinedione-induced fluid retention," *Proceedings of the National Acadamy of Sciences of the United States of America*, vol. 102, no. 26, pp. 9406–9411, 2005.

[7] Y. Guan, C. Hao, D. R. Cha et al., "Thiazolidinediones expand body fluid volume through PPARγ stimulation of ENaC-mediated renal salt absorption," *Nature Medicine*, vol. 11, no. 8, pp. 861–866, 2005.

[8] S. C. Lütken, J. Frøkiær, and S. Nielsen, "AVP-induced increase in AQP2 and p-AQP2 is blunted in heart failure during cardiac remodeling and is associated with decreased AT1R abundance in rat kidney," *PLoS ONE*, vol. 10, no. 2, Article ID 0116501, 2015.

[9] S. Tiwari, E. R. Blasi, J. R. Heyen, A. D. McHarg, and C. M. Ecelbarger, "Time course of AQP-2 and ENaC regulation in the kidney in response to PPAR agonists associated with marked edema in rats," *Pharmacological Research*, vol. 57, no. 5, pp. 383–392, 2008.

[10] Y. Fu, M. Gerasimova, F. Batz et al., "PPARγ agonist-induced fluid retention depends on aENaC expression in connecting tubules," *Nephron*, vol. 129, no. 1, pp. 68–74, 2015.

[11] H. B. Moeller, C. H. Fuglsang, and R. A. Fenton, "Renal aquaporins and water balance disorders," *Best Practice & Research Clinical Endocrinology & Metabolism*, vol. 30, no. 2, pp. 277–288, 2016.

[12] D. Zittema, N. F. Casteleijn, S. J. L. Bakker et al., "Urine concentrating capacity, vasopressin and copeptin in ADPKD and IgA nephropathy patients with renal impairment," *PLoS ONE*, vol. 12, no. 1, Article ID e0169263, 2017.

[13] T. Vukicevic, M. Schulz, D. Faust, and E. Klussmann, "The trafficking of the water channel aquaporin-2 in renal principal cells-a potential target for pharmacological intervention in cardiovascular diseases," *Frontiers in Pharmacology*, vol. 7, article 23, 2016.

[14] L. Chen, B. Yang, J. A. McNulty et al., "GI262570, a peroxisome proliferator-activated receptor γ agonist, changes electrolytes and water reabsorption from the distal nephron in rats," *The Journal of Pharmacology and Experimental Therapeutics*, vol. 312, no. 2, pp. 718–725, 2005.

[15] B. C. Rossier, "The epithelial sodium channel (ENaC): New insights into ENaC gating," *Pflügers Archiv - European Journal of Physiology*, vol. 446, no. 3, pp. 314–316, 2003.

[16] J. Wang, P. Barbry, A. C. Maiyar et al., "SGK integrates insulin and mineralocorticoid regulation of epithelial sodium transport," *American Journal of Physiology-Renal Physiology*, vol. 280, no. 2, pp. F303–F313, 2001.

[17] A. Bhargava, M. J. Fullerton, K. Myles et al., "The serum- and glucocorticoid-induced kinase is a physiological mediator of aldosterone action," *Endocrinology*, vol. 142, no. 4, pp. 1587–1594, 2001.

[18] S. Renauld, K. Tremblay, S. Ait-Benichou et al., "Stimulation of ENaC activity by rosiglitazone is pparc-dependent and correlates with SGK1 expression increase," *Journal of Membrane Biology*, vol. 236, no. 3, pp. 259–270, 2010.

[19] C. B. Kallen and M. A. Lazar, "Antidiabetic thiazolidinediones inhibit leptin (ob) gene expression in 3T3-L1 adipocytes," *Proceedings of the National Acadamy of Sciences of the United States of America*, vol. 93, no. 12, pp. 5793–5796, 1996.

[20] T. M. Willson, P. J. Brown, D. D. Sternbach, and B. R. Henke, "The PPARs: from orphan receptors to drug discovery," *Journal of Medicinal Chemistry*, vol. 43, no. 4, pp. 527–550, 2000.

[21] M. K. Moon, M. Kim, S. S. Chung et al., "S-Adenosyl-L-methionine ameliorates TNFα-induced insulin resistance in 3T3-L1 adipocytes," *Experimental & Molecular Medicine*, vol. 42, no. 5, pp. 345–352, 2010.

[22] J. H. Choi, A. S. Banks, J. L. Estall et al., "Anti-diabetic drugs inhibit obesity-linked phosphorylation of PPARγ 3 by Cdk5," *Nature*, vol. 466, no. 7305, pp. 451–456, 2010.

10

Inhibitory Effects of a Novel PPAR-γ Agonist MEKT1 on *Pomc* Expression/ACTH Secretion in AtT20 Cells

Rehana Parvin,[1] Erika Noro,[1] Akiko Saito-Hakoda,[1] Hiroki Shimada,[1] Susumu Suzuki,[1] Kyoko Shimizu,[1] Hiroyuki Miyachi,[2] Atsushi Yokoyama ⓘ,[1] and Akira Sugawara ⓘ[1]

[1]*Department of Molecular Endocrinology, Tohoku University Graduate School of Medicine, Sendai, Miyagi, Japan*
[2]*Drug Discovery Initiative, The University of Tokyo, 7-3-1 Hongo, Bunkyo-ku, Tokyo, Japan*

Correspondence should be addressed to Akira Sugawara; akiras2i@med.tohoku.ac.jp

Academic Editor: Nguan Soon Tan

Although therapeutic effects of the peroxisome proliferator-activated receptor gamma (PPAR-γ) agonists rosiglitazone and pioglitazone against Cushing's disease have been reported, their effects are still controversial and inconsistent. We therefore examined the effects of a novel PPAR-γ agonist, MEKT1, on *Pomc* expression/ACTH secretion using murine corticotroph-derived AtT20 cells and compared its effects with those of rosiglitazone and pioglitazone. AtT20 cells were treated with either 1 nM~10 μM MEKT1, rosiglitazone, or pioglitazone for 24 hours. Thereafter, their effects on proopiomelanocortin gene *(Pomc)* mRNA expression were studied by qPCR and the *Pomc* promoter (−703/+58) activity was demonstrated by luciferase assay. *Pomc* mRNA expression and promoter activity were significantly inhibited by MEKT1 at 10 μM compared to rosiglitazone and pioglitazone. SiRNA-mediated PPAR-γ knockdown significantly abrogated MEKT1-mediated *Pomc* mRNA suppression. ACTH secretion from AtT20 cells was also significantly inhibited by MEKT1. Deletion/point mutant analyses of *Pomc* promoter indicated that the MEKT1-mediated suppression was mediated via NurRE, TpitRE, and NBRE at −404/−383, −316/−309, and −69/−63, respectively. Moreover, MEKT1 significantly suppressed *Nur77*, *Nurr1*, and *Tpit* mRNA expression. MEKT1 also was demonstrated to inhibit the protein-DNA interaction of Nur77/Nurr1-NurRE, Tpit-TpitRE, and Nur77-NBRE by ChIP assay. Taken together, it is suggested that MEKT1 could be a novel therapeutic medication for Cushing's disease.

1. Introduction

Peroxisome proliferator-activated receptor gamma (PPAR-γ) is a member of the nuclear receptor superfamily also known as ligand-inducible transcription factors [1]. Ligand binding with PPAR-γ receptor acts as a switch leading to the transcription complexes mediating repression or activation of transcription on specific target genes [2]. Moreover, PPAR-γ possesses beneficial pleotropic effects including anti-inflammatory and neuroprotective actions [3, 4] and antidiabetic [5–7], antineoplastic [8], and renoprotective effects [9]. PPAR-γ is expressed in normal human anterior pituitary as well as in adrenocorticotropic hormone- (ACTH-) secreting pituitary adenomas. Moreover, PPAR-γ expression was significantly higher in pituitary adenomas than normal pituitary tissues, and its expression in ACTH-secreting adenomas was

significantly higher than any other types of pituitary adenomas [10–13]. ACTH, the product of proopiomelanocortin gene *(Pomc)*, is secreted from the corticotroph cells of the anterior pituitary. *Pomc* is exhibited in various tissues including pituitary (anterior and intermediate), hypothalamus, and skin [14].

The *Pomc* regulation is tissue-specific [15] and the regulatory mechanism of this gene has been elucidated in different tissues [16, 17] using different types of drugs. However, the PPAR-γ-mediated *Pomc* regulation mechanism has not yet been clarified in pituitary corticotroph cells. Moreover, preclinical studies conducted both *in vitro* and *in vivo* have provided the evidence of anticancer properties of particular PPAR-γ agonists, rosiglitazone and pioglitazone. Several studies demonstrating rosiglitazone and pioglitazone on *Pomc* suppression have been done [12, 18, 19], and an opposite effect of rosiglitazone was also shown by Kreutzer et al. [20]. Moreover, although rosiglitazone has been used as a therapeutic drug for the treatment of Cushing's disease due to its ability to reduce ACTH and corticosterone secretion in mouse corticotropic pituitary tumors, it has generally shown unsatisfactory results [21]. In addition, although previous studies have reported the therapeutic use of rosiglitazone and pioglitazone in Cushing's disease [11, 12, 22], there has been some controversy concerning these drugs [20, 23]. Since there have been few effective drugs for Cushing's disease, the discovery of novel drugs is very important to obtain a satisfactory treatment of Cushing's disease.

In this study, we examined the effects of a novel PPAR-γ agonist, MEKT1, on *Pomc* expression/ACTH secretion using murine pituitary corticotroph tumor-derived AtT20 cells and compared them with rosiglitazone and pioglitazone. We also examined the effects of MEKT1 on transcription factors Nur77, Nurr1, NeuroD1, and Tpit, which are known to activate *Pomc* transcription [24–26]. Our present study has indicated a possibility that MEKT1 may be a novel candidate for the therapeutic medication against Cushing's disease.

2. Materials and Methods

2.1. Reagents. MEKT1, a synthetic PPAR-γ agonist, was a gift from Okayama University. MEKT1 was dissolved in 100% DMSO at 10 mM and stored at $-20°C$. Rosiglitazone and pioglitazone hydrochloride were purchased from Sigma-Aldrich (St. Louis, MO) and Wako Pure Chemical Industries Ltd, Japan, respectively. 100% DMSO was used to dissolve rosiglitazone and pioglitazone hydrochloride at 10 mM and stored at $-20°C$. Before each experiment, these stored drugs were diluted with 100% DMSO to the desired concentration maintaining final concentration of DMSO at 0.1%.

2.2. Plasmids. Subcloned chimeric constructs which contained the rat *Pomc* genomic DNA and luciferase cDNA (pGL3-Basic, Promega, Madison, WI) were used for the studies of transient transfection: r*Pomc*-Luc ($-703/+58$-Luc: harboring the rat *Pomc* 5′-flanking region from -703 to $+58$ relative to the transcription start site upstream of the luciferase cDNA in pGL3-Basic), $-429/+58$-Luc, $-379/+58$-Luc, $-359/+58$-Luc, $-293/+58$-Luc, $-169/+58$-Luc, and $+12/+58$-Luc. Nur77/Nurr1 binding element in r*Pomc*-Luc from 5′-TGATATTTACCTCC-3′ to 5′-cagcgcccACCTCC-3′ (r*Pomc*-Luc-NurRE-Mut), Nur77 binding element in r*Pomc*-Luc from 5′-AGGTCA-3′ to 5′-gtaTCA-3′ (r*Pomc*-Luc-NBRE-Mut), and Tpit binding element in r*Pomc*-Luc from 5′-TCACACC-3′ to 5′-gacCACC-3′ (r*Pomc*-Luc-TpitRE-Mut). β-galactosidase control plasmid in pRSV (pRSV-β-gal) was purchased from Clontech (Mountain View, CA) and pcDNA3 expression plasmid from Invitrogen (Carsbad, CA). Murine Nur77, Tpit, and Nurr1 cDNA were cloned by PCR from AtT20 cells and were subcloned into the pcDNA3 expression vector (Invitrogen, Carlsbad, CA) to prepare Nur77-pcDNA3, Tpit-pcDNA3, and Nurr1-pcDNA3 [27, 28].

2.3. Cell Culture. AtT20 cells [28], obtained from the American Type Culture Collection (AtT20: CCL-89), were cultured with Dulbecco's modified Eagle medium (DMEM) added with 10% fetal bovine serum (FBS), 100 U/mL penicillin, and 100 μg/mL streptomycin. Cells were cultured in a humidified incubator at $37°C$ with 5% CO_2.

2.4. Proliferation Assay. The following procedure was outlined by Saito-Hakoda et al. [28]. Cell Counting Kit-8 (Dojindo, Kumamoto, Japan) was used for counting the cell numbers. Briefly, AtT20 cells (5×10^3 cells/well) seeded in 96-well plates were incubated in 100 μl regular media for few days. The cells were then refed with DMEM supplemented with 1% resin and charcoal-treated (stripped) FBS media containing appropriate concentrations of PPAR-γ agonist MEKT1. After 24-hour incubation, 10 μl of assay reagent was added in each well and then the plate was incubated for 4 hours at $37°C$, 5% CO_2. The generation of the colored formazan product was measured optically by measuring the absorbance at 450 nm (reference 600 nm) using a microplate reader.

2.5. Measurement of Caspase 3 Activity. Caspase 3 activity was determined using a caspase 3/CPR32 Colorimetric Assay kit, according to the manufacturer's instructions (Biovision, Mountain View, CA 94043, USA). Briefly, the AtT20 cells were lysed in caspase 3 sample lysis buffer and incubate cells on ice for 10 minutes. The homogenates were then centrifuged at 10,000 ×g and $4°C$ for 1 min and the supernatant was collected for protein estimation. The cell lysates were then exposed to the DEVD substrate conjugate provided in the kit for 1 hour at $37°C$. The sample was measured in an automatic microplate reader at an excitation of 400 nm.

2.6. RNA Isolation, cDNA Synthesis, and Quantitative Real-Time PCR. RNA isolation, cDNA synthesis, and quantitative real-time polymerase chain reaction (qPCR) were conducted as previously described [28, 29]. To confirm the amplification specificity, the PCR products from each primer pair with SYBR green were subjected to a melting curve analysis. For each sample, the expression of mRNA was normalized by dividing the expression of mouse GAPDH. The sequences of the primer sets are shown in Table 1.

2.7. Transient Transfection for Luciferase Assay. AtT20 cells were seeded to 60–70% confluence in regular medium in 24-multiwell plates and the cells were transfected (transiently) with 300 ng of each reporter plasmid and 100 or 150 ng of β-gal control plasmid. Transfection was carried out according to the manufacturer's instructions using Lipofectamine$^{(R)}$ 2000 (Invitrogen). Each expression vector is of different concentrations (200 ng and 300 ng); 135 ng of reporter plasmid and 65 ng of β-gal control plasmid were also transfected with cells in overexpression experiments. Twenty-four hours after transfection, the medium was changed to DMEM added with 1% stripped FBS, and the cells were treated without or with MEKT1 (10 μM) for the next 24 hours. Before luciferase assay, the cells were washed with 1x PBS and then the cell extracts were prepared using Glo Lysis Buffer (Promega) and β-galactosidase activity was also measured simultaneously.

TABLE 1: Primer sequences for RT-qPCR.

Mouse Pomc	Forward	5′-CAGTGCCAGGACCTCACC-3′
	Reverse	5′-CAGCGAGAGGTCGAGTTTG-3′
Mouse PPAR-γ1	Forward	5′-TTCTGACAGGACTGTGTGACAG-3′
	Reverse	5′-ATAAGGTGGAGATGCAGGTTC-3′
Mouse PPAR-α	Forward	5′-AGACACGCAGACGGGTTG-3′
	Reverse	5′-GAGGATGCCACTCCCAGA-3′
Mouse PPAR-β	Forward	5′-TGGAGCTCGATGACAGTGAC-3′
	Reverse	5′- GTACTGGCTGTCAGGGTGGT-3′
Mouse Nur77	Forward	5′-GCACAGCTTGGGTGTTGATG-3′
	Reverse	5′-CAGACGTGACAGGCAGCTG-3′
Mouse Nurr1	Forward	5′-TCAGAGCCCACGTCGATT-3′
	Reverse	5′-TAGTCAGGGTTTGCCTGGAA-3′
Mouse NeuroD1	Forward	5′-ACGCAGAAGGCAAGGTGTCC-3′
	Reverse	5′-TTGGTCATGTTTCCACTTCC-3′
Mouse Tpit	Forward	5′-GCCAGCATGTGACCTACTCTCACT-3
	Reverse	5′-AGTCCAGCTGTCAGGTCCCGAGAA-3′
Mouse Pitx1	Forward	5′-CGGTGTGGACCAACCTCACTGAA-3′
	Reverse	5′-GAGTTGCACGTGTCCCGGTAGA-3′
Mouse NFκB1	Forward	5′-GAAATTCCTGATCCAGACAAAAAC-3′
	Reverse	5′-ATCACTTCAATGGCCTCTGTGTAG-3′
Mouse NFκB2	Forward	5′ CTGGTGGACACATACAGGAAGAC-3′
	Reverse	5′-ATAGGCACTGTCTTCTTTCACCTC-3′
Mouse Pttg	Forward	5′-CTGGGCACTGGTGTCAAG-3′
	Forward	5′-GCTGTTTTGGTTGGAGGGG-3′
Mouse GAPDH	Forward	5′-ACAGTCCATGCCATCACTGCC-3′
	Reverse	5′-GCCTGCTTCACCACCTTCTTG-3′

Data were normalized by β-galactosidase activity. We followed our previously published protocol [29].

2.8. *Small Interfering RNA.* Small interfering RNAs (siRNAs) for PPAR-γ (NM_011146_stealth_342) [30] and negative control siRNA (ID: 1022076) were obtained from Qiagen (Hilden, Germany). AtT20 cells were cultured to 50% confluence in 24-multiwell plates transiently transfected with 10 pmol siRNAs using Lipofectamine(R) 2000 (Invitrogen) for 48 hours according to the manufacturer's instructions. The cells were then incubated either without or with 10 μM MEKT1 for 24 hours and then used for quantitative RT-PCR. Reporter plasmids were transfected with the cells and then incubated either without or with MEKT1 at 10 μM for 24 hours and these cells were used for luciferase assay.

2.9. *Enzyme Immunoassay (EIA).* EIA was performed for measuring of ACTH concentration. AtT20 cells were cultured to 60% confluence in regular medium in 24-multiwell plates and then incubated either without or with at appropriate concentrations of MEKT1, rosiglitazone, and pioglitazone hydrochloride in DMEM added with 1% stripped FBS for 24 hours. The ACTH concentration in the supernatants was measured by an ACTH (rat. mouse) EIA kit (Phoenix Pharmaceuticals, Burlingame, CA). Data were normalized by the total protein in each well.

2.10. *Western Blot Analyses.* AtT20 cells were grown to 70% confluence in regular medium in 6 cm dishes, and they were incubated in the presence rosiglitazone, pioglitazone, and MEKT1 (time dependently) or in the presence of 100% DMSO in DMEM supplemented with 1% stripped FBS media for 24 hours. The cells were then harvested and lysed with TNE buffer (20 mmol/L Tris-HCl, 137 mmol/L NaCl, 2 mmol/L EDTA, 1% NP-40, Protease Inhibitor Cocktail Set III (Calbiochem), pH 7.9). Thereafter, 20 μg of extracted protein was electrophoresed on a SDS-polyacrylamide gel and transferred onto PVDF membrane. For the detection of NURR1, Nur77, and TBX19 (Tpit) protein the membrane was blocked with 1% BSA for 30 minutes and probed with the primary antibody for Nur77/Nurr1 antibody (SC-990, Santa Cruz Biotechnology); anti TBX19 antibody (GTX77878, GeneTex); Nur77 (ab13851, Abcam) diluted at 1 : 1000 with 1% BSA, for overnight at 4°C, and was thereafter incubated with anti-rabbit IgG, horseradish peroxidase (HRP) linked whole antibody from donkey (NA934V, GE Healthcare Life Sciences, Pittsburgh, PA) (1 : 5000) for 1 hour at room temperature. For the detection of actin, the membrane was blocked with 1% BSA for 30 minutes at room temperature and probed with the primary antibody for actin (sc-1616, Santa Cruz Biotechnology) (diluted at 1 : 500) for overnight at 4°C and was thereafter incubated with anti-goat IgG, HRP preabsorbed from donkey (ab97120) (1 : 5000) for 1 hour at room temperature. Thereafter, the membranes were washed and were visualized using

TABLE 2: Primer sequences for ChIP-qPCR.

Mouse NurRE	Forward	5′-ACACTGGGGAAATCTGATGC-3′
	Reverse	5′-CGGTGGTCAGGAGGAACTTA-3′
Mouse TpitRE	Forward	5′-GGCAGATGGACGCACATAGG-3′
	Reverse	5′-GCGCTGGTGGTTAGGAAGAA-3′
Mouse NBRE	Forward	5′-TTTCCAGGCAGATGTGCCTTGCGCT-3′
	Reverse	5′-CAGGGTTGGGTGGGTGAGCCTTGGA-3′

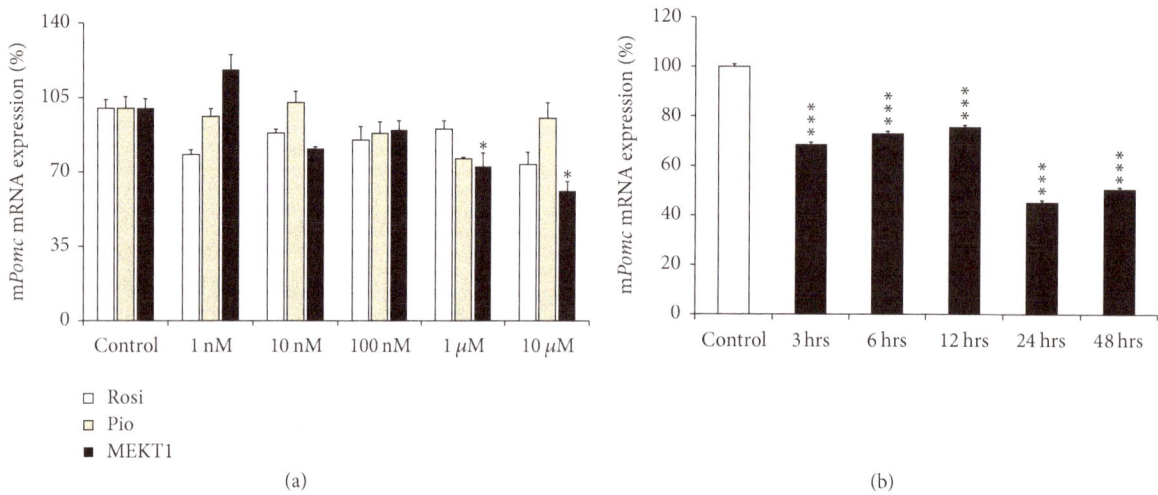

(a)   (b)

FIGURE 1: Effects of MEKT1, rosiglitazone, and pioglitazone on mRNA expression of *Pomc* in AtT20 cells. (a) Effects of MEKT1, rosiglitazone, and pioglitazone on mRNA expression of *Pomc* dose-dependently. AtT20 cells were treated with MEKT1, rosiglitazone (Rosi), and pioglitazone (Pio) (1 nM, 10 nM, 100 nM, 1 μM, or 10 μM) or 0.1% DMSO (vehicle control) for 24 hours. $^*P < 0.05$ versus control. (b) Effect of MEKT1 on *Pomc* mRNA expression time dependently. AtT20 cells were treated with 10 μM MEKT1 for 1 hour, 3 hours, 6 hours, 12 hours, or 24 hours. Vehicle control, 0.1% DMSO. Data are expressed as percentages (100%) of control. Each point indicates mean ± SEM ($n = 4$). $^{***}P < 0.001$ versus control.

ECL (Bio-Rad). Densitometric analyses of the membranes were performed using Image J.

2.11. Chromatin Immunoprecipitation (ChIP) Assay. ChIP assay was performed using anti-Nur77/Nurr1 antibody (SC-990, Santa Cruz Biotechnology); anti TBX19 antibody (GTX77878, GeneTex); normal rabbit IgG (SC-2027, Santa Cruz Biotechnology); and NurRE (Nur response element), TpitRE (Tpit response element), and NBRE (Nur77 response element) region containing primers of mouse *Pomc* promoter. ChIP assay was conducted as described previously [29]. DNA fragments were treated with Proteinase K (Wako, Osaka, Japan) and Qiagen DNA Extraction kit was used for purification of DNA. Immunoprecipitated DNA was analyzed by qPCR when KAPA SYBR FAST Universal 2x qPCR Master Mix (KAPA Biosystems) reagent was used for qPCR. Data were represented as enrichment of the immunoprecipitated DNA compared to 1% input DNA. NurRE, TpitRE, and NBRE region specific primer pairs of mouse *Pomc* promoter were designed to amplify by qPCR. The sequences of the primer sets are shown in Table 2.

2.12. Statistical Analyses. Data are displayed as means ± standard errors of means (SEM). Statistical analysis was performed with one way ANOVA followed by Tukey's post hoc test among the groups and Paired Sample *t* test between the groups. *P* value < 0.05 was considered as statistically significant. Statistical details are found in the Figures and Figure legends.

3. Results

3.1. Effects of PPAR-γ Agonists Rosiglitazone, Pioglitazone, and MEKT1 on mRNA Expression/Promoter Activity of Pomc. We first analyzed the effects of rosiglitazone, pioglitazone, and MEKT1 on mRNA expression of *Pomc* at various concentrations in AtT20 cells. After treatment of the cells with various concentrations (1 nM, 10 nM, 100 nM, 1 μM, and 10 μM) of rosiglitazone, pioglitazone, and MEKT1, *Pomc* mRNA was significantly decreased at 1 μM and 10 μM of MEKT1, but no significant suppressive effects were observed when rosiglitazone and pioglitazone were added (Figure 1(a)). Next we examined the MEKT1-mediated effect on *Pomc* mRNA expression using different durations of incubation in the cells. After treatment of the cells with MEKT1 (10 μM) for 3 hours, 6 hours, 9 hours, 24 hours, or 48 hours, the *Pomc* mRNA expression was significantly decreased from 3 hours to 48 hours in a time dependent manner (Figure 1(b)). These results

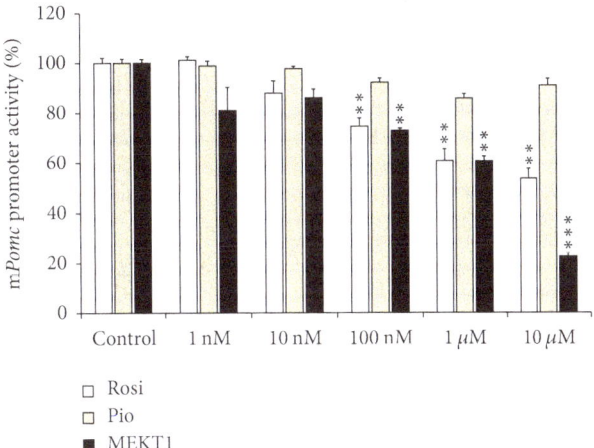

FIGURE 2: Effects of MEKT1, rosiglitazone, and pioglitazone on *Pomc* promoter activity in AtT20 cells. AtT20 cells transiently transfected with 300 ng full length r*Pomc*-Luc (−703/+58-luc) and 100 ng pRSV-β-gal were treated with MEKT1, rosiglitazone (Rosi), and pioglitazone (Pio) (1 nM, 10 nM, 100 nM, 1 μM, or 10 μM) or 0.1% DMSO (vehicle control) for 24 hours. Data are expressed as percentages (100%) of control. Each point represents mean ± SEM ($n = 4$). $^{**}P < 0.01$, $^{***}P < 0.001$ versus control.

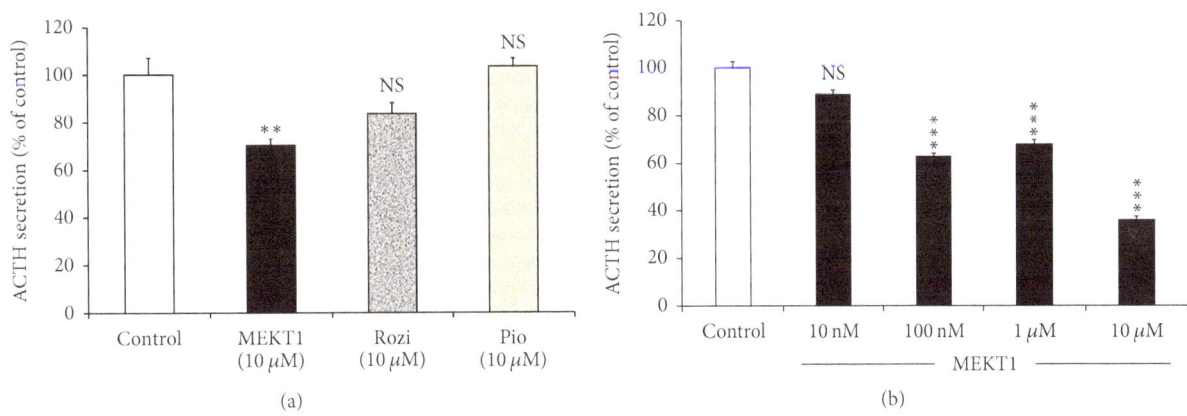

FIGURE 3: Effects of MEKT1, rosiglitazone, and pioglitazone on ACTH secretion from AtT20 cells. (a) Effects of MEKT1, rosiglitazone, and pioglitazone on ACTH secretion into the media from AtT20 cells. AtT20 cells were treated with MEKT1, rosiglitazone (Rosi), and pioglitazone (Pio) (10 μM) or DMSO (0.1%) as a control. After 24-hour incubation of the cells, the ACTH secreted to the media was determined by EIA. (b) Dose-dependent effects of MEKT1 on ACTH secretion into the media from AtT20 cells. AtT20 cells were treated with MEKT1 (10 nM, 100 nM, 1 μM, or 10 μM) or 0.1% DMSO (vehicle control) for 24 hours. After 24-hour incubation of the cells, the ACTH secreted to the media was determined by EIA. Data are expressed as percentages (100%) of control. Each point represents mean ± SEM ($n = 4$). NS means "not significant." $^{***}P < 0.001$, $^{**}P < 0.01$ versus control.

indicated that MEKT1 decreased mRNA expression of *Pomc* both dose- and time dependently. In contrast, MEKT1 dose-dependently increased PPAR-γ mRNA expression (Figure S1).

We next examined the effects of rosiglitazone, pioglitazone, and MEKT1 on the promoter activity of *Pomc* using AtT20 cells. In this experiment, the full length (−703/+58) *Pomc* promoter was used with different concentrations of rosiglitazone, pioglitazone, and MEKT1. As shown in Figure 2, MEKT1 significantly suppressed the promoter activity of *Pomc* dose-dependently, whereas pioglitazone had no suppressive effect. Though rosiglitazone had a suppressive effect on *Pomc* promoter activity, the effect was less strong than that of MEKT1. These results indicated that MEKT1-mediated

negative regulation of *Pomc* transcription is most effective than rosiglitazone and pioglitazone.

3.2. Effects of PPAR-γ Agonists MEKT1, Rosiglitazone, and Pioglitazone on ACTH Secretion.

We identified the effects of PPAR-γ agonists MEKT1, rosiglitazone, and pioglitazone at 10 μM on ACTH secretion of AtT20 cells in the supernatant and observed that only MEKT1 significantly suppressed ACTH secretion (Figure 3(a)), whereas there was no significant effect of rosiglitazone and pioglitazone on it. Due to the significant suppression of MEKT1 on ACTH secretion, we then examined the dose-dependent effects of MEKT1 on ACTH secretion. In this experiment, AtT20 cells were treated with different concentrations of MEKT1 (10 nM,

100 nM, 1 μM, and 10 μM) in Figure 3(b). MEKT1 significantly suppressed ACTH secretion from 100 nM to 10 μM.

3.3. Effects of MEKT1 on AtT20 Cell Proliferation and Apoptosis in AtT20 Cells.
We examined the effects of MEKT1 on proliferation of AtT20 cells using a WST-8 assay after incubation with various concentrations from 1 nM to 10 μM for 96 hours. MEKT1 did not exert any inhibitory effect on the proliferation of AtT20 cells from 1 nM to 10 μM (Figure 4(a)). Although treatment of rosiglitazone and pioglitazone for 24 hours did not exhibit (Figures 4(b) and 4(c)) inhibitory effect on AtT20 cell proliferation, treatment of rosiglitazone for 48 hours inhibited the cell proliferation of corticotroph tumor cells [12]. These data indicated that the MEKT1 had no toxic effect on the AtT20 cells at concentrations of 10 μM. Next we examined the effect of MEKT1 on AtT20 cell apoptosis by caspase-3 assay and observed no apoptotic activity of MEKT1 in Figure 4(e) on AtT20 cells. Moreover, we also demonstrated the effect of MEKT1 on the mRNA expression of the proliferative marker, pituitary tumor transforming gene (Pttg) in Figure 4(d), and observed no effect of MEKT1 on Pttg.

3.4. The Involvement of PPAR-γ in the MEKT1-Mediated Suppression of mRNA Expression/Promoter Activity of Pomc.
We examined the involvement of PPAR-γ in the MEKT1-mediated suppression of mRNA expression and promoter activity of Pomc by knocking down its small interfering RNA (siRNA). The decrease of endogenous PPAR-γ mRNA expression by its siRNA was confirmed by qPCR, as shown in Figure 5(a). Moreover, endogenous PPAR-α and PPAR-β mRNA expression were not observed in Figures 5(b) and 5(c), respectively. The decrease of PPAR-γ protein expression by its siRNA was confirmed by western blot analysis, as shown in Figure 5(d). PPAR-γ siRNA significantly abrogated the suppression of Pomc mRNA expression by MEKT1 (Figure 5(e)). Moreover, PPAR-γ siRNA significantly abrogated the MEKT1-mediated suppression of Pomc promoter activity (Figure S2). These results indicate that the negative regulation of Pomc expression by MEKT1 is most likely mediated via PPAR-γ.

3.5. Effects of MEKT1 on the Pomc Promoter Deletion Mutants, and the Involvement of NurRE, TpitRE, and NBRE in the MEKT1-Mediated Suppression of Pomc Promoter Activity.
We next examined the molecular mechanisms of Pomc transcription regulation by MEKT1. Therefore, we analyzed the promoter activity of Pomc 5′-flanking region deletion mutants series and it was observed that transcription suppression of Pomc promoter activity by MEKT1 was found in constructs from −703/+58 to −169/+58, but not in −12/+58 (Figure 6(a)). The luciferase activity of pGL3-Basic vector was unaffected by MEKT1 (Figure 6(a)). Pomc promoter constructs from −703/+58 to −169/+58 contained the NurRE, TpitRE, and NBRE, whereas the −12/+58 construct contained no responsive elements of Pomc promoter. It is plausible that NurRE, TpitRE, and NBRE probably exert an influential role in transcription suppression of Pomc, which occurred by MEKT1. To confirm the role of NurRE, TpitRE, and NBRE in the

suppression of Pomc transcription, we further demonstrated the impact of MEKT1 on the NurRE, TpitRE, and NBRE mutants (Figure 6(b)). As shown in Figure 6(b), NurRE and TpitRE mutants completely abrogated the MEKT1-mediated repression of Pomc promoter activity, while NBRE mutant partially abrogated the MEKT1-mediated repression of Pomc promoter activity. Therefore, NurRE and TpitRE are important for the transcription suppression of Pomc promoter activity, which was mediated by MEKT1. These data suggest that NurRE and TpitRE play a prominent role in the MEKT1-mediated negative regulation of Pomc transcription. Figure 6(c) represents the structure of the rat Pomc promoter. Since Nur77/Nurr1 [31] is known to bind to NurRE, and Tpit is known to bind to TpitRE [32], Nur77/Nurr1 and Tpit may be involved in the MEKT1-mediated suppression of Pomc promoter activity.

3.6. Effects of MEKT1 on mRNA Expression of Nur77, Nurr1, NeuroD1, Tpit, Pitx, NFkB1, and NFkB2.
We next examined the effect of MEKT1 on mouse Nur77, Nurr1, NeuroD1, Tpit, Pitx, NFkB1, and NFkB2 mRNA expression in AtT20 cells. As shown in Figures 7(a), 7(b), and 7(d), MEKT1 decreased mRNA expression of Nur77, Nurr1, and Tpit at the concentration of 10 μM but not that of NeuroD1, Pitx, NFkB1, and NFkB2 (Figures 7(c), 7(e), 7(f), and 7(g)). We also demonstrated the effect of MEKT1 on Nurr1, Nur77, and Tpit protein expression (Figure 8) in AtT20 cells. As shown in Figures 7(a), 7(b), and 7(d), results suggest that the MEKT1-mediated suppression of Pomc transcription probably was implicated via the suppression of Nur77, Nurr1, and Tpit mRNA expression which was confirmed by suppression of Nurr1, Nur77, and Tpit protein expression in Figure 8. We next examined the effects of MEKT1 at several concentrations (1 nM, 10 nM, 100 nM, 1 μM, and 10 μM) on mouse Nur77, Nurr1, and Tpit mRNA expression as shown in Figures S3A, S3B, and S3C, and observed its dose-dependent effects.

3.7. Effects of Nur77, Tpit, and Nurr1 Overexpression on the MEKT1-Mediated Suppression of mRNA Expression/Promoter Activity of Pomc.
We next performed the overexpression of Nur77, Tpit, and Nurr1 to examine the role of Nur77, Tpit, and Nurr1 in the MEKT1-mediated suppression of mRNA expression and promoter activity of Pomc. As shown in Figures 9(a) and 9(b), overexpression of Nur77 and Tpit recovered the MEKT1-mediated repression of Pomc mRNA expression, when respective control plasmid (pcDNA3) could not recover. As shown in Figures S4A and S4B, overexpression of Nur77 and Tpit recovered the MEKT1-mediated suppression of Pomc promoter activity, while respective control plasmid (pcDNA3) could not. Overexpression of Nurr1 did not recover the MEKT1-mediated suppression of Pomc mRNA expression (Figure 9(c)) and Pomc promoter activity (Figure S4C). These data suggest the involvement of Nur77 and Tpit transcription factor in the MEKT1-mediated suppression of Pomc.

3.8. Effects of MEKT1 on the Interaction between Nur77/Nurr1 and NurRE, Tpit and TpitRE, and Nur77 and NBRE on the Pomc Promoter.
Since Tpit, Nur77/Nurr1, and Nur77

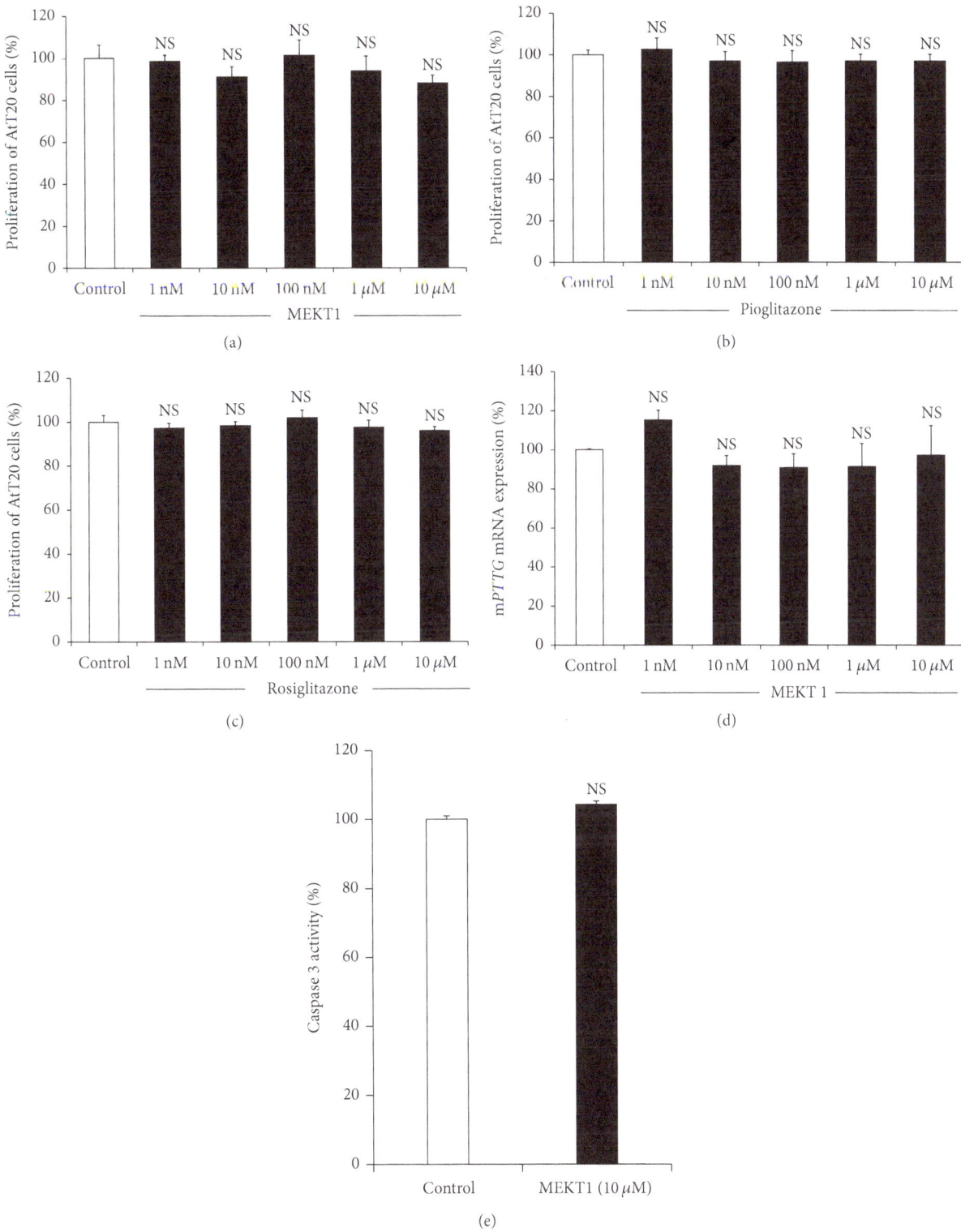

FIGURE 4: MEKT1-mediated effect on AtT20 cell proliferation and apoptosis. (a) AtT20 cells were incubated for 96 hours either in the presence of MEKT1 (1 nM, 10 nM, 100 nM, 1 μM, or 10 μM) or DMSO (0.1%) as a control for 24 hours before assay. (b) AtT20 cells were incubated for 96 hours either in the presence of pioglitazone (1 nM, 10 nM, 100 nM, 1 μM, or 10 μM) or DMSO (0.1%) as a control for 24 hours before assay. (c) AtT20 cells were incubated for 96 hours either in the presence of rosiglitazone (1 nM, 10 nM, 100 nM, 1 μM, or 10 μM) or DMSO (0.1%) as a control for 24 hours before assay. Data are expressed as percentages (100%) of control. (d) Effects of MEKT1 on mRNA expression of m*Pttg* dose-dependently. AtT20 cells were treated with MEKT1 (1 nM, 10 nM, 100 nM, 1 μM, or 10 μM) or 0.1% DMSO (vehicle control) for 24 hours. (e) Effects on MEKT1 (10 μM) on AtT20 cell apoptosis. Each point indicates mean ± SEM ($n = 4$). NS stands for "not significant."

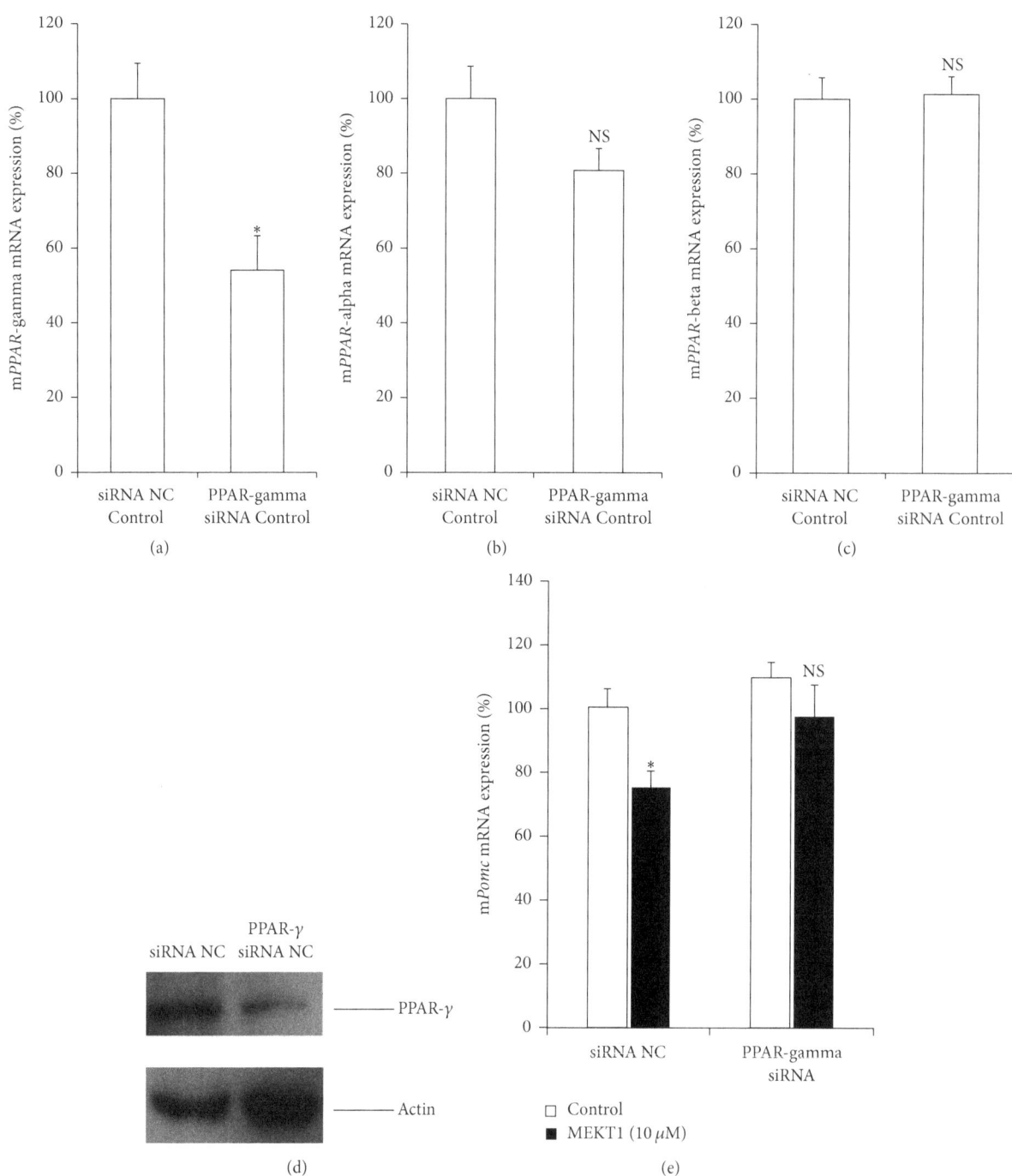

FIGURE 5: Involvement of PPAR-γ in the MEKT1 effects on *Pomc* mRNA expression. Effects of PPAR-γ knockdown by its siRNA on (a) *PPAR-γ* mRNA expression, (b) *PPAR-α* mRNA expression, and (c) *PPAR-β* mRNA expression. AtT20 cells transiently transfected with siRNA (negative control; NC or PPAR-γ) for 48 hours were incubated with 0.1% DMSO (control) for 24 hours. Results are expressed as percentages of each control. Each point represents mean ± SEM ($n = 4$). *$P < 0.05$ versus basal negative control siRNA. NS stands for "not significant." (d) Effects of PPAR-γ knockdown by its siRNA on the PPAR-γ protein expression. (e) Effects of PPAR-γ knockdown by its siRNA on the *Pomc* mRNA expression. AtT20 cells transiently transfected with siRNA (negative control; NC or PPAR-γ) for 48 hours were incubated in the presence of either MEKT1 (10 μM) or 0.1% DMSO (control) for 24 hours, respectively. Data are expressed as percentages (100%) of control. Each point represents mean ± SEM ($n = 4$). NS stands for "not significant." *$P < 0.05$ versus negative control siRNA at 10 μM MEKT1.

transcription factors are known to bind to NurRE, TpitRE, and NBRE, respectively, on the *Pomc* promoter [25, 31, 33], we next analyzed the influence of MEKT1 on the interaction between Nur77/Nurr1 and NurRE, Tpit and TpitRE,

and Nur77 and NBRE on its promoter of by ChIP assay using primers comprising NurRE, TpitRE, and NBRE (Figure 10(a)). As shown in Figures 10(b)–10(d), MEKT1 significantly suppressed the interaction between Nur77/Nurr1 and

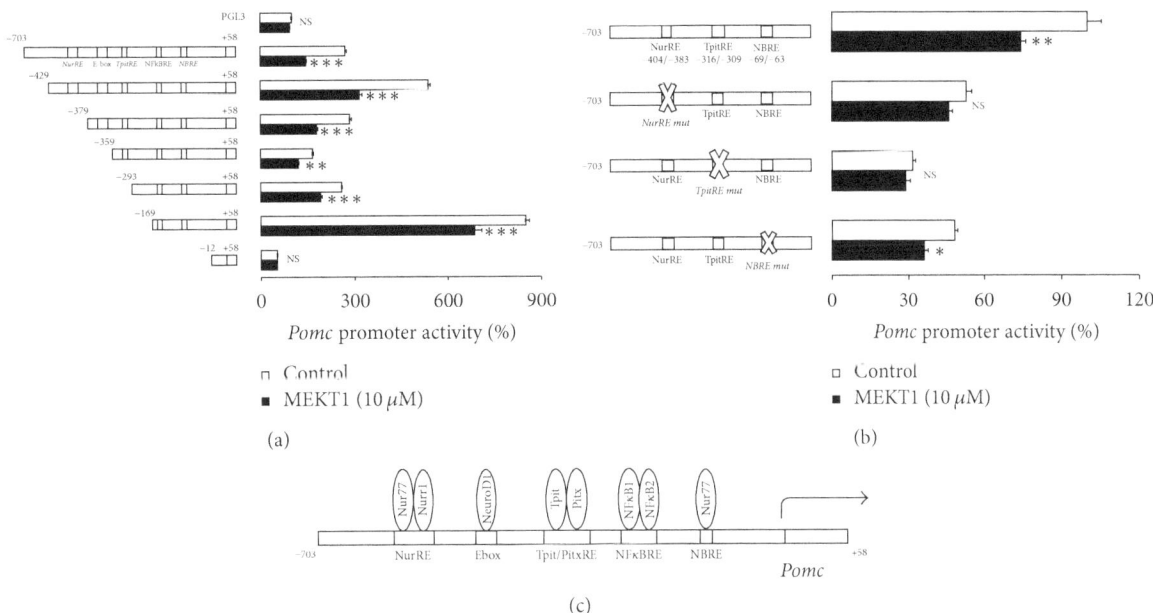

FIGURE 6: Effects of MEKT1 on *Pomc* promoter deletion mutants and role of NurRE, TpitRE, and NBRE on MEKT1-mediated effect on *Pomc* promoter activity in AtT20 cells. (a) MEKT1-mediated effect on *Pomc* promoter deletion mutants. AtT20 cells transiently transfected with 300 ng rPomc-Luc (−703/+58-luc) or each deletion mutant reporter plasmid (−429/+58-Luc, −379/+58-Luc, −359/+58-Luc, −293/+58, −169/+58, and +12/+58) and 100 ng pRSV-β-gal were incubated in the presence (10 μM) or absence of MEKT1 for 24 hours before the luciferase assay. Data are expressed as percentages of each control (100% in pGL3-Basic). (b) MEKT1-mediated effect on *Pomc* promoter activity using NurRE mut, TpitRE mut, and NBRE mut. AtT20 cells transiently transfected with 300 ng rPomc-Luc (−703/+58-luc) or NurRE mut (rPomc-Luc- NurRE -Mut), TpitRE mutant (rPomc-Luc- TpitRE -Mut), NBRE mutant of *Pomc* promoter (rPomc-Luc- NBRE -Mut) of *Pomc* full length promoter and 150 ng pRSV-β-gal were incubated in the presence (10 μM) or absence of MEKT1 for 24 hours before the luciferase assay. Data are expressed as percentages of each control (100% in rPomc-Luc). Data represent mean ± SEM ($n = 4$). NS denotes "not significant." $^*P < 0.05$, $^{**}P < 0.01$, and $^{***}P < 0.001$ versus control. (c) Graphical representation of responsive elements on the promoter of *Pomc* and transcription factors which bind to the responsive elements of *Pomc* promoter.

NurRE, Tpit and TpitRE, and Nur77 and NBRE on the *Pomc* promoter (24 hours), while it did not affect their interaction when IgG control was used. These data suggest that MEKT1 specifically inhibited their protein-DNA interactions.

4. Discussion

More than a decade ago, PPAR-γ agonist has been discovered as a new therapeutic medication for Cushing's disease [11, 12, 22]. Furthermore, it was reported that the PPAR-γ agonists rosiglitazone and pioglitazone target pituitary tumors *in vitro* and *in vivo* in Cushing's disease [11, 12, 22, 34, 35]. In the present study, we found that MEKT1 significantly suppressed the *Pomc* mRNA expression (Figure 1) and *Pomc* promoter activity after 24 hours of treatment at 10 μM (Figure 2). In addition, comparing the effects of the three PPAR-γ agonists MEKT1, rosiglitazone, and pioglitazone on ACTH secretion in AtT20 cells (Figure 3), it was clearly shown that MEKT1 more significantly suppressed the *Pomc* expression and the ACTH secretion than rosiglitazone and pioglitazone. However, Heaney et al. [12] showed that rosiglitazone can suppress *Pomc* promoter activity significantly after 48 hours. Taken together it was shown that MEKT1 is more effective than rosiglitazone and pioglitazone in suppressing *Pomc* expression. It was also determined that the potency of MEKT1

was much greater than rosiglitazone in HEK293 cells [36]. We also confirmed using PPAR-γ siRNA that the MEKT1-mediated effect on *Pomc* expression was mediated via PPAR-γ.

However, the negative regulatory mechanism of the *Pomc* transcription by PPAR-γ is still unknown. Therefore, we also attempted to elucidate the molecular mechanism of the MEKT1-mediated suppression of *Pomc* transcription regulation. To clarify the molecular mechanism, we firstly demonstrated the effects of MEKT1 on *Pomc* promoter deletion mutants of different lengths −703/+58 (full length), −429/+58, −379/+58, −359/+58, −169/+58, and −12/+58, which possess different responsive elements (Figure 6). Moreover, although we also examined the effects of MEKT1 on the promoter activity of *Pomc* using −62/+12 deletion mutants (data not shown), we did not observe any MEKT1-mediated suppression of *Pomc* promoter activity, most likely due to the lack of NurRE/TpitRE/NBRE elements. This experiment showed the importance of the responsive elements NurRE, TpitRE, and NBRE in the MEKT1-mediated suppression of *Pomc* promoter activity. In this study, we first demonstrated the molecular mechanism of the PPAR-γ-mediated negative regulation of *Pomc*.

Moreover, it is already established that Nur77/Nurr1, NeuroD1, Tpit, Pitx, NFκB1, and NFκB2 are important

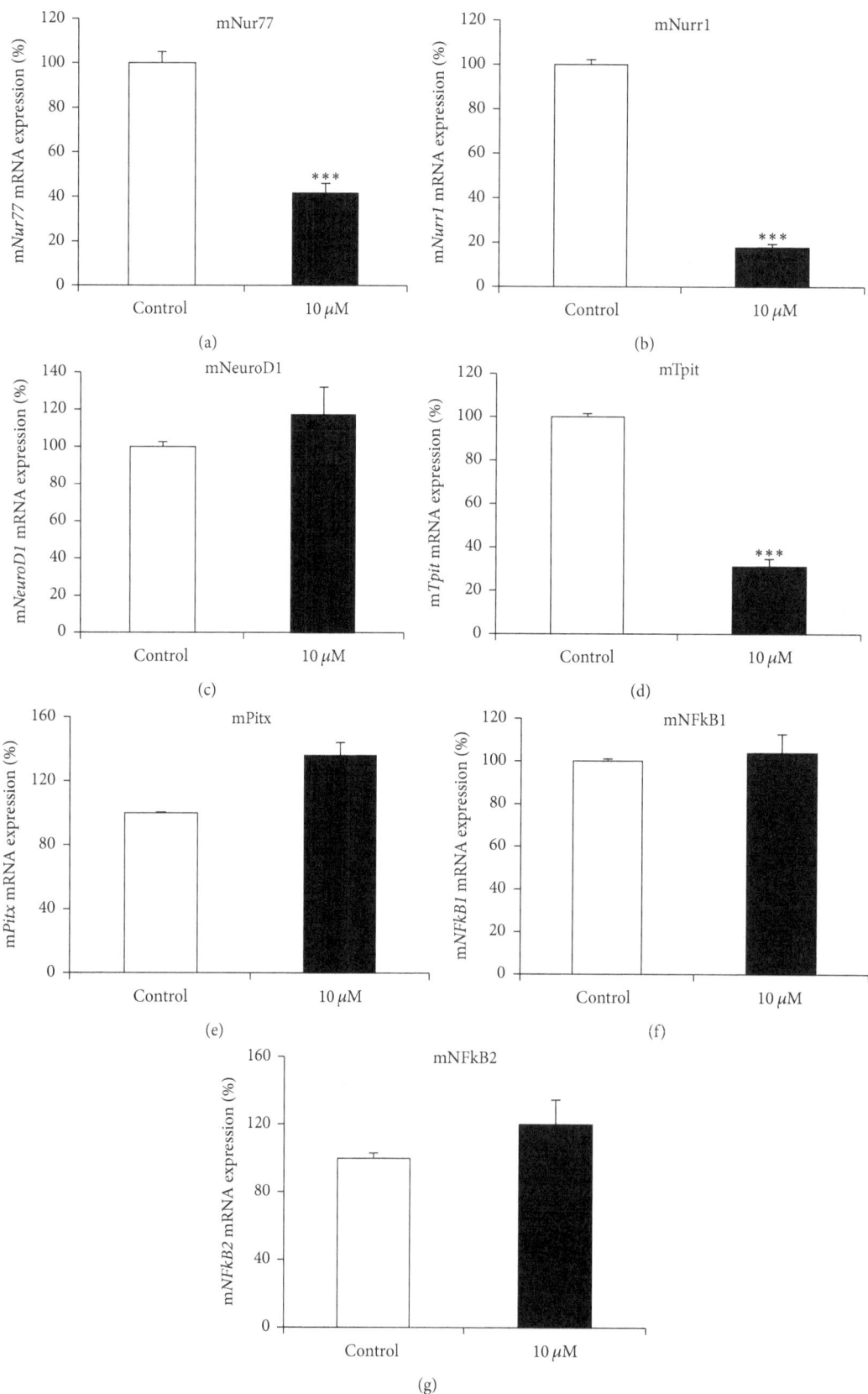

FIGURE 7: MEKT1-mediated effects on the mRNA expression of mouse *Nur77*, *Nurr1*, *NeuroD1*, *Tpit*, *Pitx*, *NFkB1*, and *NFkB2* in AtT20 cells. AtT20 cells treated with MEKT1 (10 μM) or 0.1% DMSO (vehicle control) for 24 hours. (a) *Nur77* mRNA expression, (b) *Nurr1* mRNA expression, (c) *NeuroD1* mRNA expression, (d) *Tpit* mRNA expression, (e) *Pitx* mRNA expression, (f) *NFκB1* mRNA expression, and (g) *NFκB2* mRNA expression. Data are expressed as percentages (100%) of control. Data represent mean ± SEM ($n = 4$). ***$P < 0.001$ versus control.

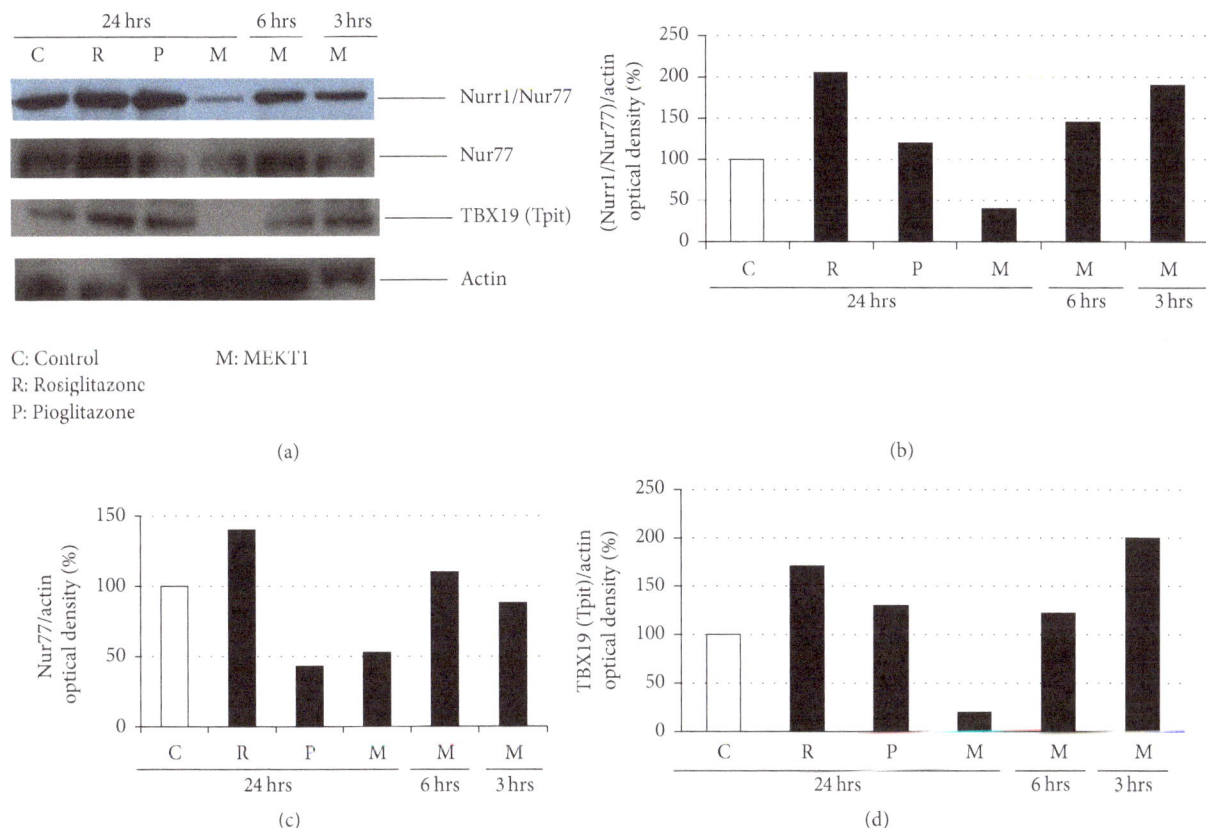

FIGURE 8: Effects of MEKT1 (time dependently), rosiglitazone, and pioglitazone on Nurr1, Nur77, and Tpit protein expression. (a) AtT20 cells treated with MEKT1 (M) at 10 μM for 24 hours, 6 hours, and 3 hours, rosiglitazone (R) at 10 μM for 24 hours, and pioglitazone (P) at 10 μM for 24 hours, or 0.1% DMSO as control (C) for 24 hours. Optical density (OD) of Nurr1/Nur77 was shown in figure (b), Nur77 in figure (c), and TBX19 (Tpit) in figure (d). OD of Nurr1/Nur77, Nur77, and TBX19 (Tpit) were normalized by OD of actin. Results are expressed as percentages of control (100%).

transcription factors for *Pomc* expression [25, 26, 33, 37–40]. Therefore, we next examined the effects of MEKT1 on these transcription factors. Although *Nur77*, *Nurr1*, and *Tpit* mRNA expression and Nur77, Nurr1, and Tpit protein expression were significantly suppressed by MEKT1 in AtT20 cells, *NeuroD1*, *Pitx*, *NFκB1*, and *NFκB2* mRNA expression were not affected by MEKT1 (Figures 7(a)–7(g), and 8). Therefore, it was predicted that the MEKT1-mediated suppression of *Nur77*, *Nurr1*, and *Tpit* mRNA expression was possibly implicated in the MEKT1-mediated suppression of *Pomc* transcription and Pomc translation. Since several transcription factor binding sites are present on the *Pomc* promoter [40], simultaneous interactions among these regulatory elements are needed for *Pomc* transcription in the pituitary [41]. The proximal binding sequence termed NBRE (−69/−63) is known to be bound by the Nur77 monomer [31, 33] and the distal NurRE, composed of two inverted NBRE related sites (−404/−397 and −390/−383) is recognized to be bound by the Nur77/Nurr1 heterodimer or Nur77 homodimer. Compared to the proximal NBRE, distal NurRE responds to Nur77 in much stronger fashion [31, 33, 40].

In addition, NF-κB RE (−151/−142) [39, 40], Tpit/PitxRE (−316/−309 and −302/−297) [32, 40], and E-box (−377/−370) [29, 38, 40] are known to be involved in regulation of *Pomc*.

Based on these data, we again examined the transcriptional activity of the site directed mutation of NurRE (NurRE mut), TpitRE (TpitRE mut), and NBRE (NBRE mut). NurRE and TpitRE mutants completely abolished the MEKT1-mediated suppressive effect of the *Pomc* promoter activity. Therefore, it can be assumed that NurRE and TpitRE are the most important responsive elements for the MEKT1-mediated suppression of the *Pomc* promoter activity. Although NBRE mutant partially abolished the MEKT1-mediated suppressive effect due to the weak interaction of Nur77 monomer and NBRE [31], it is still noteworthy that MEKT1 significantly inhibited the interaction between Nur77 and NBRE on *Pomc* promoter in the ChIP assay (Figure 10). To verify the importance of transcriptional factors Nur77, Nurr1, and Tpit, we also performed an overexpression experiment and observed that the MEKT1-mediated suppression of *Pomc* promoter activity was attenuated by the Nur77 and Tpit overexpression (Figure 9).

5. Conclusion

We can conclude as shown in Figure 11 that Nur77/Nurr1 heterodimer binding element NurRE (−383/−404), Tpit responsive element TpitRE (−309/−316), and Nur77 monomer

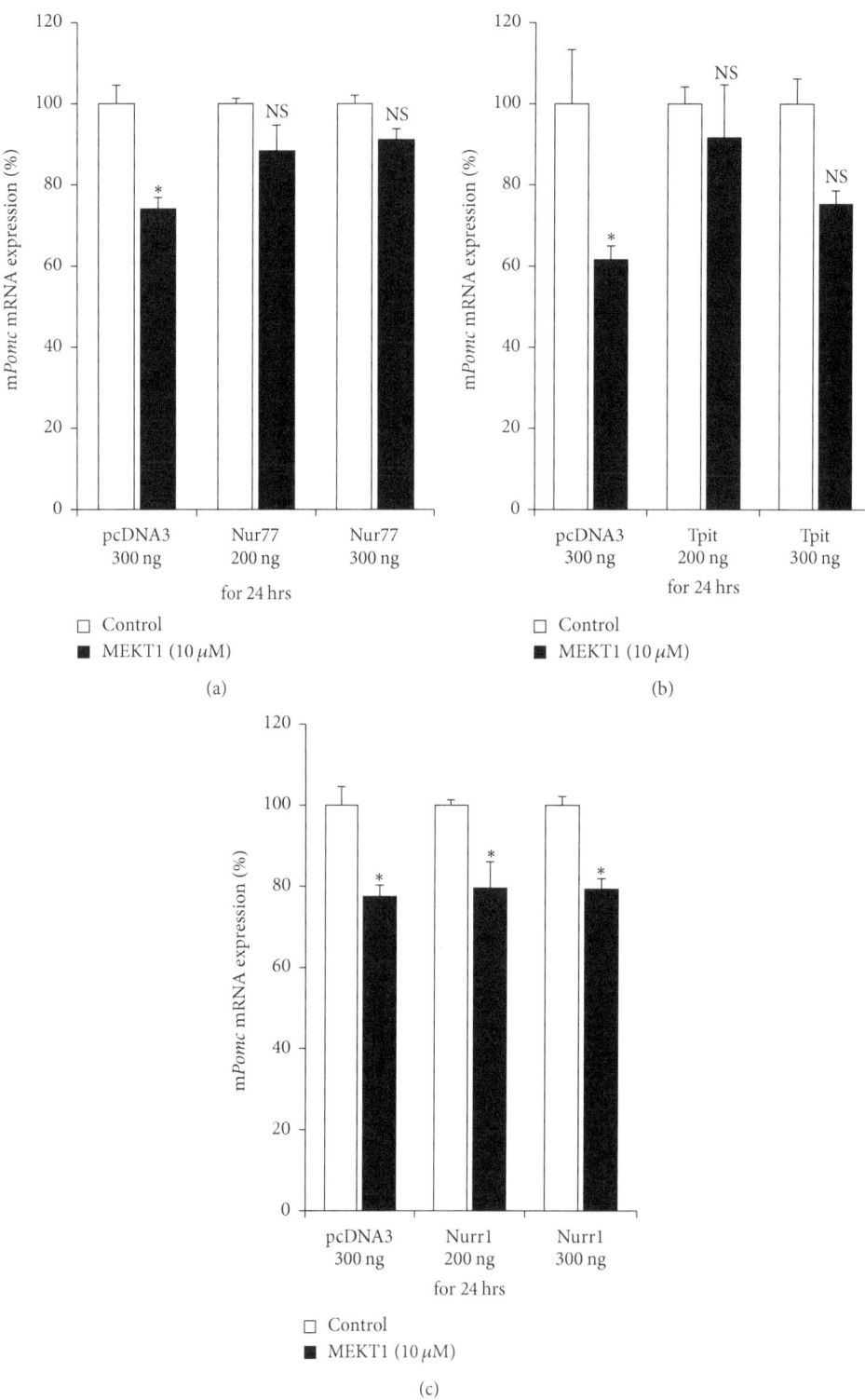

FIGURE 9: Effects of Nur77, Tpit, and Nurr1 overexpression on MEKT1-mediated effect of *Pomc* mRNA expression. (a) Nur77 overexpression effect on the MEKT1-mediated suppression of *Pomc* mRNA expression in AtT20 cells. AtT20 cells transiently transfected with pcDNA3 and Nur77 overexpression plasmid were incubated either in the presence of MEKT1 at $10\,\mu$M or DMSO at 0.1% (control) for 24 hours. (b) Tpit overexpression effect on the MEKT1-mediated suppression of *Pomc* mRNA expression. AtT20 cells transiently transfected with pcDNA3 and Tpit overexpression plasmid were incubated either in the presence of MEKT1 at $10\,\mu$M or DMSO at 0.1% (control) for 24 hours. (c) Nurr1 overexpression on the MEKT1-mediated suppression of *Pomc* mRNA expression. AtT20 cells transiently transfected with pcDNA3 and Nurr1 overexpression plasmid were incubated either in the presence of MEKT1 at $10\,\mu$M or DMSO at 0.1% (control) for 24 hours. Each overexpression plasmid volume was maintained to 300 ng adding pcDNA3 empty vector. Results are expressed as percentages (100%) of control. Data represent mean $\pm$ SEM ($n = 4$). NS stands for "not significant." $^*P < 0.05$, versus control.

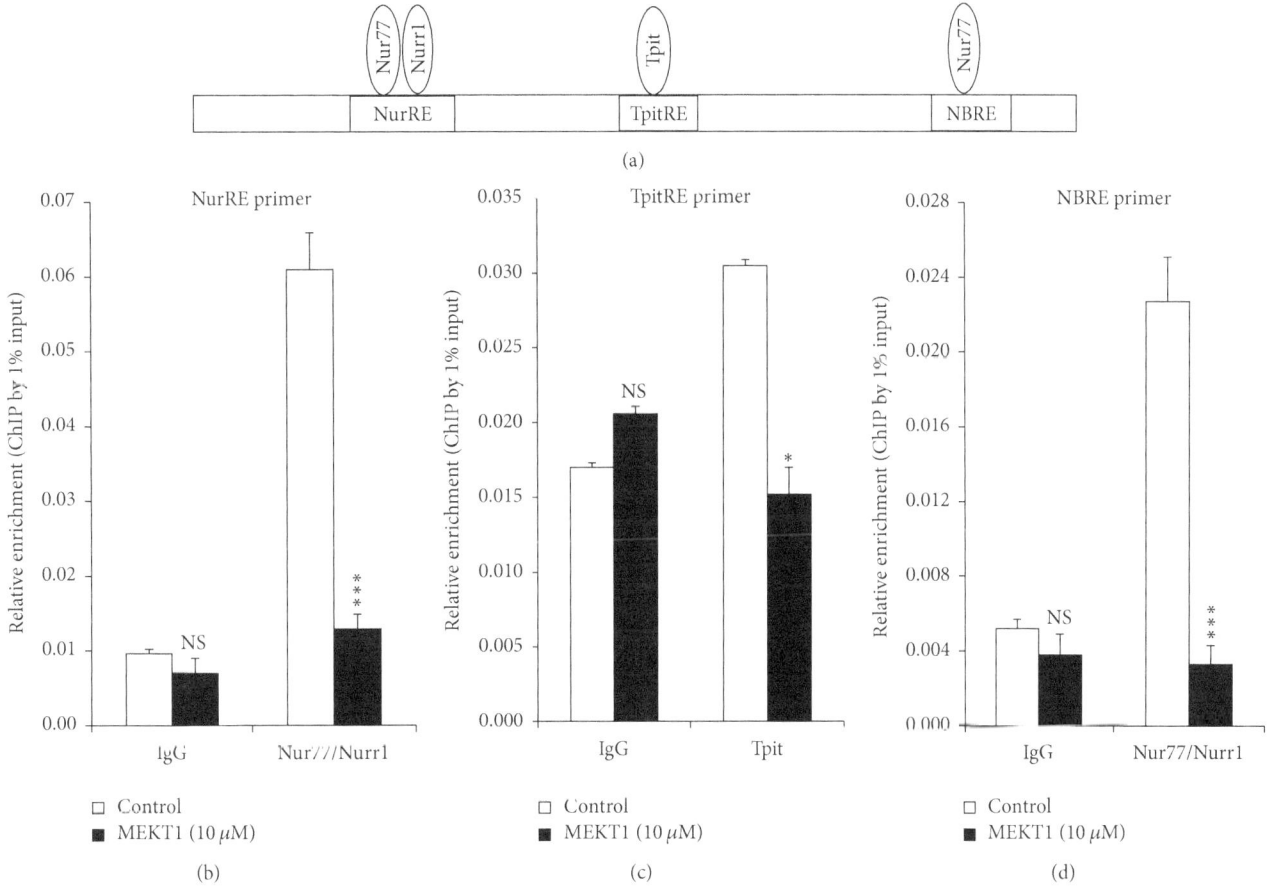

FIGURE 10: Effects of MEKT1 on the interaction between Nur77/Nurr1 and NurRE, Tpit and TpitRE, and Nur77 and NBRE on *Pomc* promoter (a) in AtT20 cells. Effects of MEKT1 on the interaction between Nur77/Nurr1 and NurRE (b), Tpit and TpitRE (c), and Nur77 and NBRE (d) on *Pomc* promoter examined by ChIP assay using NurRE, TpitRE, and NBRE primer. ChIP assay was carried out using digested chromatin extracted from the cells cultured in the presence of either 10 μM MEKT1 or 0.1% DMSO (control) for 24 hours. Chromatin fragments were immunoprecipitated either by normal rabbit IgG (negative control), anti-Nur77/Nurr1 antibody, or anti-Tpit (anti TBX 19) antibody. Purified DNA was analyzed by qPCR using primers specific for NurRE, TpitRE, and NBRE containing sequence on *Pomc* promoter. The primer product sizes of NurRE, TpitRE, and NBRE were 211 bp, 146 bp, and 102 bp, respectively. Immunoprecipitated DNA was amplified by qPCR and then normalized to the values obtained after amplification of immunoprecipitated 1% input DNA. Data represent mean ± SEM ($n = 3$). NS means "not significant." $^{*}P < 0.05$, and $^{***}P < 0.001$ significantly different from the level of control group.

responsive element NBRE (−63/−69) play important roles in *Pomc* expression [32, 33, 40]. When PPAR-γ agonist MEKT1 is added, it decreases *Nur77*, *Nurr1*, and *Tpit* mRNA expression and then probably inhibits the interactions between Nur77/Nurr1 heterodimer and NurRE, Tpit and TpitRE, and Nur77 monomer and NBRE (Figure 11), resulting the suppression of *Pomc* expression. Therefore, it can be concluded that Nur77, Nurr1, and Tpit probably play a vital role in the MEKT1-mediated negative regulation of *Pomc* expression in AtT20 cells. Furthermore, although clinical trials of MEKT1 are needed to determine its drug efficacy in the future, it can be speculated that MEKT1 is much more effective than the previously recognized PPAR-γ agonists, rosiglitazone, and pioglitazone, for the suppression of *Pomc* expression/ACTH secretion from our *in vitro* research. Therefore, MEKT1 could be a novel therapeutic medication for the treatment of Cushing's disease.

Conflicts of Interest

The authors have declared that no conflicts of interest exist.

Authors' Contributions

Conceptualization was done by Rehana Parvin, Hiroyuki Miyachi, and Akira Sugawara. Data analysis was done by Rehana Parvin, Atsushi Yokoyama, and Akiko Saito-Hakoda. Investigation was done by Rehana Parvin, Susumu Suzuki, Hiroki Shimada, Erika Noro, and Kyoko Shimizu. Writing and original draft preparation were by Rehana Parvin. Writing, review, and editing were by Akira Sugawara. Rehana Parvin and Erika Noro contributed equally to this work.

Acknowledgments

The authors thank Ms. Ikuko Sato for her technical assistance. This work was supported by Japan Society for the Promotion

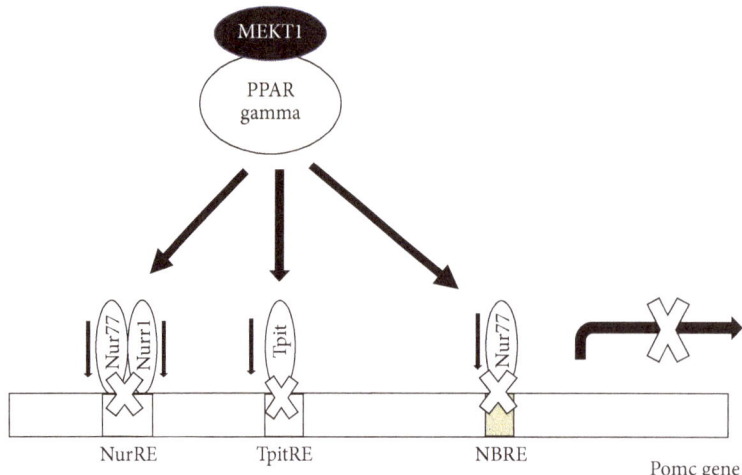

Figure 11: Involvement of Nur77, Nurr1, and Tpit transcription factors in the MEKT1 (PPAR-γ agonist)-mediated suppression of *Pomc*.

of Science (JSPS) KAKENHI Grant nos. 16H03252 (for Akira Sugawara), 16K15492 (for Akira Sugawara), and 15K09420 (for Akiko Saito-Hakoda).

Supplementary Materials

Figure S1: MEKT1-mediated effect of *PPAR-γ* mRNA expression in AtT20 cells in a dose-dependent manner. AtT20 cells were treated with MEKT1 (1 nM, 10 nM, 100 nM, 1 μM, or 10 μM) or 0.1% DMSO (vehicle control) for 24 hours. Data are expressed as percentages (100%) of control. Data represent mean ± SEM ($n = 4$). $^{**}P < 0.01$ versus control. Figure S2: involvement of PPAR-γ in the MEKT1 effects on *Pomc* promoter activity. AtT20 cells transiently transfected with rPomc-luc, pRSV-β-gal, and siRNA (negative control; NC or PPAR-γ) for 48 hours were incubated in the presence of either MEKT1 (10 μM) or 0.1% DMSO (control) for 24 hours, respectively. Results are expressed as percentages (100%) of control. Each point represents mean ± SEM ($n = 4$). NS stands for "not significant." $^{**}P < 0.01$ versus negative control of siRNA at 10 μM MEKT1. Figure S3: MEKT1-mediated effects on the mRNA expression of Nur77, *Nurr1*, and *Tpit* in AtT20 cells are dose-dependent. (A) Dose-dependent effect of MEKT1 of *Nur77* mRNA expression. AtT20 cells were treated with MEKT1 (1 nM, 10 nM, 100 nM, 1 μM, or 10 μM) or 0.1% DMSO (vehicle control) for 24 hours. (B) Dose-dependent effect of MEKT1 on *Nurr1* mRNA expression. AtT20 cells were treated with MEKT1 (1 nM, 10 nM, 100 nM, 1 μM, or 10 μM) or 0.1% DMSO (vehicle control) for 24 hours. (C) Dose-dependent effect of MEKT1 on *Tpit* mRNA expression. AtT20 cells were treated with MEKT1 (1 nM, 10 nM, 100 nM, 1 μM, or 10 μM) or 0.1% DMSO (vehicle control) for 24 hours. Each point represents mean ± SEM ($n = 4$). Data are presented as percentages of control (100%). $^{*}P < 0.05$, $^{**}P < 0.01$, and $^{***}P < 0.001$ versus control. Figure S4: effects of Nur77, Tpit, and Nurr1 overexpression on MEKT1-mediated effect of promoter activity of *Pomc*. AtT20 cells were transiently transfected with pcDNA3 and Nur77 overexpression plasmid in (A),

Tpit overexpression plasmid in (B), and Nurr1 overexpression plasmid in (C) and 135 ng of rPomc-Luc and 65 ng of pRSV-β-gal were incubated either in the presence of MEKT1 at 10 μM or DMSO at 0.1% (control) for 24 hours before the luciferase assay. Each overexpression plasmid volume was maintained at 300 ng adding pcDNA3 empty vector. Results are expressed as percentages of each control (100%). Data represent mean ± SEM ($n = 4$). NS means "not significant." $^{*}P < 0.05$ versus control. *(Supplementary Materials)*

References

[1] S. Tyagi, P. Gupta, A. S. Saini, C. Kaushal, and S. Sharma, "The peroxisome proliferator-activated receptor: a family of nuclear receptors role in various diseases," *Journal of Advanced Pharmaceutical Technology & Research*, vol. 2, no. 4, pp. 236–240, 2011.

[2] C. K. Glass and M. G. Rosenfeld, "The coregulator exchange in transcriptional functions of nuclear receptors," *Genes & Development*, vol. 14, no. 2, pp. 121–141, 2000.

[3] S. Villapol, "Roles of peroxisome proliferator-activated receptor gamma on brain and peripheral inflammation," *Cellular and Molecular Neurobiology*, vol. 38, no. 1, pp. 121–132, 2018.

[4] R. Kapadia, J.-H. Yi, and R. Vemuganti, "Mechanisms of anti-inflammatory and neuroprotective actions of PPAR-gamma agonists," *Frontiers in Bioscience*, vol. 13, no. 5, pp. 1813–1826, 2008.

[5] A. Goto, Y. Tagawa, Y. Kimura, A. Kogame, Y. Moriya, and N. Amano, "Influence of the pharmacokinetic profile on the plasma glucose lowering effect of the PPARγ agonist pioglitazone in Wistar fatty rats," *Biopharmaceutics & Drug Disposition*, vol. 38, no. 6, pp. 381–388, 2017.

[6] E. Filipova, K. Uzunova, K. Kalinov, and T. Vekov, "Effects of pioglitazone therapy on blood parameters, weight and BMI: a meta-analysis," *Diabetology & Metabolic Syndrome*, vol. 9, no. 1, 2017.

[7] R. M. Evans, G. D. Barish, and Y.-X. Wang, "PPARs and the complex journey to obesity," *Nature Medicine*, vol. 10, no. 4, pp. 355–361, 2004.

[8] S. M. Ferrari, G. Materazzi, E. Baldini et al., "Antineoplastic effects of PPARγ agonists, with a special focus on thyroid

cancer," *Current Medicinal Chemistry*, vol. 23, no. 7, pp. 636–649, 2016.

[9] A. Sugawara, A. Uruno, K. Matsuda et al., "Effects of PPARγ agonists against vascular and renal dysfunction," *Current Molecular Pharmacology*, vol. 5, no. 2, pp. 248–254, 2012.

[10] F. Bogazzi, D. Russo, M. T. Locci et al., "Peroxisome proliferator-activated receptor (PPAR)γ is highly expressed in normal human pituitary gland," *Journal of Endocrinological Investigation*, vol. 28, no. 10, pp. 899–904, 2005.

[11] A. P. Heaney, "Novel pituitary ligands: peroxisome proliferator activating receptor-γ," *The Pituitary Society*, vol. 6, no. 3, pp. 153–159, 2003.

[12] A. P. Heaney, M. Fernando, W. H. Yong, and S. Melmed, "Functional PPAR-γ receptor is a novel therapeutic target for ACTH-secreting pituitary adenomas," *Nature Medicine*, vol. 8, no. 11, pp. 1281–1287, 2002.

[13] Y. Ma, X. W. Xia, C. B. Su, and Y. G. Kong, "Distribution and expression of peroxisome proliferator activated receptor gamma in human pituitary adenomas," *Zhongguo Yi Xue Ke Xue Yuan Xue Bao*, vol. 28, pp. 375–377, 2006.

[14] A. B. Bicknell, "The tissue-specific processing of pro-opiomelanocortin," *Journal of Neuroendocrinology*, vol. 20, no. 6, pp. 692–699, 2008.

[15] L. Jeannotte, M. A. Trifiro, R. K. Plante, M. Chamberland, and J. Drouin, "Tissue-specific activity of the pro-opiomelanocortin gene promoter," *Molecular and Cellular Biology*, vol. 7, no. 11, pp. 4058–4064, 1987.

[16] J. H. Eberwine and J. L. Roberts, "Glucocorticoid regulation of pro-opiomelanocortin gene transcription in the rat pituitary," *The Journal of Biological Chemistry*, vol. 259, no. 4, pp. 2166–2170, 1984.

[17] J. Drouin, M. A. Trifiro, R. K. Plante, M. Nemer, P. Eriksson, and O. Wrange, "Glucocorticoid receptor binding to a specific DNA sequence is required for hormone-dependent repression of pro-opiomelanocortin gene transcription," *Molecular and Cellular Biology*, vol. 9, no. 12, pp. 5305–5314, 1989.

[18] F. P. Giraldi, C. Scaroni, E. Arvat et al., "Effect of protracted treatment with rosiglitazone, a PPARγ agonist, in patients with Cushing's disease," *Clinical Endocrinology*, vol. 64, no. 2, pp. 219–224, 2006.

[19] K. Winczyk, J. Kunert-Radek, A. Gruszka, M. Radek, H. Lawnicka et al., "Effects of rosiglitazone–peroxisome proliferators-activated receptor gamma (PPARgamma) agonist on cell viability of human pituitary adenomas in vitro," *Neuro Endocrinology Letters*, vol. 30, pp. 107–110, 2009.

[20] J. Kreutzer, I. Jeske, B. Hofmann, I. Blumcke, and R. Fahlbusch, "No effect of the PPAR-gamma agonist rosiglitazone on ACTH or cortisol secretion in Nelson's syndrome and Cushing's disease in vitro and in vivo," *Clinical Neuropathology*, vol. 28, pp. 430–439, 2009.

[21] M. Mannelli, G. Cantini, G. Poli et al., "Role of the PPAR-γ System in Normal and Tumoral Pituitary Corticotropic Cells and Adrenal Cells," *Neuroendocrinology*, vol. 92, no. 1, pp. 23–27, 2010.

[22] A. P. Heaney, "PPAR-gamma in Cushing's disease," *Pituitary*, vol. 7, pp. 265–269, 2004.

[23] D. Suri and R. E. Weiss, "Effect of pioglitazone on adrenocorticotropic hormone and cortisol secretion in Cushing's disease," *The Journal of Clinical Endocrinology & Metabolism*, vol. 90, no. 3, pp. 1340–1346, 2005.

[24] S. Bilodeau, S. Vallette-Kasic, Y. Gauthier et al., "Role of Brg1 and HDAC2 in GR trans-repression of the pituitary POMC gene and misexpression in Cushing disease," *Genes & Development*, vol. 20, no. 20, pp. 2871–2886, 2006.

[25] B. Lamolet, A.-M. Pulichino, T. Lamonerie et al., "A pituitary cell-restricted T box factor, Tpit, activates POMC transcription in cooperation with Pitx homeoproteins," *Cell*, vol. 104, no. 6, pp. 849–859, 2001.

[26] G. Poulin, B. Turgeon, and J. Drouin, "NeuroD1/β2 contributes to cell-specific transcription of the proopiomelanocortin gene," *Molecular and Cellular Biology*, vol. 17, no. 11, pp. 6673–6682, 1997.

[27] A. Uruno, A. Saito-Hakoda, A. Yokoyama et al., "Retinoic acid receptor-α up-regulates proopiomelanocortin gene expression in AtT20 corticotroph cells," *Endocrine Journal*, vol. 61, no. 11, pp. 1105–1114, 2014.

[28] A. Saito-Hakoda, A. Uruno, A. Yokoyama et al., "Effects of RXR agonists on cell proliferation/apoptosis and ACTH Secretion/Pomc expression," *PLoS ONE*, vol. 10, no. 12, Article ID 0141960, 2015.

[29] R. Parvin, A. Saito-Hakoda, H. Shimada et al., "Role of NeuroD1 on the negative regulation of Pomc expression by glucocorticoid," *PLoS ONE*, vol. 12, no. 4, Article ID e0175435, 2017.

[30] A. Yamashita, T. Takada, K.-I. Nemoto, G. Yamamoto, and R. Torii, "Transient suppression of PPARγ directed ES cells into an osteoblastic lineage," *FEBS Letters*, vol. 580, no. 17, pp. 4121–4125, 2006.

[31] A. Philips, S. Lesage, R. Gingras et al., "Novel dimeric Nur77 signaling mechanism in endocrine and lymphoid cells," *Molecular and Cellular Biology*, vol. 17, no. 10, pp. 5946–5951, 1997.

[32] I. Murakami, S. Takeuchi, T. Kudo, S. Sutou, and S. Takahashi, "Corticotropin-releasing hormone or dexamethasone regulates rat proopiomelanocortin transcription through Tpit/Pitx-responsive element in its promoter," *Journal of Endocrinology*, vol. 193, no. 2, pp. 279–290, 2007.

[33] M. Maira, C. Martens, A. Philips, and J. Drouin, "Heterodimerization between members of the Nur subfamily of orphan nuclear receptors as a novel mechanism for gene activation," *Molecular and Cellular Biology*, vol. 19, no. 11, pp. 7549–7557, 1999.

[34] M. Fleseriu and S. Petersenn, "Medical management of Cushing's disease: What is the future?" *The Pituitary Society*, vol. 15, no. 3, pp. 330–341, 2012.

[35] B. Ambrosi, C. Dall'Asta, S. Cannavo et al., "Effects of chronic administration of PPAR-gamma ligand rosiglitazone in Cushing's disease," *European Journal of Endocrinology*, vol. 151, no. 2, pp. 173–178, 2004.

[36] M. Ohashi, T. Oyama, I. Nakagome et al., "Design, synthesis, and structural analysis of phenylpropanoic acid-type PPARγ-selective agonists: Discovery of reversed stereochemistry-activity relationship," *Journal of Medicinal Chemistry*, vol. 54, no. 1, pp. 331–341, 2011.

[37] T. E. Wilson, T. J. Fahrner, M. Johnston, and J. Milbrandt, "Identification of the DNA binding site for NGFI-B by genetic selection in yeast," *Science*, vol. 252, no. 5010, pp. 1296–1300, 1991.

[38] M. Therrien and J. Drouin, "Cell specific helix-loop-helix factor required for pituitary expression of the pro-opiomelanocortin gene," *Molecular and Cellular Biology*, vol. 13, no. 4, pp. 2342–2353, 1993.

[39] K. P. Karalis, M. Venihaki, J. Zhao, L. E. Van Vlerken, and C. Chandras, "NF-κB participates in the corticotropin-releasing, hormone-induced regulation of the pituitary proopiomelanocortin gene," *The Journal of Biological Chemistry*, vol. 279, no. 12, pp. 10837–10840, 2004.

[40] B. G. Jenks, "Regulation of proopiomelanocortin gene expression: an overview of the signaling cascades, transcription factors, and responsive elements involved," *Annals of the New York Academy of Sciences*, vol. 1163, pp. 17–30, 2009.

[41] M. Therrien and J. Drouin, "Pituitary pro-opiomelanocortin gene expression requires synergistic interactions of several regulatory elements," *Molecular and Cellular Biology*, vol. 11, no. 7, pp. 3492–3503, 1991.

11

Fatty Acids of CLA-Enriched Egg Yolks can Induce Transcriptional Activation of Peroxisome Proliferator-Activated Receptors in MCF-7 Breast Cancer Cells

Aneta A. Koronowicz,[1] Paula Banks,[1] Adam Master,[2] Dominik Domagała,[1] Ewelina Piasna-Słupecka,[1] Mariola Drozdowska,[1] Elżbieta Sikora,[1] and Piotr Laidler[3]

[1]*Department of Human Nutrition, Faculty of Food Technology, University of Agriculture in Krakow, Balicka 122, 30-149 Krakow, Poland*

[2]*Department of Biochemistry and Molecular Biology, Medical Centre for Postgraduate Education, Marymoncka 99, 01-813 Warsaw, Poland*

[3]*Department of Medical Biochemistry, Jagiellonian University Medical College, Kopernika 7, 31-034 Krakow, Poland*

Correspondence should be addressed to Aneta A. Koronowicz; aneta.koronowicz@gmail.com

Academic Editor: Daniele Fanale

In our previous study, we showed that fatty acids from CLA-enriched egg yolks (EFA-CLA) reduced the proliferation of breast cancer cells; however, the molecular mechanisms of their action remain unknown. In the current study, we used MCF-7 breast cancer cell line to determine the effect of EFA-CLA, as potential ligands for peroxisome proliferator-activated receptors (PPARs), on identified in silico PPAR-responsive genes: *BCAR3*, *TCF20*, *WT1*, *ZNF621*, and *THRB* (transcript TR*β*2). Our results showed that EFA-CLA act as PPAR ligands with agonistic activity for all PPAR isoforms, with the highest specificity towards PPAR*γ*. In conclusion, we propose that EFA-CLA-mediated regulation of PPAR-responsive genes is most likely facilitated by *cis9,trans11CLA* isomer incorporated in egg yolk. Notably, EFA-CLA activated PPAR more efficiently than nonenriched FA as well as synthetic CLA isomers. We also propose that this regulation, at least in part, can be responsible for the observed reduction in the proliferation of MCF-7 cells treated with EFA-CLA.

1. Introduction

Peroxisome proliferator-activated receptors (PPARs) are ligand-activated transcription factors. Various fatty acids and their metabolic derivatives act as natural ligands for PPARs [1]. Some, including linoleic, linolenic, and arachidonic acid, were found to activate PPARs even at micromolar, physiologically relevant concentrations [2]. Hydroxyoctadecadienoic acids (HODEs), products of linoleic acid oxidation as well as arachidonic acid metabolite 15d-PGJ2 (15-deoxyprostaglandin J2), were also associated with PPAR activation [3, 4].

It has been suggested that ligand-dependent activation of PPARs results in the inhibition of proliferation in some model

cancer cell lines [5–7]. In particular, PPAR*γ* isoform was shown to reduce cancer cell proliferation as well as regulate cell differentiation, activate apoptosis, and inhibit angiogenesis [8–10]. Specifically, the administration of specific PPAR*γ* agonist resulted in cells arrest in G1 phase and inhibited proliferation [5, 11]. However, available literature presents also contradicting results. In some studies, PPAR*γ* specific antagonist, T0070907, significantly reduced proliferation and migration of breast cancer cells [12, 13].

Conjugated linoleic acid (CLA) term includes several isomers of linoleic acid, with two main isomers: *cis9,trans11* (80–90% of total CLA) and *trans10,cis12*. Available literature shows that CLA acts as a potent PPARs ligand and is involved in modulating lipid metabolism through PPAR-mediated pathways [14]. However, data showed isomer-specific activity of CLA; specifically, *cis9,trans11* was characterized as PPAR agonist [15, 16] while *trans10,cis12* was shown to inhibit the activity of synthetic PPAR agonists [15]. In addition, studies showed potential antitumor properties of *cis9,trans11* [17–20] while the opposite effect was observed for *trans10,cis12* isomer [18].

PPARs act as transcription factors and regulate the expression of dependent genes by binding to their PPREs. A significant number of genes regulated by PPARs have been described; however, the list is not exhaustive and is constantly being updated as new results are being published from both experimental data and bioinformatics analyses of promoter regions and PPRE consensus sequences. In the current study, we applied those tools to identify in silico PPRE selected genes involved in cell cycle progression and proliferation. Next, we analyzed the effect of synthetic *cis9,trans11CLA* and *trans10,cis12CLA* isomers as well as a mixture of fatty acids extracted from CLA-enriched and nonenriched egg yolk on the expression of those genes. To the best of our knowledge, our study is the first to address the effect of CLA incorporated in fatty acids profile of the egg yolk; we expect that activity of CLA in such a "bioorganic" form may deviate from that of a synthetic form. The presence of other fatty acids in an egg yolk, which themselves can act as potential ligands for PPARs, may modulate the action of CLA; therefore, our data may be particularly important for the evaluation of CLA-enriched food products.

2. Materials and Methods

2.1. Production of CLA-Enriched Egg Yolks. Production of CLA-enriched egg yolks was performed in the National Research Institute of Animal Production in Krakow (Poland), as per the recommendations of the Local Animal Ethics Committee (approval number: 851/2011) as described previously [21]. Eggs were collected and stored at 4°C, and yolks were separated from albumen, homogenized, and frozen at −20°C. Samples were then lyophilized and again stored at −20°C until further analyses.

2.2. Extraction and Analysis of Fatty Acids Composition. Lipids from control and CLA-enriched yolks were extracted by using modified Folch method [22] as described previously [23]. 10 mg of each lipid extract was subjected to saponification with 0.5 M KOH/methanol followed by methylation with 14% (v/v) BF3/methanol and extraction with hexane. Fatty acid methyl esters (FAME) were analyzed by GC/MS as described previously [23].

2.3. CLA Isomers and Agonists/Antagonists of PPAR. *cis9,trans11CLA* and *trans10,cis12CLA* isomers (Nu-Chek Prep, USA) were dissolved in ethanol and stored under nitrogen in −20°C and were introduced to cell cultures at final concentrations corresponding to their concentration in CLA-enriched egg yolk: *cis9,trans11* at 30 μM and *trans10,cis12* at 12 μM.

The synthetic agonists and antagonists for PPARα (WY14643 and GW-6471), PPARδ (GW-0742 and GSK0660),

and PPARγ (pioglitazone (PIO), troglitazone, and T0070907) were prepared as per appropriate protocols of the manufacturer. Respective concentrations were selected based on their EC/IC50 characteristics and confirmed for MCF-7 cell line using Cytotoxicity LDH Test (Roche, Poland).

2.4. Cell Cultures. The human breast adenocarcinoma cell line MCF-7 (ATCC® HTB22TM) was purchased from the American Type Culture Collections. Cells were cultured in appropriate medium (Sigma-Aldrich, MO, USA) as per the ATCC protocol with the addition of 10% FBS (Sigma-Aldrich, MO, USA).

Cell viability was determined by Crystal Violet Assay (Sigma-Aldrich, MO, USA).

2.5. Fatty Acid Treatment. The experimental medium contained MEM supplemented with 10% FBS and appropriate treatment: (a) fatty acids extract at 0.5 mg/mL from CLA-enriched egg yolks (EFA-CLA), (b) fatty acids extract at 0.5 mg/mL from nonenriched egg yolks (EFA), (c) *cis9,trans11* synthetic isomer (final concentration at 35 μM), (d) *trans10,cis12* synthetic isomer (final concentration at 13 μM), (e) untreated cell control (empty control, EC), and (f) negative control (NC; ethanol at final concentration 0.1%). Synthetic PPARs agonists and antagonist were used as positive controls for PPARα (10 μM WY14643 and 10 μM GW-6471), PPARδ (2 μM GW-0742 and 1 μM GSK0660), and PPARγ (40 μM PIO, 10 μM troglitazone, and 10 μM T0070907). Each treatment included 3 biological and 3 technical replicates.

2.6. Plasmids. PPAR expression vectors were prepared using Gateway® Cloning System (Thermo Fisher, USA). Briefly, PPARA (CR456547_1), PPARD (NM_006238.4), and PPARG (NM_015869.4) ORF sequences were synthesized, optimized for the expression in human cells, and cloned into the pDONR221 Entry Vectors (GeneArt, Thermo Fisher, USA). Subsequently, the ORF inserts were transferred into pcDNA6.2/N-EmGFP-DEST Destination Vectors (Thermo Fisher, USA) under the CMV promoter control via Clonase II Recombination Reaction.

2.7. Cell Transfection with PPAR Encoding Plasmids. Cell lines with PPARA, PPARD, and PPARG overexpression were obtained via transient transfections with pcDNA6.2/N-EmGFP-DEST vectors containing respective human PPAR ORF. MCF-7 cells were seeded on 12-well plates, at 1×10^5 cells per well. 24 h after seeding, cells were transiently transfected with 1.5 μg of PPAR encoding plasmids using Lipofectamine (Thermo Fisher Scientific, MA, USA) in OPTI-MEM medium (Thermo Fisher Scientific, MA, USA). 24 h after transfection, the growth medium was replaced with selective MEM medium with 10% FBS and 5.0 μg/mL blasticidin (BioShop, Canada). Transfected cells were cultured until confluency.

Real-time PCR and western blot method were performed to confirm the presence of PPAR plasmids after transfection (Figure S1 and Table S2, Supplementary Material available online at https://doi.org/10.1155/2017/2865283).

2.8. Transfection with PPRE Plasmid. Cell lines overexpressing, respectively, PPARA, PPARD, and PPARG were seeded on the 12-well plates, at 1×10^5 cells per well. After 24 hours, cells were transfected with $0.7\,\mu$g X3 PPRE-TK-luc plasmid (Cat. # 1015, Addgene, USA) and $0.7\,\mu$g pRL control (Cat. # E2261, Promega, WI, USA) using Lipofectamine (Thermo Fisher Scientific, MA, USA) in OPTI-MEM medium (Thermo Fisher Scientific, MA, USA).

2.9. Dual-Luciferase Assay. 24 hours after transfection with PPRE plasmid, the medium was again replaced with MEM medium containing 10% FBS and appropriate experimental treatment as described above. 24 hours after treatment, cells were harvested for isolation of protein luciferase.

The luciferase protein (*Photinus pyralis* and *Renilla reniformis*) detection was performed using Dual-Luciferase® Reporter Assay System (Promega, WI, USA) in GloMax® 20/20 Single Tube Luminometer (Promega, WI, USA), according to the manufacturer's instructions.

2.10. In Silico Selection and Experimental Confirmation of PPAR-Dependent Genes (PPAR-Responsive mRNAs). PPAR-responsive genes were selected in silico by searching for peroxisome proliferator hormone response elements (PPREs, AGGTCANAGGTCA) within promoters and/or $5'$-cis-regulatory regions of the promoters of genes involved in cell cycle progression and proliferation. This search was performed with NCBI Gene and Blast tools.

Experimentally, 24 hours after transfection with respective PPAR plasmids, the medium was replaced with MEM medium containing 10% FBS and appropriate experimental treatment as described above. 48 hours after treatment, cells were harvested for mRNA isolation and RT-qPCR.

2.11. RNA Isolation, cDNA Synthesis, and RT-qPCR Analysis. Total RNA was isolated from the cells using RNA isolation kit for cell cultures (A&A Biotechnology, Poland). Reverse transcription was performed on $1\,\mu$g of total RNA using Maxima First-Strand cDNA Synthesis kit for RT-qPCR (Thermo Scientific, MA, USA). Quantitative verification of genes was performed using CFX96 Touch™ Real-Time PCR Detection System instrument (Bio-Rad, CA, USA) and SYBR Green Precision Melt Supermix kit (Bio-Rad, CA, USA). Conditions of individual PCR reactions were optimized for given pair of oligonucleotide primers (Table S1, Supplementary Material). Basic conditions were as follows: 95°C for 10 min, 45 PCR cycles at 95°C, 15 s; 59°C, 15 s; 72°C, 15 s, followed by melting curve analysis (65–97°C with 0.11°C ramp rate and 5 acquisitions per 1°C). Results were normalized using at least two reference genes (*GAPDH*, *HPRT1*, *ACTB*, or *HSP90AB1*) and were calculated using the $2^{-\Delta\Delta^C T}$ method [24].

2.12. Protein Isolation and Western Blot Analysis. Cell lysis was carried out using Cell Lysis Buffer (Cell Signaling Technology, MA, USA) as per the manufacturer's protocol. Total protein quantification was performed using Pierce BCA™ Protein Assay Kit (Thermo Fisher Scientific, MA, USA).

Each western blot followed a similar procedure. Protein extract was separated on a polyacrylamide gel and

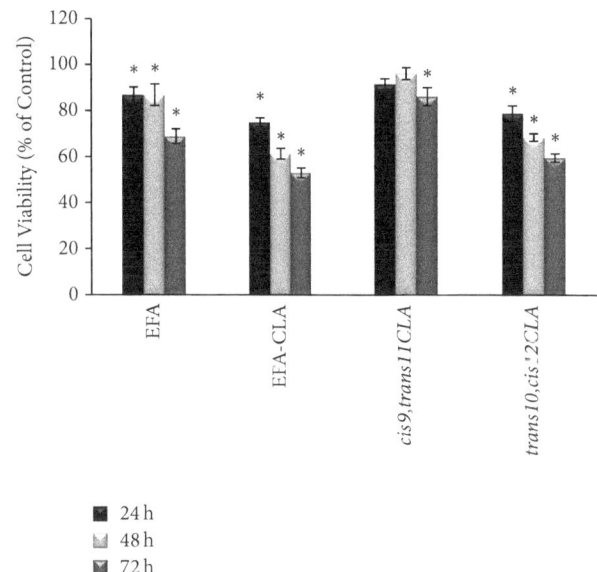

■ 24 h
▨ 48 h
▨ 72 h

FIGURE 1: Effect of fatty acids on MCF-7 cells viability. Values are expressed as means ± SD for $N \geq 9$, standardized to control (NC) as 100%. Statistical significance was based on t-test; $^*p < 0.05$ versus control.

transferred to a nitrocellulose filter (Bio-Rad, CA, USA) by wet electroblotting. Subsequently, the immobilized proteins were incubated with appropriate primary antibody, specific for PPARα (SAB2101852), PPARγ (SAB2101853), and PPARδ (AV32880) as well as for selected in silico WT1 (SAB2102716), THRB (AV36994), and TCF20 (SAB2106444) from Sigma-Aldrich, MO, USA, or β-actin (#8457) or β-tubulin (#2128) from Cell Signaling Technology, MA, USA. Finally, appropriate secondary antibody conjugated with horseradish peroxidase (#7074, Cell Signaling Technology, MA, USA) was applied. Detection was executed by chemiluminescence, using Clarity™ Western ECL Substrate (Bio-Rad, CA, USA). To remove the antibodies from the membrane, we used western blot stripping buffer (Thermo Scientific, MA, USA).

2.13. Statistical Analysis. All experiments were performed at least three independent times and measured in triplicate. Shapiro-Wilk's test was applied to assess normality of distribution. An independent samples t-test was applied to compare unpaired means between two groups. $p < 0.05$ was considered statistically significant. All analyses were performed using Statistica ver.12 (StatSoft, Tulsa, OK, USA).

3. Results

3.1. Cell Viability. Treatment with both extracts, EFA and EFA-CLA, decreased viability of MCF-7 breast cancer cell line compared to the control; however, the effect of EFA-CLA was more evident compared to EFA. 72 h after treatment, cell viability in EFA-CLA-treated group decreased by 50% while for EFA the decrease in viability reached 32% (Figure 1). Treatment with synthetic *trans10,cis12CLA* reduced cell viability in a linear manner with incubation time, reaching 43%

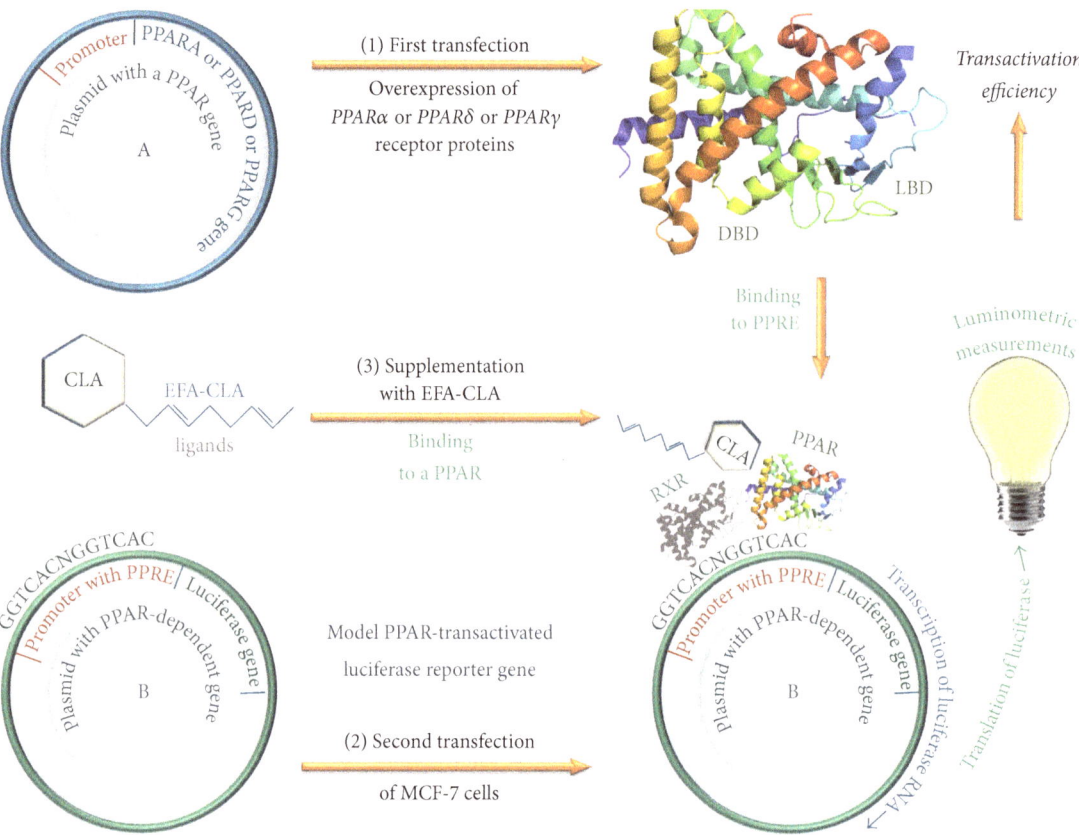

FIGURE 2: Experimental mechanism for studying the activity of EFA-CLA as a ligand for PPAR. DBD: DNA-binding domain specific for PPRE sequence in promoter regions of genes regulated by PPAR; LBD: ligand-binding domain (e.g., EFA-CLA).

at 72 h. The reductive effect of *cis9,trans11CLA* isomer was less evident and statistically significant only after 72 h (overall reduction in viability by 15%).

3.2. Effects of EFA-CLA on Transcriptional Activity of PPARs.

To analyze the activity and specificity of various CLAs as potential PPAR ligands, we applied the PPAR-dependent luciferase expression model (Figure 2). We used specific agonists and antagonists for each isoform of PPARs as positive controls. Our results confirmed the expected effects of selected agonists and antagonists (Figures 3(a)–3(c)). The effect of experimental FA extracts varied. Compared to the negative control, EFA-CLA significantly increased the activity of PPARα (202% of NC; $p < 0.05$; Figure 3(a)), PPARδ (187.10% of NC; $p < 0.01$; Figure 3(b)), and PPARγ (353% of NC; $p < 0.001$; Figure 3(c)). Compared to EFA extract, EFA-CLA also showed statistically significant activation of all PPAR isoforms (Figures 3(a)–3(c)). Synthetic *cis9,trans11* isomer also activated significantly all PPARs, PPARα (211% of NC; $p < 0.05$; Figure 3(a)), PPARδ (221.88% of NC; $p < 0.01$; Figure 3(b)), and PPARγ (237% of NC; $p < 0.01$; Figure 3(c)). *trans10,cis12CLA* isomer had little or no effect on the activation of PPARα and PPARδ (Figures 3(a) and 3(b)); however, it reduced the activity of PPARγ (85% of NC; $p < 0.05$; Figure 3(c)).

3.3. Selective Effect of FA on Transcriptional Activity of PPARs.

The selective effects of the studied FA as potential PPAR ligands are shown in Figures 4(a)–4(d). EFA-CLA was determined to be the most specific for PPARγ (3.5-fold increase in activity, $p < 0.001$; Figure 4(a)). EFA extract acted as an antagonist towards both PPARα and PPARδ, while it exhibited only negligible agonist activity on PPARδ (1.44-fold increase in activity, $p > 0.05$, Figure 4(b)). *cis9,trans11* isomer showed agonist properties towards all PPAR isoforms, with the strongest effect on PPARγ (2.37-fold increase in activity, $p < 0.005$; Figure 4(c)). *trans10,cis12* isomer showed no significant effect on transactivation of both PPARα and PPARδ ($p > 0.05$, Figure 4(d)), while it showed an antagonist activity towards PPARγ ($p < 0.01$, Figure 4(d)).

3.4. Prediction of Potential PPRE-Dependent Genes In Silico.

The prediction of potential PPRE-responsive genes was performed in silico. NCBI database was searched for the presence of specific PPRE (peroxisome proliferator response element) consensus sequences (AGGTCAAAGGTCA, AGGTCAGAGGTCA, AGGTCACAGGTCA, or AGGTCATAGGTCA) in the 5′ region of genes linked to oncogenesis and cell cycle (Figure 5). Seven genes were identified: *BCAR3, LZTS, SLC5A1, TCF20, WT1, ZNF621,* and *THRB* (transcript TRβ2), potentially regulated by PPARs (Table 1). *THRB*

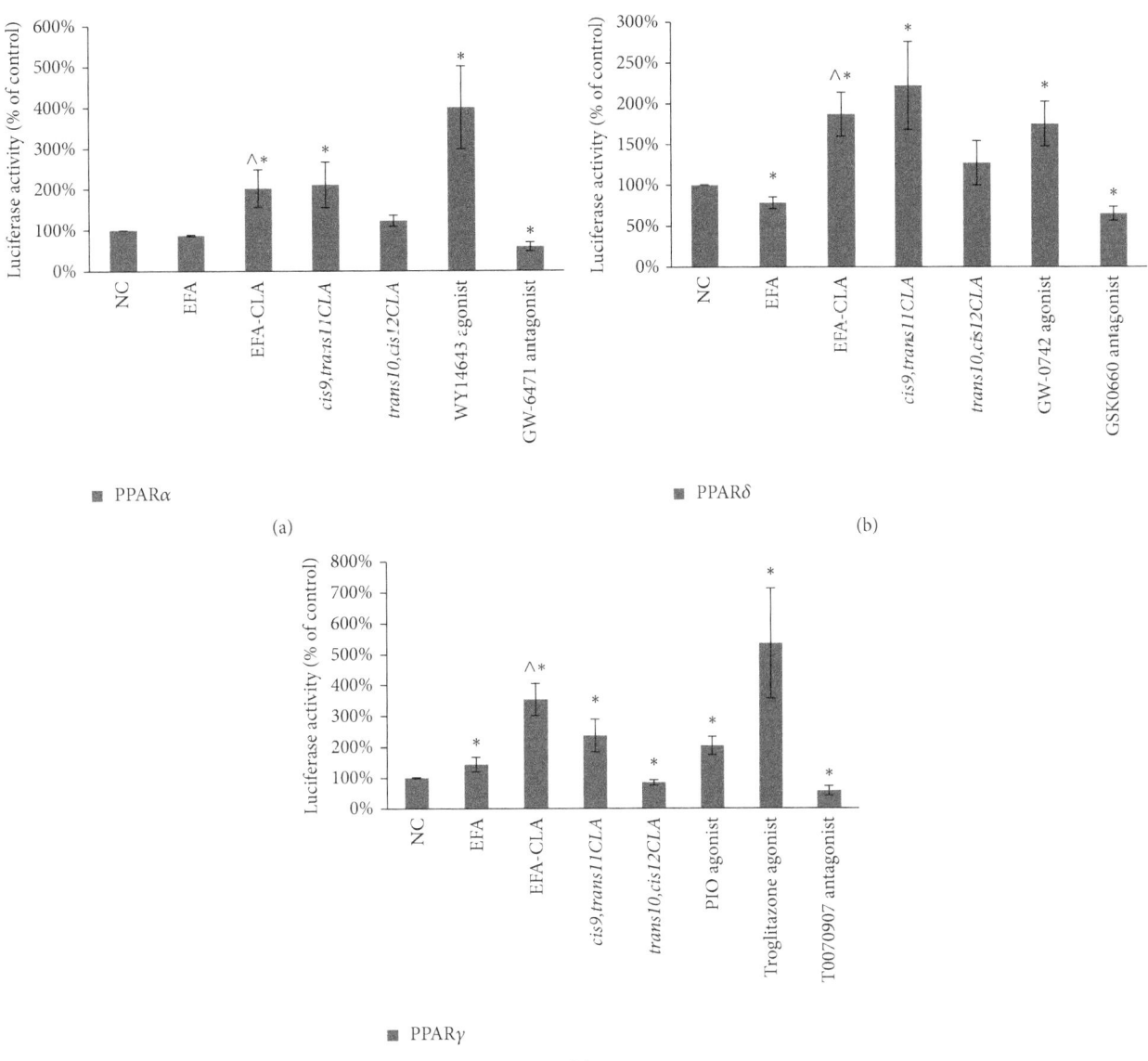

FIGURE 3: Effect of EFA-CLA on the activity of (a) PPARα, (b) PPARδ, and (c) PPARγ based on measured luciferase activity in dual-luciferase assay. *Values are expressed as means ± SEM for N ≥ 12, standardized to control (NC) as 100%. Statistical significance was based on t-test;* $^*p < 0.05$ *versus NC or* $^\wedge p < 0.05$ *versus EFA.*

TABLE 1: Identification of in silico putative PPAR-responsive genes.

Gene symbol	Transcript	Position	NCBI reference sequence
BCAR3	AGGTCAGAGGTCA	93663502–93663514	NC_000001.11
LZTS1	AGGTCAAAGGTCA	20248971–20248983	NC_000008.11
SLC5A1	AGGTCACAGGTCA	32033858–32033870	NC_000022.11
TCF20	AGGTCATAGGTCA	42271609–42271621	NC_000022.11
WT1	AGGTCAGAGGTCA	32470961–32470973 32470822–32470834	NC_000011.10
ZNF621	AGGTCAGAGGTCA	41052623–41052635	NC_000003.12
THRB (TRβ2)	AGGTCACAGGTCA	24169753–24169765	NC_000003.12

BCAR3: breast cancer antiestrogen resistance 3; *LZTS1*: leucine zipper putative tumor suppressor 1; *SLC5A*: solute carrier family 5 member 1; *TCF20*: transcription factor 20; *WT1*: Wilms tumor 1; *ZNF621*: zinc finger protein 621; *THRB*: thyroid hormone receptor beta.

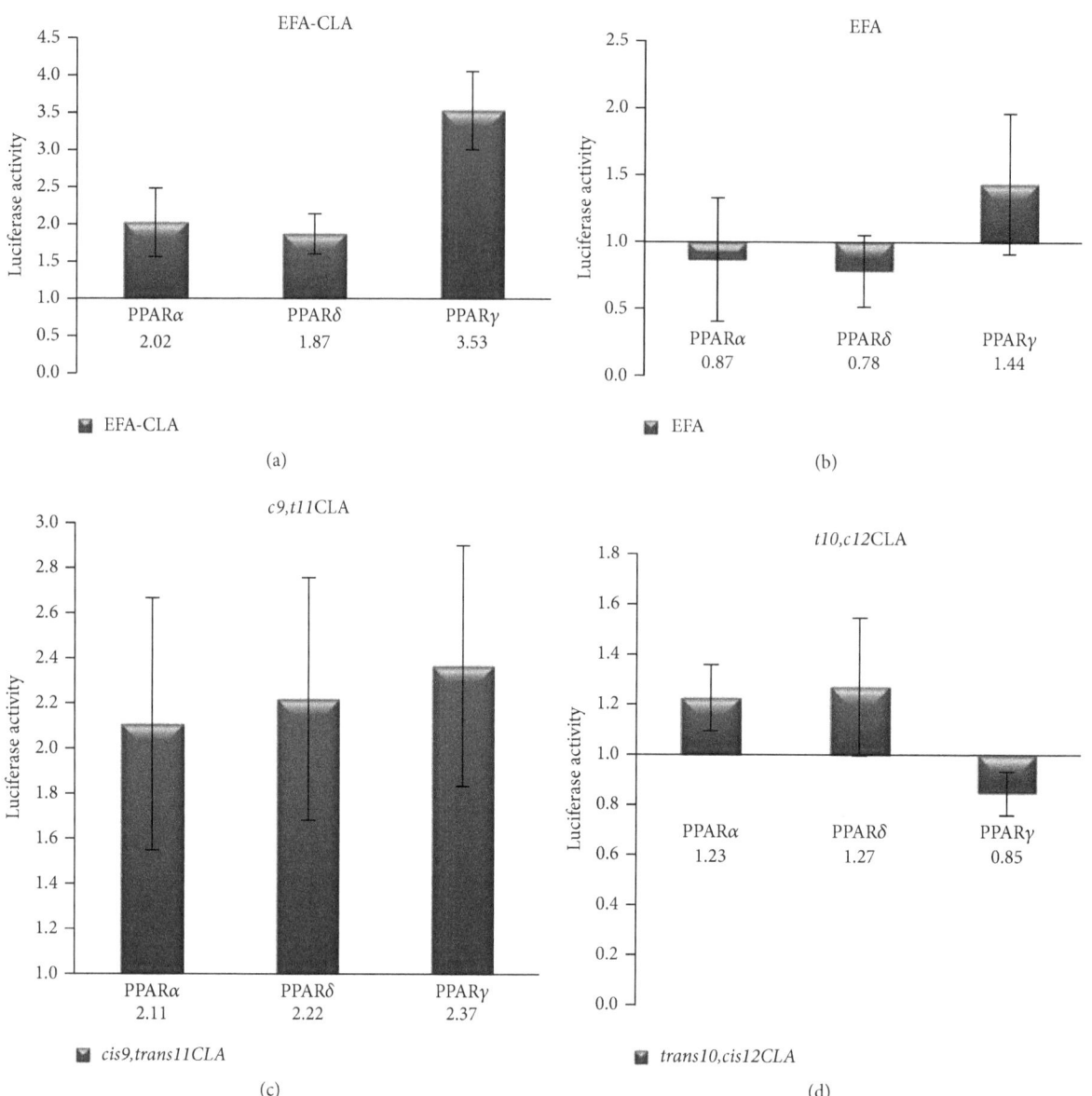

FIGURE 4: Selective effect of FA on PPARs expressed as fold difference versus control (100%), based on data from Figure 3. Values are expressed as means ± SEM for the $N \geq 12$.

gene was identified by the presence of the PPRE consensus sequence in a region of the alternative promoter for TRβ2 isoform (intron between the 4th and 5th exon). Among identified potential PPRE-dependent genes, few were selected for further experimental analyses, including *TCF20*, *WT1* *ZNF621*, and *THRB*.

3.5. Effects of EFA-CLA on the Expression of PPAR-Regulated Genes. Expression of selected PPAR-responsive genes (containing PPRE) has been tested in response to various experimental fatty acids as potential ligands for PPARA, PPARD, or PPARG. Our results showed both agonist and antagonist effects of studied experimental FA.

EFA-CLA added to the PPARγ-overexpressing cells elevated the expression of *TCF-20* over 3.2-fold and *ZNF621* over 3.1-fold, while decreasing the expression of *WT1* gene 1.2-fold. However, the latest may be explained, at least in part, from the fact that *WT1* gene is cotranscribed with interfering long, noncoding antisense RNA (WT1-AS) from the same bidirectional promoter. For cells overexpressing PPARδ, EFA-CLA treatment resulted in the elevated expression of *TCF-20* over 3-fold, while for the PPARα-overexpressing cells *ZNF621* gene was upregulated 1.8-fold.

The strongest enhancement of *TCF-20* expression (over 13-fold) was observed in PPARγ- and PPARδ-overexpressing cells after treatment with *trans10,cis12CLA*. Interestingly, the

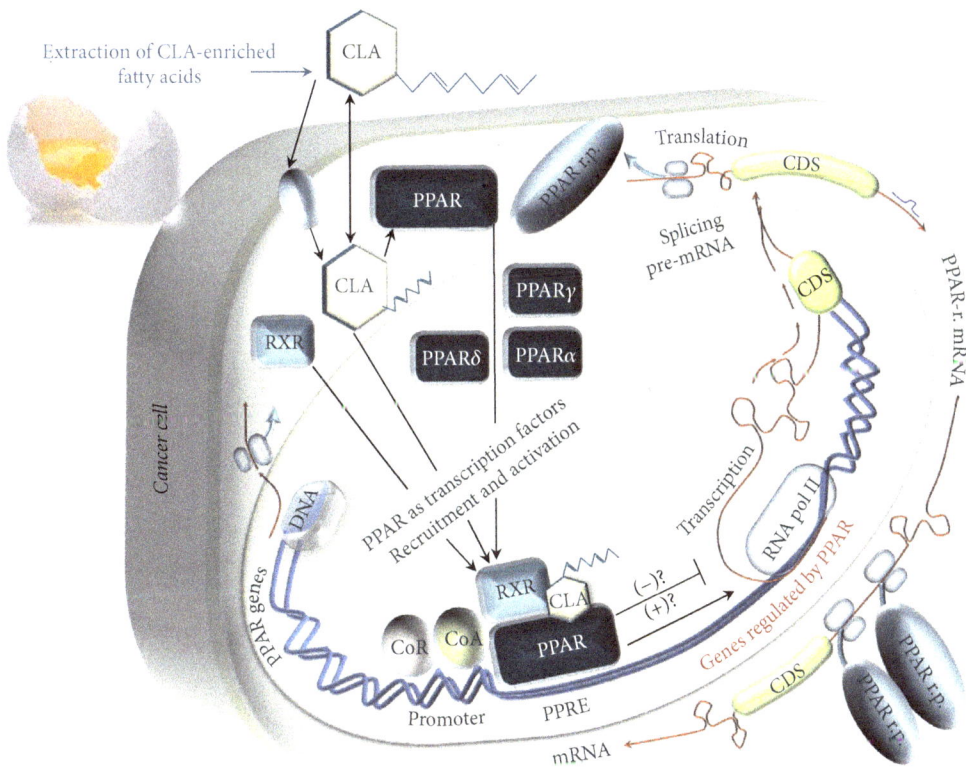

FIGURE 5: Molecular aspects of CLA-induced accumulation of PPAR-responsive transcripts. PPAR-r. mRNA: PPAR-regulated mRNAs; PPAR-r.p.: PPAR-regulated proteins; PPRE: peroxisome proliferator hormone response element (AGGTCANAGGTCA); RXR: retinoid X receptor; ORF: open reading frame (coding sequence).

expression of *THRB* (TRβ2 variant) gene was also strongly increased by the treatment with *trans10,cis12CLA* over 18.15-, 17.2-, and 7.9-fold in PPARδ-, PPARγ-, and PPARα-overexpressing cells, respectively, but not observed for EFA-CLA-treated cells. Those results show that the presence of other fatty acids in EFA-CLA mixture contributes to the overall effect of FA treatment.

It is clear that the expression of the selected genes (*TCF-20, WT1, ZNF621*, and *THRB*), which were identified for the first time in this work as putative PPAR-responsive genes, was altered in the presence of the used agents (Table 2) and that among them *TCF-20* was affected the most by EFA-CLA.

4. Discussion

Chicken egg enriched with conjugated linoleic acid (CLA) via feed modification meets the criteria of the functional food product. Based on Roberfroid's [25] classification, CLA-enriched egg can be considered as a conventional food product that is intended to be consumed as a part of a normal diet but is modified to contain biologically active substances, that is, CLA isomers. It has been shown to have a beneficial effect on physiological functions of the human body, in a way that goes beyond its nutritional value, specifically by lowering the risk of developing atherosclerosis [26]. Our previous

studies showed additional beneficial properties of CLA-enriched eggs in reducing proliferation of breast cancer and melanoma cells [23, 27]. The current manuscript supports those findings as our new results showed that fatty acids extract from CLA-enriched egg yolks (EFA-CLA) reduced the viability of MCF-7 breast cancer cell line (Figure 1). However, the molecular mechanism is not fully understood. Comparison of the effect on cancer cell proliferation between extracts from CLA-enriched and nonenriched egg yolks could lead to the conclusion that it is simply the result of the presence of CLA isomers incorporated in the egg yolk lipids. Available literature would support such a hypothesis as numerous studies showed an inhibitory effect, especially for *cis9,trans11CLA* isomer, on tumor cells [28–32]. Indeed, our analysis of FA profile of CLA-enriched egg yolk showed that *cis9,trans11CLA* was incorporated more efficiently (3 : 1 ratio) than *trans10,cis12* isomer [21] and therefore could predominate in EFA-CLA. Interestingly, comparison of the effect of synthetic CLA isomers with CLA-EFA from egg yolk showed the advantage of the latter in reducing cancer cell viability (Figure 1). The analysis of fatty acids profiles between enriched and nonenriched egg yolks revealed not only CLA incorporation but also unexpected, significant change in SFA/MUFA ratio, specifically an increase in total SFA concentration at the expense of MUFA. Thus, a question

TABLE 2: mRNA expression of PPARs-responsive genes in PPAR-transfected MCF-7 cells (with overexpression of PPARs) after treatment with experimental FA or specific agonist/antagonist of PPAR for 48 h.

Gene symbol	FC values ± SD					
	EFA versus NC	EFA-CLA versus NC	cis9,trans11CLA versus NC	trans10,cis12CLA versus NC	Agonist versus NC	Antagonist versus NC
(A) mRNA expression of PPARα-dependent genes						
TCF-20	-1.00^* ± 0.02	1.02 ± 0.03	1.10 ± 0.24	1.70^* ± 0.14	1.24 ± 0.14	-3.09^* ± 0.23
WT1	-1.32 ± 0.11	-1.49^* ± 0.11	-1.86^* ± 0.07	-1.31 ± 0.23	1.34 ± 0.26	-2.11 ± 0.18
ZNF621	1.36 ± 0.16	1.80^* ± 0.20	-2.51^* ± 0.04	1.09 ± 0.19	-1.06 ± 0.18	-1.20 ± 0.24
THRB (TRβ2)	2.49 ± 0.08	1.15 ± 0.12	1.74^* ± 0.09	7.98^* ± 0.34	2.54^* ± 0.22	-1.77^* ± 0.00
(B) mRNA expression of PPARδ-dependent genes						
TCF-20	2.03^* ± 0.04	3.08^* ± 0.03	7.05^* ± 0.11	13.02^* ± 0.08	-1.43^* ± 0.01	2.36 ± 0.08
WT1	1.18 ± 0.26	-1.38^* ± 0.03	-1.52^* ± 0.05	1.71 ± 0.29	1.90^* ± 0.04	1.81^* ± 0.01
ZNF621	1.37^* ± 0.03	-1.29^* ± 0.02	1.09 ± 0.16	-1.26 ± 0.19	-1.76 ± 0.11	-1.23^* ± 0.03
THRB (TRβ2)	1.61^* ± 0.02	1.33^* ± 0.01	6.67^* ± 0.09	18.15^* ± 0.11	1.90^* ± 0.04	1.81^* ± 0.01
(C) mRNA expression of PPARγ-dependent genes						
TCF-20	2.09^* ± 0.03	3.21^* ± 0.04	6.66^* ± 0.16	13.48^* ± 0.09	1.92^* ± 0.03	2.00^* ± 0.01
WT1	-1.02 ± 0.04	-1.24 ± 0.06	-1.32^* ± 0.03	-1.02 ± 0.08	1.48 ± 0.07	-1.47^* ± 0.03
ZNF621	2.99^* ± 0.01	3.12^* ± 0.17	-1.13 ± 0.05	1.46 ± 0.07	5.97^* ± 0.20	3.76^* ± 0.10
THRB (TRβ2)	1.09 ± 0.01	1.14 ± 0.01	9.96^* ± 0.10	17.22^* ± 0.13	-1.91^* ± 0.01	-1.58^* ± 0.00

FC: fold change; NC: negative control. Agonist/antagonist: for PPARα, WY14643/GW-6471; for PPARδ, GW-0742/GSK0660; for PPARγ, troglitazone/T0070907. * $p < 0.05$.

arises of whether it is an individual or combined effect of CLA and modified SFA/MUFA ratio in enriched egg yolks on MCF-7 cell line [23]. We observed that results of CLA-EFA are most likely achieved by the effect of both: incorporated CLA isomers and other fatty acids in eggs modified organically through hens' diet [23]; however, this issue requires further research.

It has been shown that PPAR agonists have different properties for individual PPAR isoforms, with different absorption and distinctive gene expression profiles. To our knowledge, this is the first study focused on the effect of FA from CLA-enriched egg yolks on transcriptional activation of PPARs (PPARα, PPARγ, and PPARδ). All experiments included as controls synthetic CLA isomers as well as standard agonists and antagonists of different PPARs. Our results showed that EFA-CLA extract exhibits the properties of agonists for all PPAR isoforms (Figures 3(a)–3(c)); however, those properties seem to be most selective towards PPARγ (Figure 4). Interestingly, PPARγ has been associated with the greatest impact on cancer cell proliferation, survival, and differentiation, and its ligands are associated with anticancer properties [33, 34]. In addition, as observed for EFA-CLA, transactivation of PPAR receptors is more effective compared to fatty acids extracted from a nonenriched egg yolk (EFA) (Figures 3(a)–3(c)). Since cis9,trans11CLA isomer showed PPAR agonist activity (Figures 3(a)–3(c)) and since this isomer was 3-fold more efficiently incorporated into egg yolks than trans10,cis12CLA [23], it could be hypothesized that cis9,trans11CLA plays a significant role in EFA-CLA-mediated activation of PPARs.

The effect of synthetic CLA isomers provided us with important information about their specificity. While cis9,trans11 isomer acted as a PPAR agonist (Figures 3(a)–3(c)), the antagonist effect was observed for trans10,cis12 isomer, specifically on PPARγ (Figure 3(c)). Available literature is consistent with our results. cis9,trans11 isomer has been reported to inhibit cell growth [15, 16] showing antitumor properties [17–20]. It has been found as well that the presence of trans10,cis12 isomer may abrogate the antiproliferative activity of cis9,trans11 [18] and even inhibit the activity of synthetic PPAR agonists [15]. Thus, it is even more interesting that our results showed more efficient reduction in cancer cells proliferation for EFA-CLA treatment than using a pure synthetic cis9,trans11CLA isomer that may suggest other factors including modified SFA/MUFA ratio in enriched egg yolks [23], supporting antiproliferative action of cis9,trans11CLA isomer.

PPARs act as transcription factors and regulate the expression of dependent genes by binding to their PPREs. Available literature gives a number of genes regulated by PPARs; the ligand-dependent transcription factors [35] and the expression of those genes can be both inhibited or activated depending on the ligand, suggesting selectivity [36]. CLA isomers have been found to act as PPAR ligands and shown to be involved in the inhibition of transcription of genes including TNF [37], NFKB1 [38], and NR1I3 [39] as well as transactivation: TGFB1 [40], BRCA1 [41], PTEN [42], p21/WAF1/CDKN1A [43], CEBPA [44], ABCB4 [45], and AOX [46]. Although a significant number of genes regulated by PPARs have been described, the list is not exhaustive and

is constantly updated as new results are being published from both experimental data and bioinformatics analyses of promoter regions containing PPRE consensus sequences (AGGTCANAGGTCA) (Figure 5).

In the current study, we applied bioinformatic tools to find genes with PPRE and analyze the effect of CLA on the expression of these genes. To our knowledge, we proposed several new genes that could be potentially PPAR-regulated: BCAR3, LZTS, SLC5A, TCF20, WT1, ZNF621, and THRB (transcript TRβ2) (Table 2). Since preliminary data showed that some of them were strongly regulated by PPARs, we studied the expression of TCF20, WT1, THRB (TRβ2), and ZNF621 genes in the context of various PPAR ligands, including EFA-CLA.

First one TCF20 can act as a phosphoserine-specific repressor of estrogen receptors (ER) in estrogen-dependent tumors [47]. MCF-7 human breast carcinoma cell line is estrogen receptor (ER) positive; thus, the expression of TCF20 should inhibit ER and consequently impair the viability of the tumor cells. Our results confirm these assumptions, showing elevated TCF20 mRNA level in cells treated with EFA-CLA. This effect was much stronger than for EFA (Table 2). Interestingly, the most pronounced effect was found for trans10,cis12CLA isomer (Table 2), which may explain its advantages over the cis9,trans11CLA in reducing the viability of MCF-7 (positively correlates with its effect on the reduction in cell viability) (Figure 1). In contrast to Pariza et al. [18], this result also suggests that trans10,cis12CLA isomer could support antiproliferative action of cis9,trans11CLA in EFA-CLA via transcription-enhancing effects on TCF20.

Available literature addresses the relationship between receptors encoded by PPAR and THRB genes [48–50]. THRB encodes three isoforms of human thyroid hormone receptor: TRβ1 and tissue-specific TRβ2 and TRβ4, which are thought to be engaged in cell cycle control and metabolism [51]. Recently, THRB has been studied as a tumor suppressor [52]. Although TRβ1 isoform has been found to play a role in the competitive inhibition of the PPAR transactivation [53], there is limited information on the relationships between TRβ2 and PPAR receptors. TRβ and PPAR receptors are linked by the same obligatory coreceptor, retinoid X receptor (RXR), that binds to their heterodimeric partners before binding to DNA. Although RXR plays a central role in regulating the activity of a number of nuclear hormone receptors including TRβ and PPARs by acting as a heterodimeric partner, this receptor is known to be constitutively expressed in cells [53]; therefore, focusing on PPARs, we do not show the expression of RXR in this paper. Nevertheless, it has been reported that TRβ and PPAR receptors can compete for binding to RXRs in the nucleus [54]. Since we have found PPRE within the sequence of TRβ2-specific promoter, located in intron IV of THRB gene, the bidirectional regulation of TRβ2 and PPARs is thought to be more complex. Results presented in the current manuscript indicated enhanced transactivation of TRβ2 by all PPARs isoforms in response to the treatment with experimental FA (Table 2) that may be evidence of the functional activity of the TRβ2-specific PPRE; however, this needs further studies. The most significant effect was measured for the synthetic CLA isomers, especially *trans10,cis12* (Table 2). Taken together, our findings showed that transcription levels of TRβ2 are elevated by PPARs and their agonists. Simultaneously, TRβ1 isoform has been shown to compete with PPAR for access to the RXR coreceptor or for PPRE binding sites in promoter regions of regulated genes [50] that could suggest TRβ1-mediated inhibitory role in expression of TRβ2 isoform and possibly other PPAR-responsive genes.

WT1 gene, as a transcription factor, directly or indirectly interacts with a number of genes involved in cell cycle and neoplasia, including *HIF1A, AREG, SRY, NROB1, SOX9, IGF2, MDM4, BRCA1, TP53,* and *SP1* (NCBI Gene). Available literature suggests an oncogenic nature of *WT1* and has shown its overexpression in various tumors and tumor cell lines, especially in breast cancer cells and melanoma [55, 56]. In addition, decreased levels of *WT1* gene expression correlated with reduced cell proliferation in both melanoma and breast cancer cells [57, 58]. *WT1* has also been linked with malignant transformation in breast cancer, and its overexpression associated with reduced susceptibility to drug treatment. Indeed, it has been shown for estrogen-dependent lines that *WT1* positively regulates the expression of *EGFR* and *HER2* [55], contributing to the resistance to hormone therapy [59, 60]. In melanoma, in vitro *WT1* silencing resulted in decreased cell proliferation, followed by apoptosis induction with caspase-3 activation [61], while in vivo it reduced the melanoma metastatic to lungs [56]. On the other hand, some studies indicate that pharmacologic activation of PPARδ by its agonists (GW0742 and GW501516) inhibited proliferation of the murine melanoma cells, accompanied by downregulation of *WT1* [62]. It was suggested that PPARδ can act via the PPRE in the *WT1* promoter and directly suppress its activity; however, our results do not support this hypothesis. Although the use of a known PPARδ agonist, GW0742, resulted in PPARδ activation (Figure 3(b)), no decrease in the expression of *WT1* was measured (Table 1). This contradiction may result from the use of different biological materials suggesting cell/tissue-specific regulation and/or association/dissociation of different corepressors or coactivators to transcription machinery. Interestingly, we showed that treatment with EFA-CLA and *cis9,trans11* reduced expression of *WT1* via the activation of PPARδ (Table 2). A similar effect was observed for other experimental FA (Table 2) suggesting that various PPAR ligands may exert different effects in different cells; however, this hypothesis should be studied.

5. Conclusion

In conclusion, potential tumor suppressor properties of PPAR receptors make their ligands attractive candidates for the development of new chemopreventive, anticancer agents. Here, we show for the first time a functional food product, CLA-enriched egg (EFA-CLA), that is more effective in reducing of MCF-7 cancer cells proliferation than synthetic CLA isomers. This EFA-CLA effect could result from the high content of *cis9,trans11* isomer, altered SFA/MUFA ratio in enriched egg yolks, and/or supportive role of *trans10,cis11* isomer in regulation of specific genes. Our results indicate that EFA-CLA can act as a ligand of PPARs, showing an

agonist activity, specifically towards the PPARγ isoform. Control, synthetic *cis9,trans11* isomer of CLA exerted an agonist effect on all PPAR receptors, while *trans10,cis12* showed no effects or even acted as an antagonist of PPARγ. However, this isomer was able to regulate some specific genes containing PPREs such as *TCF20* involved in cell cycle arrest. Simultaneously, *cis9,trans11* isomer upregulated *THRB* suppressor and downregulated *WT1* oncogene showing a small part of a PPAR action that in case of EFA-CLA leads to the observed reduction in proliferation of the breast cancer cells. It seems therefore that CLA-enriched eggs could be considered as food products with anticancer potential.

Conflicts of Interest

The authors report *no* financial or other *conflicts of interest* relevant to the subject of this *article*.

Acknowledgments

This work was supported by the Polish National Science Center (Grant no. 2011/03/B/NZ9/01423) "Conjugated Linoleic Acid (CLA) Induced Transcriptional Activation of PPAR: An Investigation of Molecular Mechanisms of Putative Anticancer Action of Fatty Acids of CLA-Enriched Egg Yolks" and by the Ministry of Science and Education (Grant no. N N312 236038) "The Influence of CLA-Enriched Hen's Egg Yolk Lipids on the Proliferation of Selected Tumor Cell Lines."

References

[1] B. Grygiel-Górniak, "Peroxisome proliferator-activated receptors and their ligands: nutritional and clinical implications—a review," *Nutrition Journal*, vol. 13, no. 1, article 17, 2014.

[2] G. Krey, O. Braissant, F. L'Horset et al., "Fatty acids, eicosanoids, and hypolipidemic agents identified as ligands of peroxisome proliferator-activated receptors by coactivator-dependent receptor ligand assay," *Molecular Endocrinology*, vol. 11, no. 6, pp. 779–791, 1997.

[3] L. Nagy, P. Tontonoz, J. G. A. Alvarez, H. Chen, and R. M. Evans, "Oxidized LDL regulates macrophage gene expression through ligand activation of PPARγ," *Cell*, vol. 93, no. 2, pp. 229–240, 1998.

[4] S. A. Kliewer, J. M. Lenhard, T. M. Willson, I. Patel, D. C. Morris, and J. M. Lehmann, "A prostaglandin J2 metabolite binds peroxisome proliferator-activated receptor γ and promotes adipocyte differentiation," *Cell*, vol. 83, no. 5, pp. 813–819, 1995.

[5] W. Motomura, T. Okumura, N. Takahashi, T. Obara, and Y. Kohgo, "Activation of peroxisome proliferator-activated receptor γ by troglitazone inhibits cell growth through the increase of p27^{Kip1} in human pancreatic carcinoma cells," *Cancer Research*, vol. 60, no. 19, pp. 5558–5564, 2000.

[6] M. Maggiora, M. Bologna, M. P. Cerù et al., "An overview of the effect of linoleic and conjugated-linoleic acids on the growth of several human tumor cell lines," *International Journal of Cancer*, vol. 112, no. 6, pp. 909–919, 2004.

[7] G. Martinasso, M. Oraldi, A. Trombetta et al., "Involvement of PPARs in cell proliferation and apoptosis in human colon cancer specimens and in normal and cancer cell lines," *PPAR Research*, Article ID 93416, 2007.

[8] J. N. Feige, L. Gelman, C. Tudor, Y. Engelborghs, W. Wahli, and B. Desvergne, "Fluorescence imaging reveals the nuclear behavior of peroxisome proliferator-activated receptor/retinoid X receptor heterodimers in the absence and presence of ligand," *Journal of Biological Chemistry*, vol. 280, no. 18, pp. 17880–17890, 2005.

[9] A. Margeli, G. Kouraklis, and S. Theocharis, "Peroxisome proliferator activated receptor-γ (PPAR-γ) ligands and angiogenesis," *Angiogenesis*, vol. 6, no. 3, pp. 165–169, 2003.

[10] S. Sethi, O. Ziouzenkova, H. Ni, D. D. Wagner, J. Plutzky, and T. N. Mayadas, "Oxidized omega-3 fatty acids in fish oil inhibit leukocyte-endothelial interactions through activation of PPARα," *Blood*, vol. 100, no. 4, pp. 1340–1346, 2002.

[11] H. Koga, S. Sakisaka, M. Harada et al., "Involvement of p21$^{WAF1/Cip1}$, p27^{Kip1}, and p18^{INK4c} in troglitazone-induced cell-cycle arrest in human hepatoma cell lines," *Hepatology*, vol. 33, no. 5, pp. 1087–1097, 2001.

[12] Y. Y. Zaytseva, N. K. Wallis, R. C. Southard, and M. W. Kilgore, "The PPARγ antagonist T0070907 suppresses breast cancer cell proliferation and motility via both PPARγ-dependent and -independent mechanisms," *Anticancer Research*, vol. 31, no. 3, pp. 813–823, 2011.

[13] W. Lu, P. Che, Y. Zhang et al., "HL005—a new selective PPARγ antagonist specifically inhibits the proliferation of MCF-7," *Journal of Steroid Biochemistry and Molecular Biology*, vol. 124, no. 3–5, pp. 112–120, 2011.

[14] S. Y. Moya-Camarena, J. P. Vanden Heuvel, S. G. Blanchard, L. A. Leesnitzer, and M. A. Belury, "Conjugated linoleic acid is a potent naturally occurring ligand and activator of PPARα," *Journal of Lipid Research*, vol. 40, no. 8, pp. 1426–1433, 1999.

[15] J. R. Miller, P. Siripurkpong, J. Hawes, A. Majdalawieh, H.-S. Ro, and R. S. McLeod, "The trans-10, cis-12 isomer of conjugated linoleic acid decreases adiponectin assembly by PPARγ-dependent and PPARγ-independent mechanisms," *Journal of Lipid Research*, vol. 49, no. 3, pp. 550–562, 2008.

[16] Y. Yu, P. H. Correll, and J. P. V. Heuvel, "Conjugated linoleic acid decreases production of pro-inflammatory products in macrophages: evidence for a PPARγ-dependent mechanism," *Biochimica et Biophysica Acta—Molecular and Cell Biology of Lipids*, vol. 1581, no. 3, pp. 89–99, 2002.

[17] M. F. McCarty, "Activation of PPARgamma may mediate a portion of the anticancer activity of conjugated linoleic acid," *Medical Hypotheses*, vol. 55, no. 3, pp. 187–188, 2000.

[18] M. W. Pariza, Y. Park, and M. E. Cook, "Mechanisms of action of conjugated linoleic acid: evidence and speculation," *Proceedings of the Society for Experimental Biology and Medicine*, vol. 223, no. 1, pp. 8–13, 2000.

[19] C. Ip, S. Banni, E. Angioni et al., "Conjugated linoleic acid-enriched butter fat alters mammary gland morphogenesis and reduces cancer risk in rats," *Journal of Nutrition*, vol. 129, no. 12, pp. 2135–2142, 1999.

[20] M. M. Ip, P. A. Masso-Welch, S. F. Shoemaker, W. K. Shea-Eaton, and C. Ip, "Conjugated linoleic acid inhibits proliferation and induces apoptosis of normal rat mammary epithelial cells in primary culture," *Experimental Cell Research*, vol. 250, no. 1, pp. 22–34, 1999.

[21] A. A. Koronowicz, P. Banks, B. Szymczyk et al., "Dietary conjugated linoleic acid affects blood parameters, liver morphology and expression of selected hepatic genes in laying hens," *British Poultry Science*, vol. 57, no. 5, pp. 663–673, 2016.

[22] J. Folch, M. Lees, and G. H. Sloane Stanley, "A simple method for the isolation and purification of total lipides from animal tissues," *The Journal of biological chemistry*, vol. 226, no. 1, pp. 497–509, 1957.

[23] A. A. Koronowicz, P. Banks, D. Domagala, A. Master, D. Domagała et al., "Fatty acids extract from CLA-enriched egg yolks can mediate transcriptome reprogramming of MCF-7 cancer cells to prevent their growth and proliferation," *Genes & Nutrition*, vol. 11, article 22, 2016.

[24] K. J. Livak and T. D. Schmittgen, "Analysis of relative gene expression data using real-time quantitative PCR and the $2^{-\Delta\Delta C_T}$ method," *Methods*, vol. 25, no. 4, pp. 402–408, 2001.

[25] M. B. Roberfroid, "Global view on functional foods: European perspectives," *The British Journal of Nutrition*, vol. 88, supplement 2, pp. S133–S138, 2002.

[26] M. Franczyk-Zarów, R. B. Kostogrys, B. Szymczyk et al., "Functional effects of eggs, naturally enriched with conjugated linoleic acid, on the blood lipid profile, development of atherosclerosis and composition of atherosclerotic plaque in apolipoprotein E and low-density lipoprotein receptor double-knockout mice (apoE/LDLR-/-)," *British Journal of Nutrition*, vol. 99, no. 1, pp. 49–58, 2008.

[27] A. Koronowicz, K. Żwawa, B. Szymczyk, P. Pisulewski, and P. Laidler, "Wpływ lipidów żółtka jaja kurzego naturalnie wzbogaconego w izomery sprzężonego kwasu linolowego na proliferację komórek czerniaka ludzkiego," *Bromatologia i Chemia Toksykologiczna*, vol. 42, no. 3, pp. 1047–1051, 2009.

[28] G. Lu, G. Zhang, X. Zheng, Y. Zeng et al., "c9, t11- conjugated linoleic acid induces HCC cell apoptosis and correlation with PPAR-γ signaling pathway," *American Journal of Translational Research*, vol. 7, no. 12, pp. 2752–2763, 2015.

[29] X. Wan, X. Yuan, X. Yang, Y. Li, and L. Zhong, "Studies on mechanism of cis9, trans11-CLA and trans10, cis12-CLA inducing apoptosis of human breast cancer cell line MCF-7," *Chinese-German Journal of Clinical Oncology*, vol. 9, no. 10, pp. 583–589, 2010.

[30] N. S. Kelley, N. E. Hubbard, and K. L. Erickson, "Conjugated linoleic acid isomers and cancer," *Journal of Nutrition*, vol. 137, no. 12, pp. 2599–2607, 2007.

[31] H. Chujo, M. Yamasaki, S. Nou, N. Koyanagi, H. Tachibana, and K. Yamada, "Effect of conjugated linoleic acid isomers on growth factor-induced proliferation of human breast cancer cells," *Cancer Letters*, vol. 202, no. 1, pp. 81–87, 2003.

[32] K. L. Erickson and N. E. Hubbard, "Fatty acids and breast cancer: the role of stem cells," *Prostaglandins Leukotrienes and Essential Fatty Acids*, vol. 82, no. 4–6, pp. 237–241, 2010.

[33] P. Sertznig, M. Seifert, W. Tilgen, and J. Reichrath, "Present concepts and future outlook: function of peroxisome proliferator-activated receptors (PPARs) for pathogenesis, progression, and therapy of cancer," *Journal of Cellular Physiology*, vol. 212, no. 1, pp. 1–12, 2007.

[34] J. Berger and D. E. Moller, "The mechanisms of action of PPARs," *Annual Review of Medicine*, vol. 53, pp. 409–435, 2002.

[35] A. Rogue, C. Spire, M. Brun, N. Claude, and A. Guillouzo, "Gene expression changes induced by PPAR gamma agonists in animal and human liver," *PPAR Research*, vol. 2010, Article ID 325183, 16 pages, 2010.

[36] M. Sokolowska, M. L. Kowalski, R. Pawliczak, and M. Sokołowska, "Peroxisome proliferator-activated receptors-g (PPAR-g) and their role in immunoregulation and inflammation control," *Postępy Higieny i Medycyny Doświadczalnej*, vol. 59, pp. 472–484, 2005.

[37] B. Zhang, J. Berger, E. Hu et al., "Negative regulation of peroxisome proliferator-activated receptor-γ gene expression

contributes to the antiadipogenic effects of tumor necrosis factor-α," *Molecular Endocrinology*, vol. 10, no. 11, pp. 1457–1466, 1996.

[38] X. Wang, Y. Sun, Y. Zhao et al., "Oroxyloside prevents dextran sulfate sodium-induced experimental colitis in mice by inhibiting NF-κB pathway through PPARγ activation," *Biochemical Pharmacology*, vol. 106, pp. 70–81, 2016.

[39] N. Wieneke, K. I. Hirsch-Ernst, M. Kuna, S. Kersten, and G. P. Püschel, "PPARα-dependent induction of the energy homeostasis-regulating nuclear receptor NR1i3 (CAR) in rat hepatocytes: potential role in starvation adaptation," *FEBS Letters*, vol. 581, no. 29, pp. 5617–5626, 2007.

[40] H. A. Burgess, L. E. Daugherty, T. H. Thatcher et al., "PPARγ agonists inhibit TGF-β induced pulmonary myofibroblast differentiation and collagen production: implications for therapy of lung fibrosis," *American Journal of Physiology—Lung Cellular and Molecular Physiology*, vol. 288, no. 6, pp. L1146–L1153, 2005.

[41] M. Pignatelli, C. Cocca, A. Santos, and A. Perez-Castillo, "Enhancement of BRCA1 gene expression by the peroxisome proliferator-activated receptor γ in the MCF-7 breast cancer cell line," *Oncogene*, vol. 22, no. 35, pp. 5446–5450, 2003.

[42] S. Y. Lee, G. Y. Hur, K. H. Jung et al., "PPAR-γ agonist increase gefitinib's antitumor activity through PTEN expression," *Lung Cancer*, vol. 51, no. 3, pp. 297–301, 2006.

[43] Y.-M. Sue, C.-P. Chung, H. Lin et al., "PPARδ-mediated p21/p27 induction via increased CREB-binding protein nuclear translocation in beraprost-induced antiproliferation of murine aortic smooth muscle cells," *American Journal of Physiology—Cell Physiology*, vol. 297, no. 2, pp. C321–C329, 2009.

[44] Z. Wu, E. D. Rosen, R. Brun et al., "Cross-regulation of C/EBPα and PPARγ controls the transcriptional pathway of adipogenesis and insulin sensitivity," *Molecular Cell*, vol. 3, no. 2, pp. 151–158, 1999.

[45] R. P. J. Oude Elferink and C. C. Paulusma, "Function and pathophysiological importance of ABCB4 (MDR3 P-glycoprotein)," *Pflugers Archiv European Journal of Physiology*, vol. 453, no. 5, pp. 601–610, 2007.

[46] M. Heim, J. Johnson, F. Boess et al., "Phytanic acid, a natural peroxisome proliferator-activated receptor (PPAR) agonist, regulates glucose metabolism in rat primary hepatocytes," *The Federation of American Societies for Experimental Biology Journal*, vol. 16, no. 7, pp. 718–720, 2002.

[47] V. Gburcik, N. Bot, M. Maggiolini, and D. Picard, "SPBP is a phosphoserine-specific repressor of estrogen receptor α," *Molecular and Cellular Biology*, vol. 25, no. 9, pp. 3421–3430, 2005.

[48] S. Kouidhi, I. Seugnet, S. Decherf et al., "Peroxisome proliferator-activated receptor-γ (PPARγ) modulates hypothalamic Trh regulation in vivo," *Molecular and Cellular Endocrinology*, vol. 317, no. 1-2, pp. 44–52, 2010.

[49] S. Sasaki, K. Kawai, Y. Honjo, and H. Nakamura, "Thyroid hormones and lipid metabolism," *Nihon Rinsho. Japanese Journal of Clinical Medicine*, vol. 64, no. 12, pp. 2323–2329, 2006.

[50] T. Miyamoto, A. Kaneko, T. Kakizawa et al., "Inhibition of peroxisome proliferator signaling pathways by thyroid hormone receptor. Competitive binding to the response element," *Journal of Biological Chemistry*, vol. 272, no. 12, pp. 7752–7758, 1997.

[51] A. Master and A. Nauman, "THRB (Thyroid Hormone Receptor, Beta)," *Atlas of Genetics and Cytogenetics in Oncology and Haematology*, vol. 18, no. 6, pp. 400–433, 2014.

[52] A. Master, A. Wójcicka, K. Giżewska, P. Popławski, G. R. Williams, and A. Nauman, "A novel method for gene-specific

enhancement of protein translation by targeting 5′UTRs of selected tumor suppressors," *PLoS ONE*, vol. 11, no. 5, Article ID e0155359, 2016.

[53] L. Al-Alem, R. C. Southard, M. W. Kilgore, and T. E. Curry, "Specific thiazolidinediones inhibit ovarian cancer cell line proliferation and cause cell cycle arrest in a PPARγ independent manner," *PLoS ONE*, vol. 6, no. 1, Article ID e16179, 2011.

[54] C. Lu and S.-Y. Cheng, "Thyroid hormone receptors regulate adipogenesis and carcinogenesis via crosstalk signaling with peroxisome proliferator-activated receptors," *Journal of Molecular Endocrinology*, vol. 44, no. 3, pp. 143–154, 2010.

[55] L. Wang and Z.-Y. Wang, "The Wilms' tumor suppressor WT1 induces estrogen-independent growth and anti-estrogen insensitivity in ER-positive breast cancer MCF7 cells," *Oncology Reports*, vol. 23, no. 4, pp. 1109–1117, 2010.

[56] D. E. Zamora-Avila, P. Zapata-Benavides, M. A. Franco-Molina et al., "WT1 gene silencing by aerosol delivery of PEI-RNAi complexes inhibits B16-F10 lung metastases growth," *Cancer Gene Therapy*, vol. 16, no. 12, pp. 892–899, 2009.

[57] N. Wagner, J. Panelos, D. Massi, and K.-D. Wagner, "The Wilms' tumor suppressor WT1 is associated with melanoma proliferation," *Pflügers Archiv—European Journal of Physiology*, vol. 455, no. 5, pp. 839–847, 2008.

[58] P. Zapata-Benavides, M. Tuna, G. Lopez-Berestein, and A. M. Tari, "Downregulation of Wilms' tumor 1 protein inhibits breast cancer proliferation," *Biochemical and Biophysical Research Communications*, vol. 295, no. 4, pp. 784–790, 2002.

[59] G. Arpino, L. Wiechmann, C. K. Osborne, and R. Schiff, "Crosstalk between the estrogen receptor and the HER tyrosine kinase receptor family: molecular mechanism and clinical implications for endocrine therapy resistance," *Endocrine Reviews*, vol. 29, no. 2, pp. 217–233, 2008.

[60] R. I. Nicholson, I. R. Hutcheson, M. E. Harper et al., "Modulation of epidermal growth factor receptor in endocrine-resistant, oestrogen receptor-positive breast cancer," *Endocrine-Related Cancer*, vol. 8, no. 3, pp. 175–182, 2001.

[61] D. E. Zamora-Avila, M. A. Franco-Molina, L. M. Trejo-Avila, C. Rodríguez-Padilla, D. Reséndez-Pérez, and P. Zapata-Benavides, "RNAi silencing of the WT1 gene inhibits cell proliferation and induces apoptosis in the B16F10 murine melanoma cell line," *Melanoma Research*, vol. 17, no. 6, pp. 341–348, 2007.

[62] J.-F. Michiels, C. Perrin, N. Leccia, D. Massi, P. Grimaldi, and N. Wagner, "PPARß activation inhibits melanoma cell proliferation involving repression of the Wilms' tumour suppressor WT1," *Pflugers Archiv European Journal of Physiology*, vol. 459, no. 5, pp. 689–703, 2010.

12

Transcriptome-Wide Analysis Reveals the Role of PPARγ Controlling the Lipid Metabolism in Goat Mammary Epithelial Cells

Hengbo Shi,[1,2] Wangsheng Zhao,[3,4] Changhui Zhang,[3] Khuram Shahzad,[5] Jun Luo,[3] and Juan J. Loor[5]

[1]*College of Life Science, Zhejiang Sci-Tech University, Hangzhou, Zhejiang 310018, China*
[2]*Zhejiang Provincial Key Laboratory of Silkworm Bioreactor and Biomedicine, Hangzhou, Zhejiang 310018, China*
[3]*Shaanxi Key Laboratory of Molecular Biology for Agriculture, College of Animal Science and Technology, Northwest A&F University, Yangling, Shaanxi 712100, China*
[4]*School of Life Science and Engineering, Southwest University of Science and Technology, Mianyang 621010, China*
[5]*Mammalian NutriPhysioGenomics, Department of Animal Sciences and Division of Nutritional Sciences, University of Illinois, Urbana, IL 61801, USA*

Correspondence should be addressed to Jun Luo; luojun@nwsuaf.edu.cn and Juan J. Loor; jloor@illinois.edu

Academic Editor: Marcelo H. Napimoga

To explore the large-scale effect of peroxisome proliferator-activated receptor γ (*PPARG*) in goat mammary epithelial cells (GMEC), an oligonucleotide microarray platform was used for transcriptome profiling in cells overexpressing *PPARG* and incubated with or without rosiglitazone (ROSI, a PPARγ agonist). A total of 1143 differentially expressed genes (DEG) due to treatment were detected. The Dynamic Impact Approach (DIA) analysis uncovered the most impacted and induced pathways "fatty acid elongation in mitochondria," "glycosaminoglycan biosynthesis-keratan sulfate," and "pentose phosphate pathway." The data highlights the central role of *PPARG* in milk fatty acid metabolism via controlling fatty acid elongation, biosynthesis of unsaturated fatty acid, lipid formation, and lipid secretion; furthermore, its role related to carbohydrate metabolism promotes the production of intermediates required for milk fat synthesis. Analysis of upstream regulators indicated that *PPARG* participates in multiple physiological processes via controlling or cross talking with other key transcription factors such as *PPARD* and *NR1H3* (also known as liver-X-receptor-α). This transcriptome-wide analysis represents the first attempt to better understand the biological relevance of PPARG expression in ruminant mammary cells. Overall, the data underscored the importance of PPARG in mammary lipid metabolism and transcription factor control.

1. Introduction

Ruminant milk products are now common and popular throughout the world. Milk fat is an important component of dairy products and is a major contributor to dietary energy density. The higher concentrations of unsaturated and medium-chain fatty acids are responsible for the characteristic "goaty" odour of goat milk and also confer unique organoleptic properties [1]. Therefore, understanding the mechanisms for altering the milk fatty acid composition of goat milk may lead to further improvements in nutritional value. Recent evidence indicates that milk fat biosynthesis is

regulated by key transcription factors including peroxisome proliferator-activated receptor γ (*PPARG*) [2, 3].

It is well established that *PPARG* is a critical transcription factor controlling adipogenesis and glucose metabolism in various cells in nonruminants [4–6]. After binding of ligands (e.g., rosiglitazone (ROSI) or pioglitazone), *PPARG* causes conformational changes in the receptor [7, 8] and then forms a heterodimeric complex with RXR proteins and binds to PPAR response element (PPRE) upstream of target genes [9]. Through controlling the downstream genes, *PPARG* regulates adipocyte differentiation and promotes insulin sensitivity in human and rodents [7]. The activation of PPARG also enhances macrophage lipid uptake as well as lipid export and has anti-inflammatory effects [10].

In bovine cells, the activation of *PPARG* with rosiglitazone provided a demonstration that PPARG could control expression of genes involved in milk fat synthesis [11]. The current data from goats indicates that *PPARG* regulates genes involved in triacylglycerol synthesis and secretion in mammary gland epithelial cells [12]. It was also demonstrated that *PPARG* stimulates the synthesis of monounsaturated fatty acids in dairy goat mammary epithelial cells (GMEC) via the control of stearoyl-coenzyme A desaturase (*SCD*) [2]. Furthermore, our recent data revealed that PPARG could modulate lipid accumulation via regulation of Perilipin 2 (*PLIN2*) gene expression in GMEC [13]. Although some work [2, 3] has been performed to study the function of *PPARG* in ruminant mammary cells, a comprehensive dataset on gene profiles altered by *PPARG* is not available.

Microarray analysis provides an efficient tool to simultaneously study the expression of multiple genes in tissues or cells in response to a given treatment or physiological condition. It has been widely used in the bovine to study the differential gene expression among different treatments or physiological conditions [14–16]. Structural genomic studies of domestic animals have indicated that goats are closely related to bovine species [17]. Previous evidences were highly suggestive that cross-species hybridization is possible using a bovine cDNA microarray to study goat gene expression [18–20].

The primary aim of this study was to assess the potential role of *PPARG* in GMEC at global scale. To that aim, a microarray analysis was used to detect the transcriptome alterations of GMEC after overexpression of *PPARG*. The results indicated that *PPARG* gain of function induced more than 1,000 differentially expressed genes (DEG), most of which are related to metabolism pathways.

2. Experimental Section

2.1. Cell Culture and Treatments. The mammary epithelial cells were isolated from peak lactation Xinong Saanen goats as described previously [21]. Details of cell culture were described recently [3, 12]. Cultures of GMEC at approximately 80% confluence were transfected with one of the adenovirus supernatants (Ad-PPARG or Ad-GFP). Transfected GMEC were cultured with the PPARG-specific ligand ROSI (BioVision, USA) (PPARG+ROSI) or control [dimethyl sulfoxide (DMSO)] (Sigma, St. Louis, MO, USA) (PPARG+DMSO and Ad-GFP+DMSO) at 50 μM after 24 h of the initial culture and then harvested at 48 h (24 h later) for RNA extraction. The generation and application of the adenovirus expression PPARG (Ad-PPARG) were described elsewhere [2]. Each treatment was performed in triplicate.

2.2. Total RNA Extraction. The procedures for total RNA extraction, purification, and qPCR were recently described [22]. Total RNA from GMEC was extracted using the RNA Prep pure cell kit (Tiangen Biotech Co. Ltd., Beijing, China) according to the manufacturer's protocol. The RNA used in

the qPCR was treated with DNAase (Tiangen Biotech Co. Ltd., Beijing, China) to remove genomic DNA contamination. Synthesis of cDNA was conducted using the Prime Script™ RT kit (Takara Bio Inc., Otsu, Japan) according to the manufacturer's instructions.

2.3. Microarray. An Agilent platform was chosen to conduct the microarray experiment (44K Bovine (V2) gene expression microarray chip, Agilent Technologies Inc.) following the manufacturer's protocols. Briefly, a total of 200 ng of RNA per sample were used to generate first-strand cDNA, which was reverse transcribed to cRNA using the low-input quick amp labeling kit (Agilent Technologies Inc.). The resulting cRNA was labeled with either Cy3 or Cy5 fluorescent dye, purified using RNeasy minispin columns (Qiagen), and subsequently eluted in 30 μL of DNase-RNase-free water. The NanoDrop ND-1000 (Thermo Fisher Scientific Inc., Waltham, MA) and a Bioanalyzer 2100 (Agilent Technologies) were used to confirm the manufacturer's recommended criteria for yield of at least 0.825 μg/μL and RNA integrity $\geq$ 6, respectively.

2.4. Quantitative Real-Time PCR (qPCR). The results from microarray were validated via qPCR for a selected panel of 15 genes considered important for fatty acid metabolism. The gene names and primers used in this study are reported in Supporting File 1 (in Supplementary Material available online at http://dx.doi.org/10.1155/2016/9195680). Methods for primer pair design and validation and qPCR were as previously described [12]. Data of qPCR were normalized to three internal control genes, Ubiquitously Expressed, Prefoldin-Like Chaperone (*UXT*), Mitochondrial Ribosomal Protein L39 (*MRPL39*), and Ribosomal Protein S9 (*RPS9*).

2.5. Data Analysis. Data from microarrays were normalized using Lowess prior to statistical analysis using ANOVA in GeneSpring (Agilent Technologies). Differences in relative expression between PPARG versus CON, PPARG+ROSI versus CON, and PPARG+ROSI versus PPARG were considered significant at an unadjusted $P < 0.05$ and a fold change greater or lower than 2 [23]. The qPCR data were log$_2$ transformed prior to statistical analysis. The data were analyzed using a Generalized Linear Model (GLM) using SAS with treatments (CON, PPARG, and PPARG+ROSI) as the main effect. Significance was declared at $P < 0.05$.

2.6. Data Mining. Data were mined by an integrative systems biology approach applying the newly developed Dynamic Impact Approach (DIA) [24] and an upstream gene network analysis using Ingenuity Pathway Analysis (IPA) [14]. The Kyoto Encyclopedia of Genes and Genomes (KEGG) pathways and Gene Ontology (GO) biological process category database of bovine were used for functional analysis with the DIA. The detailed methodology for data analysis using DIA was described previously [14]. The IPA Knowledgebase is used to predict the expected causal effects between upstream regulators and targets (i.e., DEG).

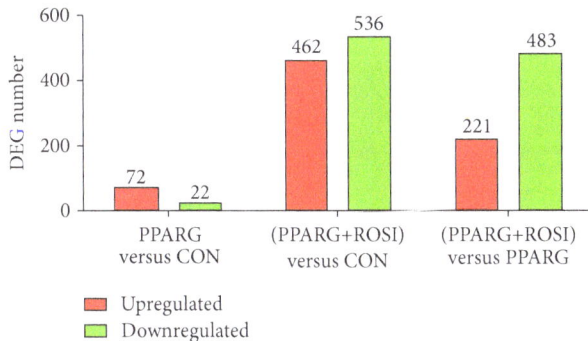

FIGURE 1: Differentially expressed genes in goat mammary epithelial cells across different treatment comparisons. Cells overexpression of peroxisome proliferator-activated receptor-γ (PPARG) with rosiglitazone (ROSI) (PPARG+ROSI) versus CON (cells treated with adenovirus expressing GFP), PPARG versus CON, and PPARG+ROSI versus PPARG.

3. Results

3.1. Number of Differentially Expressed Genes (DEG) in the Microarray Data.

Overall, there were more than 1,398 DEG detected by microarray. Among these, only the genes (1143) annotated with a bovine Entrez gene ID with a significant difference ($P < 0.05$) and 2-fold change ratio were used for the analysis. The number of DEG indicated a marked difference in expression in the cells overexpressing PPARG with ROSI compared with cells without ROSI (Figure 1). Compared with control, there were 464 DEG upregulated and 536 DEG downregulated in PPARG+ROSI versus CON. The overexpression of PPARG alone did not markedly alter the transcriptome, but there were 72 upregulated and 22 downregulated genes. When compared with cells expressing PPARG with and without ROSI, the analysis indicated that the number of upregulated and downregulated DEG was 221 and 483, respectively.

3.2. Overall Summary of KEGG Categories.

Using the DIA, the estimate of the perturbation in a biological pathway is represented by the "impact" while the overall direction of the perturbation is represented by the "flux" (or Direction of the Impact) [24]. The DIA provides a summary of the KEGG pathways in the form of categories and subcategories (Figure 3) which are altered by treatments. The details of each pathway are reported in Supporting File S3.

In accordance with the number of DEG in Figure 1, KEGG pathway categories were more impacted in the two comparisons related to cells treated with ROSI. Among these pathways, the category "metabolism" was the most impacted (Figure 2). With the exception of the subcategories of pathways within "biosynthesis of other second metabolites," "nucleotide metabolism," and "amino acid metabolism," all the other subcategories within metabolism had an impact value >25 in the comparison of PPARG+ROSI with CON.

A similar induction effect was uncovered in the comparison of PPARG+ROSI with PPARG. Except for the minor inhibition of "glycan biosynthesis and metabolism,"

in the comparison of PPARG+ROSI with CON, most of the metabolic pathways were markedly activated including "carbohydrate metabolism," "energy metabolism," "lipid metabolism," "amino acid metabolism," "metabolism of other amino acids," "glycan biosynthesis and metabolism," "metabolism of cofactors and vitamins," "metabolism of terpenoids and polyketides," and "xenobiotics biodegradation and metabolism." Compared with the control group, only the overexpression of PPARG had a weaker impact on pathway categories except "metabolism."

According to the impact value, the categories "genetic information processing," "environment information processing," "cellular process," and "organismal system" also were altered in the comparison of PPARG+ROSI with CON. However, most of their flux values were slightly activated or did not change. In PPARG+ROSI versus PPARG, the fluxes in the four categories were inhibited or exhibited no change.

3.3. Most Impacted KEGG Pathways.

The DIA analysis revealed that the most impacted pathway was "fatty acid elongation in mitochondria" with flux >60, followed by "glycosaminoglycan biosynthesis" (Figure 3). The categories containing "fatty acid elongation in mitochondria," "pentose phosphate pathway," "glyoxylate and dicarboxylate metabolism," "riboflavin metabolism," "nicotinate and nicotinamide metabolism," "PPAR signaling pathway," and "pantothenate and CoA biosynthesis" were highly activated. In contrast, the pathways "glycosphingolipid biosynthesis-globoseries" and "folate biosynthesis" were inhibited.

Even though "glycosaminoglycan biosynthesis" was the second most impacted pathway, it was slightly inhibited by the activation of PPARG. "Glycosphingolipid biosynthesis" was highly inhibited with the activation of PPARG. Among the top ten overall most impacted terms, only PPARG belonged to "endocrine system"; the rest of them belonged to "metabolism" (Figure 3).

3.4. Expression of Selected Genes by qPCR.

Fifteen genes considered important for fatty acid metabolism were selected to assess the reliability of the microarray data. Overall, >80% of genes measured by qPCR had a result deemed similar to microarray data. Compared with the control group, the cells overexpressing PPARG plus ROSI altered more genes compared with PPARG without ROSI. Among the genes involved in the upstream transcription factor regulation network, the expression level of NR1H3, PPARG, SREBF2, and PPARD by qPCR was similar to microarray, whereas data of SREBF1 and PPARGC1A were less sensitive by microarray compared with qPCR (Figure 4). A contrasting response between microarray and qPCR was also observed for FASN.

3.5. Upstream Regulators.

Consistent with the number of DEG, there were a high number of upstream transcription regulators in the comparisons of PPARG+ROSI versus CON and PPARG+ROSI versus PPARG. All the upstream upregulated transcription regulators and their potential targets are depicted in Figures 5, 6, and 7. Among the

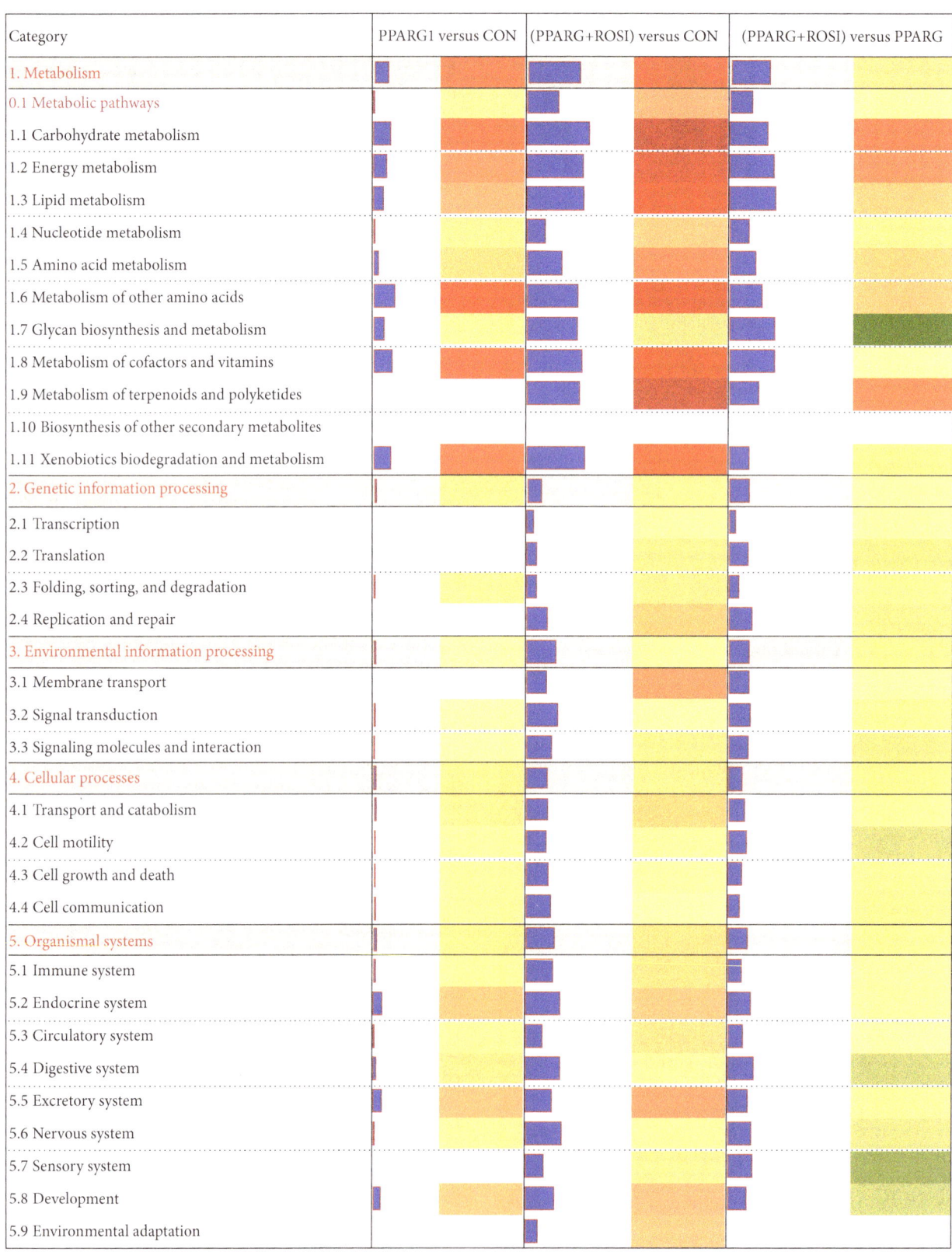

FIGURE 2: The summary of KEGG pathways provided by the Dynamic Impact Approach (DIA). The "impact" is represented by the horizontal blue bars (the larger the bar, the larger the impact) and the "flux" (Direction of the Impact) is represented by green (more inhibited) to red (more activated) rectangles.

10 most overall impacted terms	Impact	Flux	Rank
Fatty acid elongation in mitochondria			1
Glycosaminoglycan biosynthesis-keratan sulfate			2
Pentose phosphate pathway			3
Glyoxylate and dicarboxylate metabolism			4
Riboflavin metabolism			5
Glycosphingolipid biosynthesis-globoseries			6
Nicotinate and nicotinamide metabolism			7
PPAR signaling pathway			8
Pantothenate and CoA biosynthesis			9
Folate biosynthesis			10

Bar	0	25	50
Shade	−50	0	50

(a)

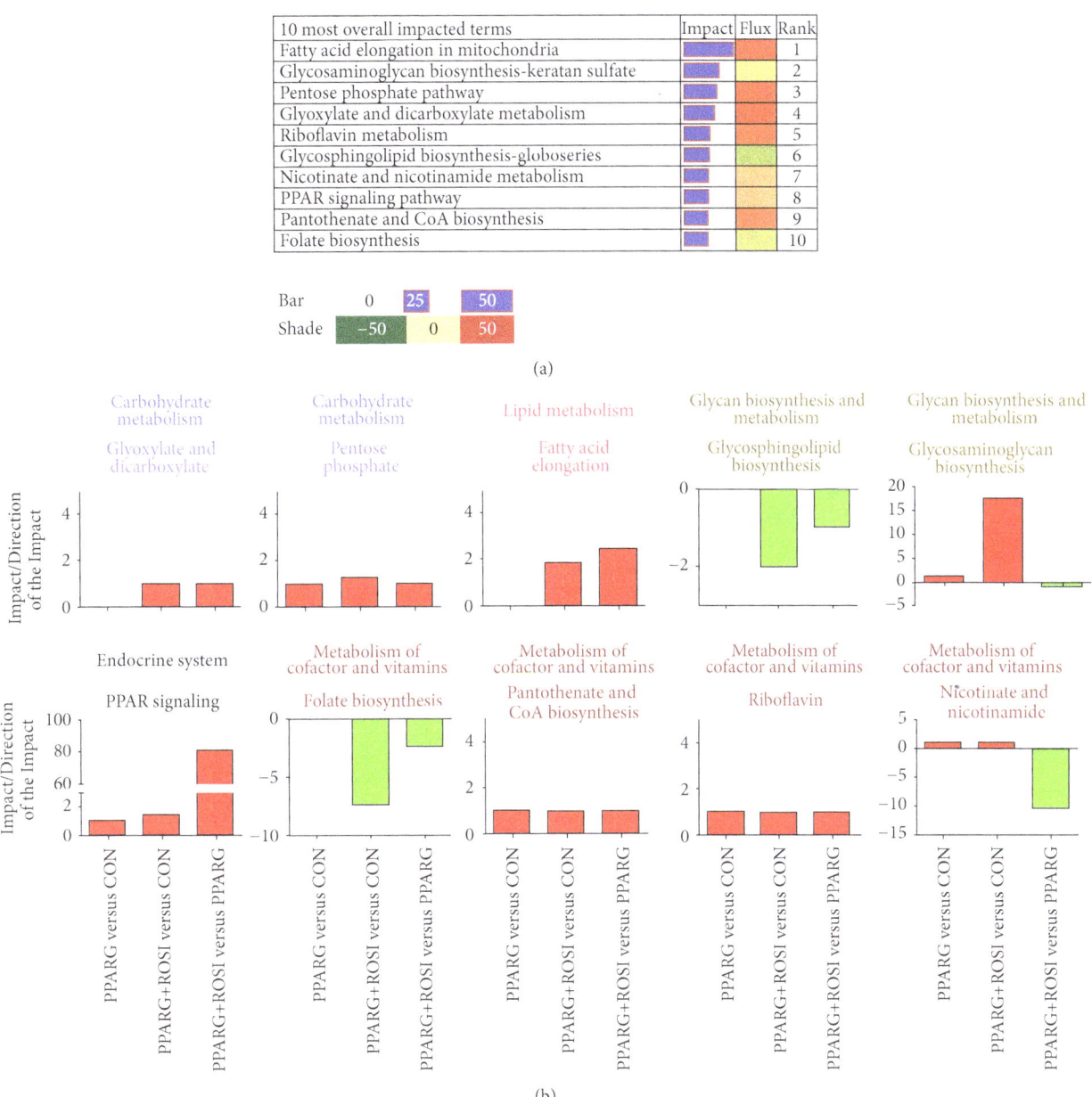

(b)

FIGURE 3: Dynamic Impact Approach (DIA) results for the 10 most impacted KEGG pathways. (a) The overall 10 most impacted pathways and rank. (b) The impact/Direction of the Impact of 10 most impacted pathways in each comparison.

upsteam transcription regulators with PPARG versus CON, there were two related to lipid metabolism including *PPARG* and CCAAT/enhancer binding protein (*C/EBP*), alpha (*CEBPA*). Comparing PPARG+ROSI with CON, eight upstream transcription regulators were upregulated: activating transcription factor 3 (*ATF3*), *CEBPA*, Jun protooncogene (*JUN*), homeobox A9 (*HOXA9*), hypoxia inducible factor 1, alpha (*HIF1A*), NR1H3, peroxisome proliferator-activated receptor delta (*PPARD*), and *PPARG* (Figure 6). Among them, *CEBPA*, *NR1H3*, *PPARD*, and *PPARG* are classical transcription factors related to lipid metabolism. Compared with PPARG+ROSI versus CON, the comparison of PPARG+ROSI with PPARG had a lower number

of upregulated upstream transcription regulators including HIFA, nuclear factor, erythroid 2-like 3 (*NFE2L3*), *NR1H3*, and *PPARG* (Figure 7).

A few upstream transcription regulators were inhibited in the comparison of PPARG+ROSI versus CON and PPARG+ROSI versus PPARG (Figures S1 and S2). In comparison of PPARG+ROSI with CON, the transcription regulators early growth response 1 (*EGR1*), CXXC finger protein 1 (*CXXC1*), neurogenin 1 (*NEUROG1*), Protein Inhibitor of Activated STAT, 1 (*PIAS1*), pleomorphic adenoma gene-like 1 (*PLAGL1*), Kruppel-Like factor 4 (*KLF4*), *RXRA*, *GFI1B*, *KLF5*, *KLF6*, *RARG*, *MYOD1*, and *SOX2* were inhibited. Similar to PPARG+ROSI versus CON, the genes expression

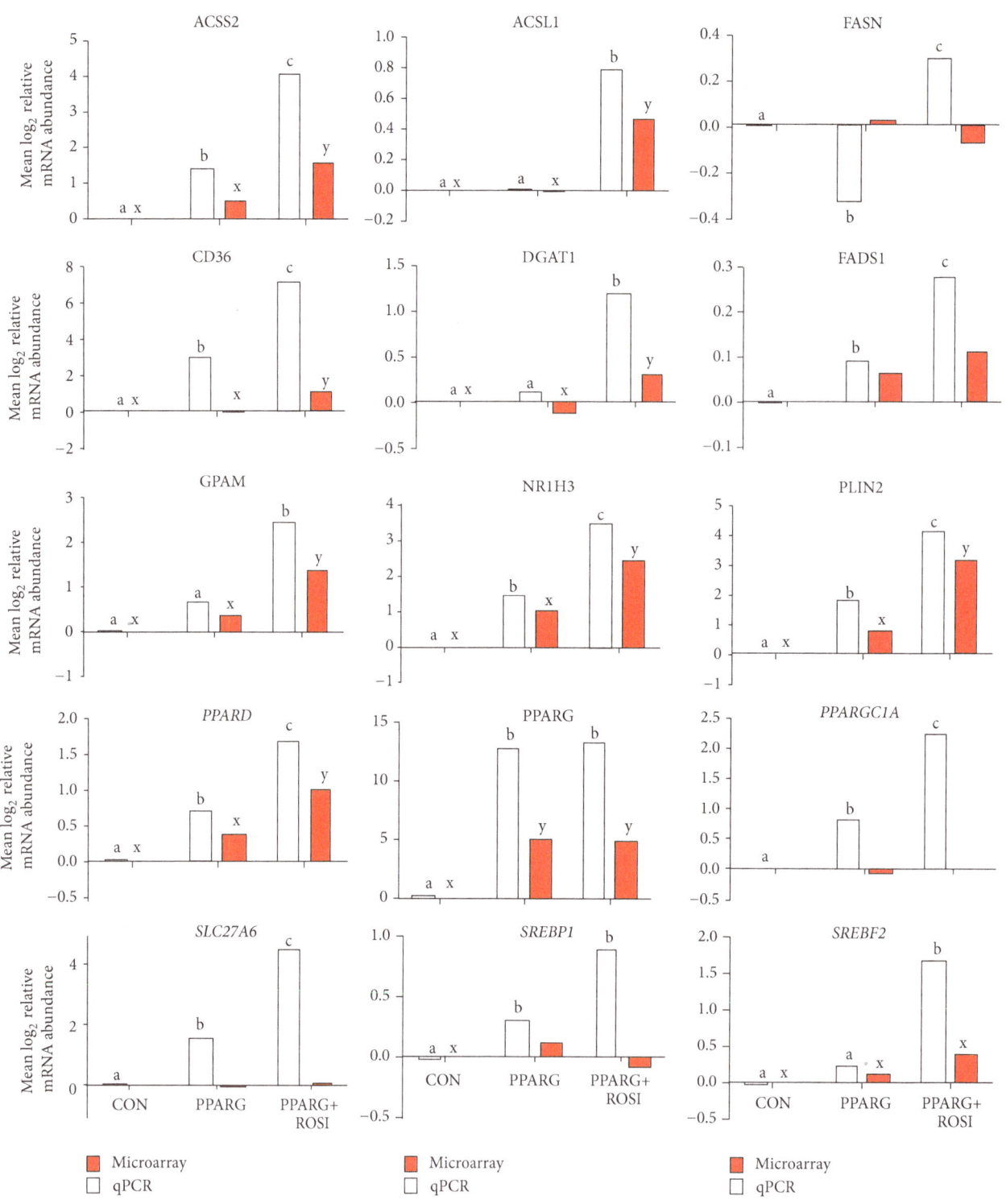

FIGURE 4: qPCR analysis of selected transcripts and comparison with microarray data. Several of selected transcripts were present and differentially expressed among the comparison in the microarray data and qPCR. a, b, and c denote differences with $P < 0.05$ in qPCR data and x and y denote differences with $P < 0.05$ in microarray data.

of *NEUROD1*, *KLF4*, *KLF6*, *CXXC1*, *KLF5*, *RXRA*, myogenic differentiation 1 (*MYOD1*), PIAS1, sex determining region Y box 2 (SOX2), and growth factor independent 1B transcription repressor (GFI1B) was also inhibited in the comparison of PPARG+ROSI with PPARG.

4. Discussion

Due to the unavailability of goat microarrays and the fact that structural genome of goats is closely related to that of bovine species, bovine arrays have been successfully

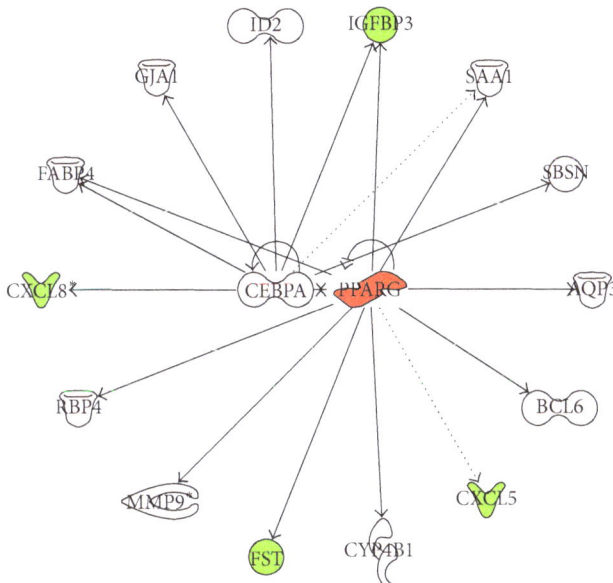

FIGURE 5: Ingenuity pathway upstream network analysis of differentially expressed genes (DEG) between cells treated with Ad-PPARG and those with Ad-GFP. Upstream regulators are located at the center of the network and downstream genes are located in the periphery. In the network, their downstream genes are also reported. Genes with red background are upregulated: red color (high upregulation) to light red color (moderate upregulation). Genes with green background were downregulated: green color (highly inhibited) to light red color (moderately highly inhibited). Arrows denote direct (solid lines) or indirect (dotted lines) interactions among genes.

adapted and applied in studies with goat mammary tissue [20, 25], goat ovary [26], and goat milk leukocytes [27]. To further explore the transcriptome alteration by PPARG gain of function, a commercial whole-transcriptome bovine microarray was used in the present study. The data revealed close to 1,000 DEG altered by overexpression of PPARG plus the chemical agonist ROSI. The most impacted category by PPARG was related to metabolism, which agrees with the previous findings demonstrating that PPARG plays a central role in adipogenesis [28]. Furthermore, analysis of a subset of genes by qPCR revealed a high degree of agreement with microarray data.

The DIA is efficient for the analysis of data from multiple treatment comparisons [24, 29]. Among the overall most impacted pathways in present study, the "fatty acid elongation in mitochondria," "glycosaminoglycan biosynthesis-keratan sulfate," and "glycosphingolipid biosynthesis-globo series" are novel and of biological interest. In adipose cells, PPARG promotes the uptake of fatty acids and storage as energy [7]. Our previous data also revealed that PPARG stimulated the expression of genes related to triacylglycerol (TAG) synthesis in GMEC [3, 12]. Thus, we expected to find that TAG synthesis would be the most impacted pathway in the present study. The finding that "fatty acid elongation in mitochondria" was the most impacted is supported by the high expression of hydroxyacyl-CoA dehydrogenase, alpha subunit (HADHA), and hydroxyacyl-CoA dehydrogenase,

beta subunit (HADHB), both of which are the rate-limiting enzymes for fatty acid elongation. Further, these genes appear to be potential PPARG target genes in GMEC. Consistent with promoting fatty acid elongation, the uptake of long-chain fatty acid was also induced because CD36 [3] and solute carrier family 27 (fatty acid transporter), member 6 (SLC27A6), were upregulated (Figure 2).

Both qPCR and microarray revealed that the expression of long-chain acyl-CoA synthetase 1 (ACSL1) was enhanced by overexpression of PPARG with ROSI (Figure 2). ACSL1 catalyzes the conversion of free fatty acids (FFAs) into their activated acyl-CoA derivatives, which are in turn used in the cell for β-oxidation, synthesis, or reacylation of many different cellular lipids or other cellular processes. Previous data suggested that FA activation in bovine mammary tissue occurs primarily via ACSL1 due to the fact that its mRNA is the most predominant among ACSL isoforms [30, 31].

Synthesis of very-long-chain FA is carried out by fatty acid desaturases 1 (FADS1) and 2 (FADS2), which add double bonds at the Δ5 and Δ6 position of PUFA and synthesize eicosapentaenoic acid (20:5n-3) and docosahexaenoic acid (22:6n-3). In this study, the fact that the expression of FADS1 was significantly upregulated in PPARG-overexpressing cells indicated that this nuclear receptor may enhance the biosynthesis of polyunsaturated fatty acids. These data suggested that FADS1 may be a target of PPARG. Hence, we hypothesize that the increase of omega-3/omega-6 ratio in milk fat could be achieved through the activation of PPARG in mammary cells. In fact, the hypothesis is supported by the fact that the subcategory "biosynthesis of unsaturated fatty acid" was among the top 30 categories in this study (File S3).

The perilipin (PAT) family [32–34] and cell death-inducing DFF45 like effector (CIDE) family [35, 36] play a pivotal role in lipid formation. In the present study, the marked upregulation of PLIN2 in PPARG-overexpressing GMEC is consistent with recent data indicating that PPARG could directly bind to the promoter of PLIN2 and modulate the lipid formation in GMEC [13]. Less is known about the role of CIDEA in lipid droplet formation in ruminant mammary cells; however, it was the only CIDE isoform which was upregulated significantly after overexpression of PPARG plus ROSI. This indicates that CIDEA is a target of PPARG.

In addition to the PPAR family, the key transcription factors SREBF1, NR1H3, CEBPA, H1F1A, JUN, and HOXA9 also had a significant change in response to the PPARG gain of function with or without ROSI. The cross talk between PPARG and SREBF1 and NR1H3 was described in our recent papers [2, 3, 12] and completely agrees with the present data that expression of SREBF1 and NR1H3 was enhanced by the overexpression of PPARG plus ROSI. The data from the IPA analysis indicating that overexpression of PPARG down- or upregulated these upstream transcription factors further supports our previous hypothesis that PPARG regulates the gene network related to fatty acid metabolism in a direct or indirect manner [3, 12]. Overall, the results indicated that goat mammary tissue relies heavily on PPARG regulation of genes to induce copious milk fat synthesis and secretion.

The pathway "glycosaminoglycan biosynthesis-keratan sulfate" is involved in the synthesis of keratan sulfate (KS);

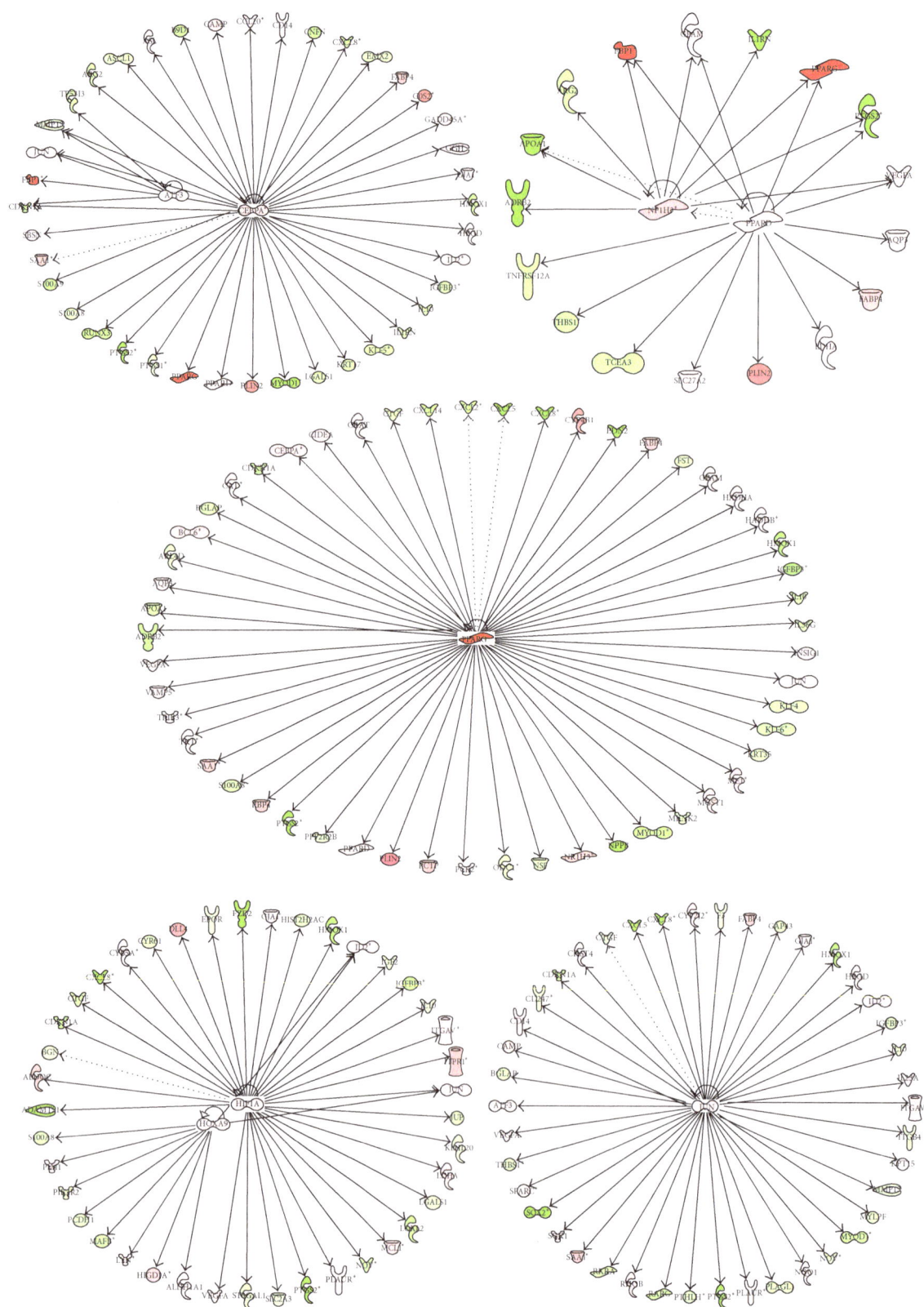

FIGURE 6: Ingenuity pathway upstream network analysis of differentially expressed genes (DEG) between cells treated with Ad-PPARG and rosiglitazone and those with Ad-GFP. Only upregulated transcription factors are shown in this network. Upstream regulators are located at the center of the network and downstream genes are located in the periphery. In the network, their downstream genes are also reported. The description of the color background and arrows in this figure is the same as Figure 5.

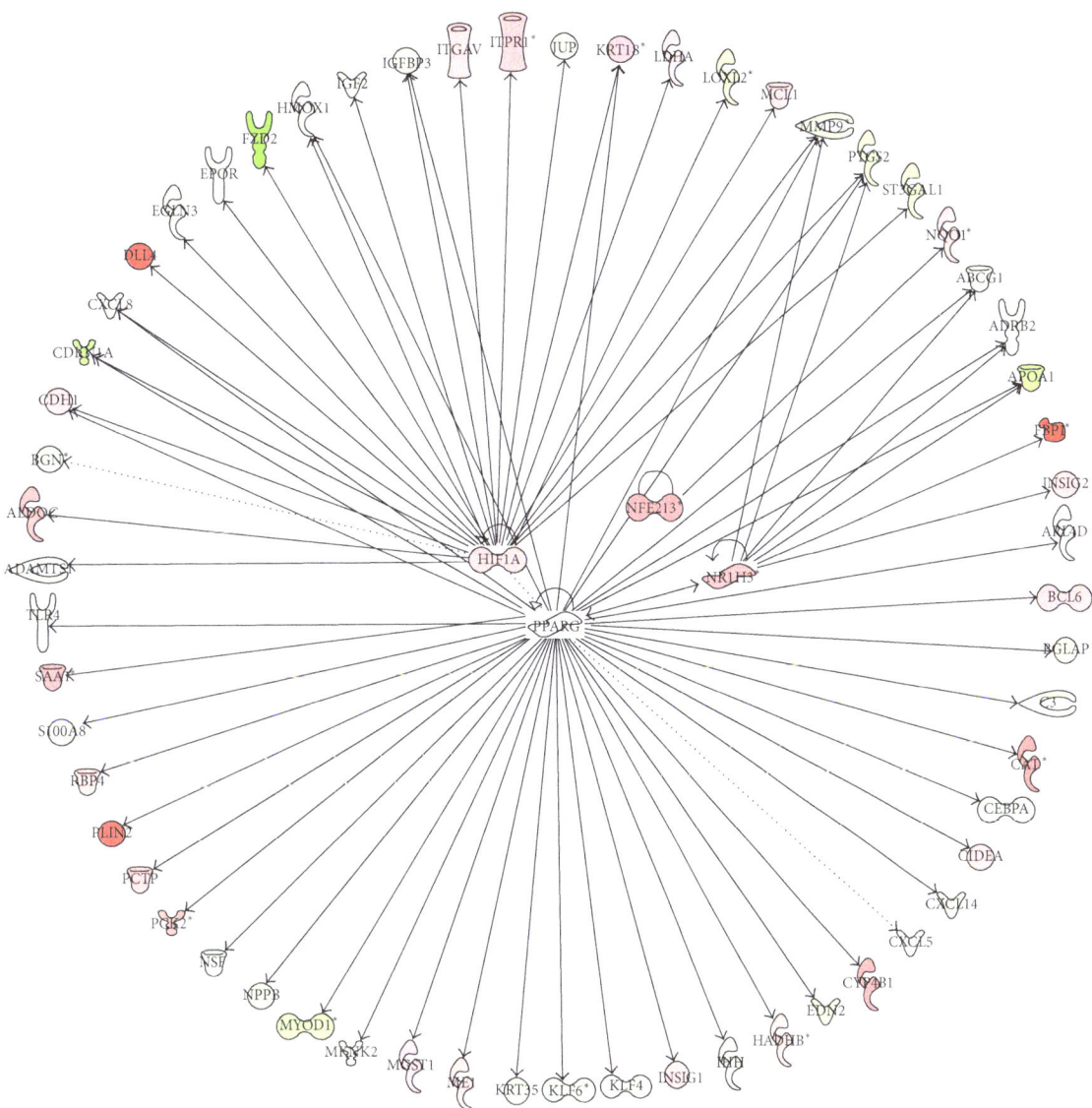

FIGURE 7: Ingenuity pathway upstream network analysis of differentially expressed genes (DEG) between cells treated with Ad-PPARG and rosiglitazone and those with Ad-PPARG. Only upregulated transcription factors are shown in this network. Upstream regulators are located at the center of the network and downstream genes are located in the periphery. In the network, their downstream genes are also reported. The description of the color background and arrows in this figure is the same as Figure 5.

thus, its marked activation indicated that *PPARG* could control inflammatory response via regulating the synthesis of keratan sulfate. The hypothesis is consistent with the role of *PPARG* in inflammation in nonruminants [37–40]. Thus, this finding is novel and more research on KS synthesis seems warranted to better understand its role in the process inflammation, for example, during onset of mastitis.

The high activation of "pentose phosphate pathway" after overexpression of *PPARG* suggests that it promoted the efficient utilization of glucose in GMEC to generate substrates supporting other cellular processes. The high activation of glucose oxidation or other carbohydrate metabolism pathways in PPARG-overexpressing GMEC supports the view of a mechanism whereby *PPARG* alters metabolic pathways in lactating mammary gland; that is, *PPARG* promotes

carbohydrate metabolism to produce intermediates to serve other aspects of milk fatty acid metabolism and lactose synthesis [41].

Due to the limitation of the microarray platform used [29], the interpretation of the findings from the present study has some limitations. For instance, the microarray platform used could not completely cover the genes with functional annotation in the goat genome. In addition, the difference between the goat and bovine genome will unavoidably miss some genes. In the future, goat specific oligo microarrays or next-generation sequencing should be used to confirm the transcriptome alterations caused by the *PPARG* gain of function. In that context, however, the present transcriptome analysis provides an initial global insight into the biological processes altered by *PPARG* in ruminant mammary cells.

5. Conclusions

Using cross-species hybridization microarray data, the present data support a role for *PPARG* activation on biological processes including and going beyond milk fat synthesis. The data indicated an overall increase in metabolism with large increase in anabolism, particularly involving fatty acid synthesis and glucose utilization. Most impacted terms underscored the regulatory role of *PPARG* in fatty acid elongation. The fact that pentose phosphate pathway was highly activated by *PPARG* suggests an important role in carbohydrate metabolism to produce intermediates for milk fatty metabolism.

The upstream regulator analysis indicated that *PPARG* controls molecular processes through an extensive level of cross talk with other signaling pathways, for example, *JUN* and *CEBPA*. All these data support our previous hypothesis that *PPARG* plays a central role in milk fatty metabolism in GMEC. In addition, the data also uncovered a likely role of *PPARG* in the GMEC response to inflammation via the "glycosaminoglycan biosynthesis-keratan sulfate" pathway. In conclusion, the data highlighted a strong transcriptional regulation of *PPARG* in the metabolism in GMEC.

Competing Interests

The authors declare that there is no conflict of interests regarding the publication of this paper.

Authors' Contributions

Hengbo Shi and Wangsheng Zhao contributed equally to this paper.

Acknowledgments

This work is jointly supported by the Transgenic New Species Breeding Program of China (2014ZX08009-051B).

References

[1] G. F. W. Haenlein, "Goat milk in human nutrition," *Small Ruminant Research*, vol. 51, no. 2, pp. 155–163, 2004.

[2] H. B. Shi, J. Luo, D. W. Yao et al., "Peroxisome proliferator-activated receptor-γ stimulates the synthesis of monounsaturated fatty acids in dairy goat mammary epithelial cells via the control of stearoyl-coenzyme A desaturase," *Journal of Dairy Science*, vol. 96, no. 12, pp. 7844–7853, 2013.

[3] H. B. Shi, W. S. Zhao, J. Luo et al., "Peroxisome proliferator-activated receptor γ1 and γ2 isoforms alter lipogenic gene networks in goat mammary epithelial cells to different extents," *Journal of Dairy Science*, vol. 97, no. 9, pp. 5437–5447, 2014.

[4] M. Kawai and C. J. Rosen, "PPARγ: a circadian transcription factor in adipogenesis and osteogenesis," *Nature Reviews Endocrinology*, vol. 6, no. 11, pp. 629–636, 2010.

[5] P. Tontonoz and B. M. Spiegelman, "Fat and beyond: the diverse biology of PPARγ," *Annual Review of Biochemistry*, vol. 77, pp. 289–312, 2008.

[6] S. Heikkinen, J. Auwerx, and C. A. Argmann, "PPARγ in human and mouse physiology," *Biochimica et Biophysica Acta (BBA)—Molecular and Cell Biology of Lipids*, vol. 1771, no. 8, pp. 999–1013, 2007.

[7] M. Lehrke and M. A. Lazar, "The many faces of PPARγ," *Cell*, vol. 123, no. 6, pp. 993–999, 2005.

[8] G. Lee, F. Elwood, J. McNally et al., "T0070907, a selective ligand for peroxisome proliferator-activated receptor γ, functions as an antagonist of biochemical and cellular activities," *Journal of Biological Chemistry*, vol. 277, no. 22, pp. 19649–19657, 2002.

[9] R. Zou, G. Xu, X.-C. Liu et al., "PPARγ agonists inhibit TGF-β-PKA signaling in glomerulosclerosis," *Acta Pharmacologica Sinica*, vol. 31, no. 1, pp. 43–50, 2010.

[10] J. Glas, J. Seiderer, C. Markus et al., "Role of PPARG gene variants in inflammatory bowel disease," *Inflammatory Bowel Diseases*, vol. 17, no. 4, pp. 1057–1058, 2011.

[11] A. K. G. Kadegowda, M. Bionaz, L. S. Piperova, R. A. Erdman, and J. J. Loor, "Peroxisome proliferator-activated receptor-γ activation and long-chain fatty acids alter lipogenic gene networks in bovine mammary epithelial cells to various extents," *Journal of Dairy Science*, vol. 92, no. 9, pp. 4276–4289, 2009.

[12] H. B. Shi, J. Luo, J. J. Zhu et al., "PPARγ regulates genes involved in triacylglycerol synthesis and secretion in mammary gland epithelial cells of dairy goats," *PPAR Research*, vol. 2013, Article ID 310948, 10 pages, 2013.

[13] Y. Kang, S. Hengbo, L. Jun et al., "PPARG modulated lipid accumulation in dairy GMEC via regulation of ADRP gene," *Journal of cellular biochemistry*, vol. 116, no. 1, pp. 192–201, 2015.

[14] K. Shahzad, M. Bionaz, E. Trevisi, G. Bertoni, S. L. Rodriguez-Zas, and J. J. Loor, "Integrative analyses of hepatic differentially expressed genes and blood biomarkers during the peripartal period between dairy cows overfed or restricted-fed energy prepartum," *PLoS ONE*, vol. 9, no. 6, Article ID e99757, 2014.

[15] S. J. Moisá, D. W. Shike, D. E. Graugnard et al., "Bioinformatics analysis of transcriptome dynamics during growth in Angus cattle longissimus muscle," *Bioinformatics and Biology Insights*, vol. 7, pp. 253–270, 2013.

[16] J. J. Loor, R. E. Everts, M. Bionaz et al., "Nutrition-induced ketosis alters metabolic and signaling gene networks in liver of periparturient dairy cows," *Physiological Genomics*, vol. 32, no. 1, pp. 105–116, 2007.

[17] L. Schibler, D. Vaiman, A. Oustry, C. Giraud-Delville, and E. P. Cribiu, "Comparative gene mapping: a fine-scale survey of chromosome rearrangements between ruminants and humans," *Genome Research*, vol. 8, no. 9, pp. 901–915, 1998.

[18] S. Ollier, C. Robert-Granié, L. Bernard, Y. Chilliard, and C. Leroux, "Mammary transcriptome analysis of food-deprived lactating goats highlights genes involved in milk secretion and programmed cell death," *The Journal of Nutrition*, vol. 137, no. 3, pp. 560–567, 2007.

[19] G. Pisoni, B. Castiglioni, A. Stella et al., "Microarray analysis of gene expression of milk leukocytes in healthy goats," *Veterinary Research Communications*, vol. 32, no. 1, pp. S219–S221, 2008.

[20] S. Ollier, C. Leroux, A. de la Foye, L. Bernard, J. Rouel, and Y. Chilliard, "Whole intact rapeseeds or sunflower oil in high-forage or high-concentrate diets affects milk yield, milk composition, and mammary gene expression profile in goats," *Journal of Dairy Science*, vol. 92, no. 11, pp. 5544–5560, 2009.

[21] Z. Wang, J. Luo, W. Wang, W. Zhao, and X. Lin, "Characterization and culture of isolated primary dairy goat mammary gland epithelial cells," *Chinese Journal of Biotechnology*, vol. 26, no. 8, pp. 1123–1127, 2010.

[22] X.-Z. Lin, J. Luo, L.-P. Zhang, W. Wang, H.-B. Shi, and J.-J. Zhu, "MiR-27a suppresses triglyceride accumulation and affects gene mRNA expression associated with fat metabolism in dairy goat mammary gland epithelial cells," *Gene*, vol. 521, no. 1, pp. 15–23, 2013.

[23] H. Akbar, F. C. Cardoso, S. Meier et al., "Postpartal subclinical endometritis alters transcriptome profiles in liver and adipose tissue of dairy cows," *Bioinformatics and Biology Insights*, vol. 8, pp. 45–63, 2014.

[24] M. Bionaz, K. Periasamy, S. L. Rodriguez-Zas, W. L. Hurley, and J. J. Loor, "A novel dynamic impact approach (DIA) for functional analysis of time-course omics studies: validation using the bovine mammary transcriptome," *PLoS ONE*, vol. 7, no. 3, Article ID e32455, 2012.

[25] F. Faucon, E. Rebours, C. Bevilacqua et al., "Terminal differentiation of goat mammary tissue during pregnancy requires the expression of genes involved in immune functions," *Physiological Genomics*, vol. 40, no. 1, pp. 61–82, 2009.

[26] D. M. Magalhães-Padilha, J. Geisler-Lee, A. Wischral et al., "Gene expression during early folliculogenesis in goats using microarray analysis," *Biology of Reproduction*, vol. 89, no. 1, article 19, 2013.

[27] G. Pisoni, P. Moroni, S. Genini et al., "Differentially expressed genes associated with *Staphylococcus aureus* mastitis in dairy goats," *Veterinary Immunology and Immunopathology*, vol. 135, no. 3-4, pp. 208–217, 2010.

[28] B. B. Lowell, "PPARγ: an essential regulator of adipogenesis and modulator of fat cell function," *Cell*, vol. 99, no. 3, pp. 239–242, 1999.

[29] M. Bionaz, K. Periasamy, S. L. Rodriguez-Zas et al., "Old and new stories: revelations from functional analysis of the bovine mammary transcriptome during the lactation cycle," *PLoS ONE*, vol. 7, no. 3, Article ID e33268, 2012.

[30] D. G. Mashek and R. A. Coleman, "Cellular fatty acid uptake: the contribution of metabolism," *Current Opinion in Lipidology*, vol. 17, no. 3, pp. 274–278, 2006.

[31] M. Bionaz and J. J. Loor, "Gene networks driving bovine milk fat synthesis during the lactation cycle," *BMC Genomics*, vol. 9, no. 1, article 366, 2008.

[32] B. M. Chong, P. Reigan, K. D. Mayle-Combs, D. J. Orlicky, and J. L. McManaman, "Determinants of adipophilin function in milk lipid formation and secretion," *Trends in Endocrinology and Metabolism*, vol. 22, no. 6, pp. 211–217, 2011.

[33] P. E. Bickel, J. T. Tansey, and M. A. Welte, "PAT proteins, an ancient family of lipid droplet proteins that regulate cellular lipid stores," *Biochimica et Biophysica Acta—Molecular and Cell Biology of Lipids*, vol. 1791, no. 6, pp. 419–440, 2009.

[34] F. Wilfling, J. T. Haas, T. C. Walther, and R. V. Farese Jr., "Lipid droplet biogenesis," *Current Opinion in Cell Biology*, vol. 29, pp. 39–45, 2014.

[35] H. Yang, A. Galea, V. Sytnyk, and M. Crossley, "Controlling the size of lipid droplets: lipid and protein factors," *Current Opinion in Cell Biology*, vol. 24, no. 4, pp. 509–516, 2012.

[36] R. Singaravelu, R. K. Lyn, P. Srinivasan et al., "Human serum activates CIDEB-mediated lipid droplet enlargement in hepatoma cells," *Biochemical and Biophysical Research Communications*, vol. 441, no. 2, pp. 447–452, 2013.

[37] Y. Wan, A. Saghatelian, L.-W. Chong, C.-L. Zhang, B. F. Cravatt, and R. M. Evans, "Maternal PPARγ protects nursing neonates by suppressing the production of inflammatory milk," *Genes & Development*, vol. 21, no. 15, pp. 1895–1908, 2007.

[38] S. Genini, B. Badaoui, G. Sclep et al., "Strengthening insights into host responses to mastitis infection in ruminants by combining heterogeneous microarray data sources," *BMC Genomics*, vol. 12, article 225, 2011.

[39] P. Ji, J. K. Drackley, M. J. Khan, and J. J. Loor, "Inflammation- and lipid metabolism-related gene network expression in visceral and subcutaneous adipose depots of Holstein cows," *Journal of Dairy Science*, vol. 97, no. 6, pp. 3441–3448, 2014.

[40] M. Masoodi, O. Kuda, M. Rossmeisl, P. Flachs, and J. Kopecky, "Lipid signaling in adipose tissue: connecting inflammation & metabolism," *Biochimica et Biophysica Acta—Molecular and Cell Biology of Lipids*, vol. 1851, no. 4, pp. 503–518, 2015.

[41] M. Bionaz, S. Chen, M. J. Khan, and J. J. Loor, "Functional role of PPARs in ruminants: potential targets for fine-tuning metabolism during growth and lactation," *PPAR Research*, vol. 2013, Article ID 684159, 28 pages, 2013.

13

Interactions between PPAR Gamma and the Canonical Wnt/Beta-Catenin Pathway in Type 2 Diabetes and Colon Cancer

Yves Lecarpentier,[1] Victor Claes,[2] Alexandre Vallée,[3,4] and Jean-Louis Hébert[5]

[1]Centre de Recherche Clinique, Hôpital de Meaux, Meaux, France
[2]Department of Pharmaceutical Sciences, University of Antwerp, Wilrijk, Belgium
[3]CHU Amiens Picardie, Université Picardie Jules Verne, Amiens, France
[4]Experimental and Clinical Neurosciences Laboratory, INSERM U1084, University of Poitiers, France
[5]Institut de Cardiologie, Hôpital de la Pitié-Salpêtrière, Assistance Publique-Hôpitaux de Paris, Paris, France

Correspondence should be addressed to Yves Lecarpentier; yves.c.lecarpentier@gmail.com

Academic Editor: Richard P. Phipps

In both colon cancer and type 2 diabetes, metabolic changes induced by upregulation of the Wnt/beta-catenin signaling and downregulation of peroxisome proliferator-activated receptor gamma (PPAR gamma) may help account for the frequent association of these two diseases. In both diseases, PPAR gamma is downregulated while the canonical Wnt/beta-catenin pathway is upregulated. In colon cancer, upregulation of the canonical Wnt system induces activation of pyruvate dehydrogenase kinase and deactivation of the pyruvate dehydrogenase complex. As a result, a large part of cytosolic pyruvate is converted into lactate through activation of lactate dehydrogenase. Lactate is extruded out of the cell by means of activation of monocarboxylate lactate transporter-1. This phenomenon is called Warburg effect. PPAR gamma agonists induce beta-catenin inhibition, while inhibition of the canonical Wnt/beta-catenin pathway activates PPAR gamma.

1. Introduction

In numerous mammalian living cells, PPAR gamma and the canonical Wnt/beta-catenin pathway behave in an opposite manner [1–5]. Beta-catenin and PPAR gamma interact with each other in a mechanism that alters each of their activities [6]. In several diseases, PPAR gamma is upregulated while canonical Wnt/beta-catenin is downregulated [7] such as in arrhythmogenic right ventricular cardiomyopathy (ARVC), osteoporosis, and certain neurodegenerative diseases (Alzheimer's disease [8], bipolar disorder, and schizophrenia). Conversely, in other diseases, PPAR gamma is downregulated while canonical Wnt/beta-catenin is upregulated such as in type 2 diabetes, cancers, and certain neurodegenerative diseases (amyotrophic lateral sclerosis [9], Parkinson's disease, Huntington's disease, multiple sclerosis, and Friedreich's ataxia). PPAR gamma agonists induce beta-catenin inhibition in several cellular systems [1, 3, 4, 10].

Moreover, inhibition of canonical Wnt/beta-catenin pathway induces activation of PPAR gamma [11–13]. Nonsteroidal anti-inflammatory drug inhibition of beta-catenin in malignant cells requires a high level expression of PPAR gamma and its coreceptor retinoid-X-receptor alpha [14]. In terms of PPAR gamma and Wnt/beta-catenin signaling, both type 2 diabetes and colon cancer share several similarities from a metabolic point of view. In the two diseases, upregulation of the canonical Wnt system leads to activation of pyruvate dehydrogenase kinase (PDK), which decreases the activity of the pyruvate dehydrogenase complex (PDH). Thus, pyruvate cannot be totally converted into acetyl-coenzyme which does not the mitochondrial TCA cycle. Conversely, PPAR gamma activation selectively decreased PDK mRNA [15]. The multiple and complex properties of these two major pathways, particularly in glucose regulation and cell proliferation, may partly account for the association frequently observed between type 2 diabetes and colon cancer.

2. Link between Type 2 Diabetes and Colon Cancer

The association between type 2 diabetes and cancer, including pancreatic and endometrial carcinoma, breast cancer, and colorectal and bladder cancers, has been known for many years. Epidemiological studies have reported a link between type 2 diabetes, obesity, and cancer, especially colon cancer [16–19]. Type 2 diabetes associated with obesity represents a major risk factor for cancer [20–24]. Shared risk factors for colorectal cancer and type 2 diabetes include obesity, physical inactivity, and ageing. Patients with type 2 diabetes present a 30–40% higher risk of developing colon cancer compared to those without diabetes. Type 2 diabetes risk variants also contribute to the risk of colorectal cancer [25]. Metformin, an antidiabetic agent, decreases cancer mortality in diabetic patients [26].

3. Underlying Molecular Basis for the Link between Diabetes and Colon Cancer

The underlying molecular basis for the link between type 2 diabetes and colon cancer is not fully understood. Hyperinsulinemia provides a link between diabetes, obesity, and cancer. Hyperinsulinemia and/or insulin resistance represent major factors in cancer pathogenesis [27]. The hypothesis for the association between diabetes and cancer is based on the fact that, in type 2 diabetes, hyperinsulinemia promotes the growth of cancer cells [28]. In colon cancer, the hyperinsulinemia hypothesis suggests that elevated levels of both insulin and free insulin growth factor (IGF-1) promote cell proliferation and enhancement of cell transformation, ultimately resulting in colorectal cancer [29]. High insulin levels represent an adaptive process to insulin resistance at the onset of type 2 diabetes. Cancers overexpress receptors for insulin, including insulin receptor A and IGF-1 receptor. Increased insulin/IGF signaling favors the proliferative properties of the two hormones. Moreover, hyperglycemia and chronic inflammation may also play a role in promoting cancer growth [30].

4. Activation of Canonical Wnt Signaling Induces Aerobic Glycolysis or Warburg Effect

4.1. Canonical Wnt/Beta-Catenin Pathway (Figures 1 and 2). The Wnt/beta-catenin signaling plays an important role in cell fate, epithelial-mesenchymal transition (EMT) signaling, and embryonic development. Its dysfunction is involved in several pathologies such as carcinogenesis [31–34]. The major effector of the canonical Wnt pathway is the transcription factor beta-catenin/T-cell factor/lymphoid enhancer factor (TCF/LEF). In the absence of Wnt, the free cytosolic beta-catenin is phosphorylated and is tightly controlled by a destruction complex, consisting of AXIN, tumor suppressor adenomatous polyposis coli (APC), and glycogen synthase kinase-3 (GSK-3beta). The destruction complex interacts with beta-catenin and phosphorylates it. The phosphorylated

beta-catenin is then degraded in the proteasome (beta-catenin proteasomal degradation: CPD). In the presence of ligands, the Wnt receptor interacts with the Frizzled (Fzd) receptor and LDL receptor-related protein 5/6 (LRP5/6) coreceptors. The Wnt receptor associates with Dishevelled protein (Dsh). This triggers the disruption of the destruction complex and prevents CPD. Beta-catenin then translocates to the nucleus and interacts with TCF/LEF which stimulates the beta-catenin downstream target genes (PDK, MTC-1, cMyc, cyclin D1, Cox 2, AXIN 2, etc.) [35–38] (Figures 1 and 2).

4.2. Canonical Wnt Pathway and Glucose. Importantly, glucose itself can directly impact the canonical Wnt pathway [39]. In cancer cells, glucose-induced beta-catenin acetylation favors the Wnt pathway. High glucose level enhances the nuclear translocation of beta-catenin in response to Wnt signaling. Increased glucose consumption is characteristic of cancer cells and high serum glucose levels may modulate cancer-related signaling.

4.3. Aerobic Glycolysis in Cancer Cells: The Warburg Effect. The role of the Wnt pathway in driving cell proliferation during oncogenesis and especially colon cancer is well-known [40]. On the one hand, overactivation of canonical Wnt/beta-catenin signaling via TCF/LEF leads to cell proliferation, migration, angiogenesis, and EMT signaling [41–43]. On the other hand, the Wnt pathway induces aerobic glycolysis allowing glucose utilization for cancer cell proliferation [38, 44]. In cancer cells, a large proportion of the glucose supply is fermented in lactate regardless of the availability of oxygen. This phenomenon is called aerobic glycolysis or Warburg effect [45] and ultimately leads to anabolic production of biomass, that is, nucleotide synthesis [46, 47]. As a consequence, in the Warburg effect, a large part of cytosolic pyruvate is not converted into acetyl-CoA which does not enter the TCA cycle. PDK1, a key regulator of glycolysis, phosphorylates the PDH complex which partially inhibits the conversion of pyruvate to acetyl-CoA into mitochondria [48]. PDK1 is upregulated in colon cancer [38]. Thus, cytosolic pyruvate is converted into lactate through activation of LDH-A. Moreover, upregulation of MCT-1 diverts pyruvate towards lactate secretion from the cell. Aerobically derived lactate stimulates angiogenesis [49]. Thus, most of the cytosolic pyruvate is converted into lactate, which is secreted from the cell, and not oxidized in the mitochondrial TCA cycle, despite the availability of oxygen.

In colon cancer, it has recently been shown that activation of the canonical Wnt/beta-catenin pathway partly decreases the oxidative metabolism in the TCA cycle and promotes cell proliferation [38]. Both PDK1 and the lactate transporter MCT-1 are Wnt/beta-catenin targets and are overexpressed in cancer cells. Moreover, the Wnt pathway induces the transcription of genes involved in cell proliferation, that is, cMyc (through glutaminolysis, nucleotide synthesis, and LDH-A activation) and cyclin D1 (through G1) [50–55]. The Wnt target gene cMyc drives aerobic glycolysis and glutaminolysis [52, 54, 56]. Myc also induces LDH-A activation (for conversion of cytosolic pyruvate into lactate). cMyc

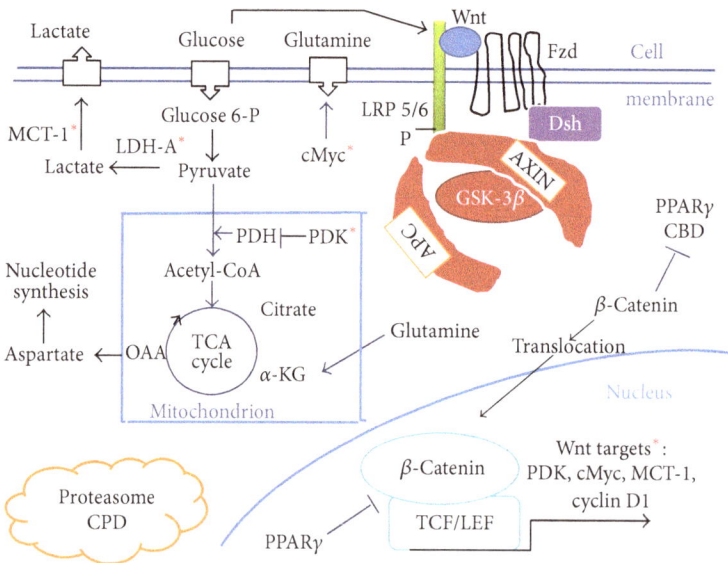

FIGURE 1: A model of interactions between the canonical Wnt/beta-catenin pathway and PPAR gamma under aerobic glycolysis conditions in colon cancer. In the absence of the Wnt ligand ("off state"), cytosolic beta-catenin is phosphorylated by GSK-3 beta. APS and AXIN combine with GSK-3 beta and beta-catenin to enhance the destruction process in the proteasome (beta-catenin proteasomal degradation: CPD). In the presence of the Wnt ligand ("on state"), Wnt binds both Frizzled and LRP5/6 receptors to initiate LRP phosphorylation and dishevelled-mediated Frizzled internalization. This leads to dissociation of the AXIN/APC/GSK-3 beta complex. Beta-catenin phosphorylation is inhibited. Thus, beta-catenin accumulates in the cytosol and then translocates to the nucleus to bind TCF-LEF cotranscription factors, which induce the Wnt-response gene transcription (PDK, MCT-1, cMyc, and cyclin D1). Glucose itself activates the Wnt pathway. PPAR gamma via APC activates CPD. PPAR gamma inhibits the beta-catenin-TCF/LEF complex. Beta-catenin binds PPAR gamma CBD. PDK inhibits the PDH complex in mitochondria. Thus pyruvate cannot be converted into acetyl-CoA and enters the TCA cycle. Myc activates LDH-A which converts cytosolic pyruvate into lactate. MCT-1 favors lactate secretion from the cytosol which favors angiogenesis. cMyc increases glutamine entry in the cytosol and mitochondria. Myc-induced glutamine enhances nucleotide synthesis. Abbreviations are as follows: adenomatous polyposis coli (APC); alpha ceto-glutarate (a-KG); beta-catenin proteasomal degradation: CPD; catenin binding domain (CBD); Dishevelled (Dsh); Frizzled (Fzd); glycogen synthase kinase-3beta (GSK-3beta); lactate dehydrogenase (LDH); low-density lipoprotein receptor-related protein 5/6 (LRP5/6); monocarboxylate lactate transporter-1 (MCT-1); peroxisome proliferator-activated receptor gamma (PPAR gamma); pyruvate dehydrogenase complex (PDH); pyruvate dehydrogenase kinase (PDK); T-cell factor/lymphoid enhancer factor (TCF/LEF); tricarboxylic acid (TCA); *: Wnt targets: PDK, cMyc, MCT-1, and cyclin D1.

induces glutamine uptake into the cell and the mitochondria and favors aspartate synthesis [52] (Figures 1 and 2). Through the Warburg effect, cMyc-induced glutaminolysis favors nucleotide synthesis. cMyc also increases the hypoxia-inducible factor-1 alpha- (HIF-1alpha-) mediated control of PDK1 [57].

Thus, in colon cancer, activation of canonical Wnt signaling directly acts on aerobic glycolysis and increases vessel development via the Wnt target gene PDK1 [38]. Part of the pyruvate is converted into acetyl-CoA which enters the TCA cycle and is converted into citrate, which promotes protein synthesis. Cellular accumulation of metabolic intermediates (aspartate, serine, glycine, and ribose) allows de novo nucleotide synthesis, which contributes to growth and proliferation (Figure 1). Moreover, blocking Wnt reduces PDK1 levels via the transcription regulation and reduces in vivo tumor growth. PDK1 is upregulated in several cancers, especially colon cancer [58–60]. Likewise, PDK1 and PDK2 enhance angiogenesis [61, 62]. PDK1 favors vascularization [38]. Angiogenesis is also favored by lactates [63]. MCTs are also upregulated in colon cancer [64].

5. Pyruvate Dehydrogenase Kinases (PDKs) and Diseases

Metabolic disorders combined with abnormal PDK activity are often associated with numerous diseases, such as type 2 diabetes, obesity, metabolic disorders, cardiomyopathies, neuropathies, and several types of cancer. PDKs play a key role in metabolic flexibility [65]. They are transcriptionally regulated by insulin, glucocorticoids, thyroid hormone, and fatty acids and play an important role in diabetes and obesity [66]. In type 2 diabetes, the two isoforms PDK2 and PDK4 are induced in a tissue-specific manner. Transcriptional upregulation of PDKs [67–69] decreases the PDH activity in several metabolic disorders, such as diabetes [70–72]. In type 2 diabetes, decreased levels of insulin promote an increase in both PDK4 gene expression and PDK2 mRNA levels. PDK2 and PDK4 mRNAs are upregulated in response to glucose deprivation and fatty acid supplementation. This is reversed by insulin treatment as insulin directly downregulates PDK2 and PDK4 mRNA transcripts [15].

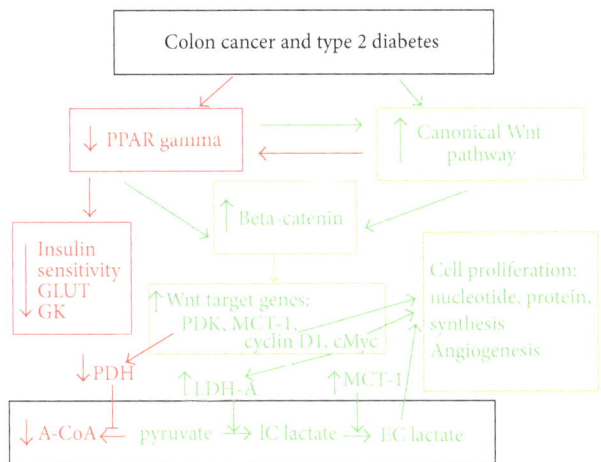

FIGURE 2: A schematic representation of interactions between PPAR gamma and the canonical Wnt/beta-catenin pathway in type 2 diabetes and colon cancer. Green arrow: activation; red arrow: inhibition; abbreviations are as follows: acetyl-CoA (A-CoA); glucokinase (GK); glucose transporter (GLUT); intracellular lactate (IC lactate); extracellular lactate (EC lactate); lactate dehydrogenase-A (LDH-A); monocarboxylate lactate transporter-1 (MCT-1); pyruvate dehydrogenase (PDH); pyruvate dehydrogenase kinase (PDK); peroxisome proliferator-activated receptor gamma (PPAR gamma).

6. Interactions between PPAR Gamma and the Canonical Wnt/Beta-Catenin Pathway

6.1. PPAR Gamma (Figures 1 and 2). PPAR alpha, beta/delta, and gamma are ligand-activated transcriptional factors which belong to the nuclear hormone receptor superfamily. PPARs heterodimerize with the retinoid X receptor (RXR). PPAR gamma is expressed in various cell types, such as adipose tissues, muscles, brain, and immune cells. PPAR gamma is involved in the expression of many genes and contributes to glucose homeostasis, insulin sensitivity, lipid metabolism, immune responses, inflammation, and cell fate [73–75]. The net result of the pleiotropic effects of thiazolidinediones (TZDs), a class of PPAR gamma agonists, is improvement of insulin sensitivity [76] in peripheral tissues together with an increase in the glucose-sensing ability of pancreatic beta-cells in diabetic subjects. They improve glucose tolerance and insulin sensitivity in type 2 diabetic patients and in animal models of insulin resistance [77, 78]. Enhanced insulin sensitivity improves peripheral glucose disposal, which decreases the demand for insulin secretion from beta-cells and hepatic glucose production. Effects of TZDs result in increased peripheral glucose use, reduced hepatic glucose output, and, consequently, improvement in overall glycemic control. They act on the promoters of GLUT2 and beta-glucokinase (GK) in pancreatic beta-cells and liver. In adipose tissue, several genes are under the transcriptional control of PPAR gamma, including lipoprotein lipase, acyl-CoA synthetase, fatty acid translocase, and fatty acid transport protein [75]. Dysfunction of PPAR gamma is implied in numerous pathological states such as diabetes, obesity, cancers, and atherosclerosis.

TZDs directly activate PPAR gamma and are insulin sensitizing drugs. Some TZDs have been used for treating type 2 diabetes. PPAR gamma also regulates circadian cardiovascular rhythms of blood pressure and heart rate by means of BMAL1 [79, 80]. In cultured muscle cells, PPAR alpha and delta agonists specifically upregulate the expression of PDK4 mRNA, whereas PPAR gamma activation selectively decreases PDK2 mRNA [15]. The PPAR alpha agonist WY-14,643 increases PDK4 mRNA levels in Morris hepatoma 7800 C1 cells [67]. In the diabetic heart, PPAR alpha activity and its downstream targets are upregulated, which leads to a dramatic increase in both fatty acid uptake and oxidation [81] and decreases the mitochondrial pyruvate degradation by upregulating PDK2 and 4.

6.2. PPAR Gamma Agonists Induce Beta-Catenin Inhibition in Several Cellular Systems. The functional crosstalk between PPAR gamma and the canonical Wnt/beta-catenin signaling involves the TCF/LEF binding domain of beta-catenin and a catenin binding domain (CBD) within PPAR gamma. In cells that express an APC-containing destruction complex, activation of PPAR gamma induces CPD (Figure 1). TZDs induce a reduction in the cytoplasmic level of beta-catenin in both adipocytes [1] and hepatocytes [3]. PPAR gamma inhibits osteoblastogenesis, promotes adipogenesis, and suppresses the Wnt/beta-catenin pathway during adipogenesis [4, 10]. Conversely Wnt/beta-catenin signaling activation inhibits PPAR gamma and leads to osteogenesis [4].

6.3. Inhibition of Canonical Wnt/Beta-Catenin Pathway Induces Activation of PPAR Gamma in Several Cellular Systems. Inhibition of Wnt/beta-catenin signaling and upregulation of PPAR gamma have been reported in ARVC [12, 13]. Gamma-catenin presents structural similarities with beta-catenin [31]. In transgenic mice, gamma-catenin translocates to the nucleus, competes with beta-catenin, and inhibits the canonical Wnt/beta-catenin signaling through the TCF/LEF transcription factors [82, 83]. This results in enhancing adipogenesis, thus summarizing the phenotype of the human ARVC [11–13].

6.4. Inactivation of PPAR Gamma and Activation of the Wnt/Beta-Catenin Pathway in Colon Cancer. Beta-catenin-TCF/LEF signaling is activated in colon cancer [84]. Nuclear accumulation of beta-catenin, a marker of poor prognosis, drives cancer cell proliferation. Activation of Wnt signaling can occur via *APC* gene mutations and this enables development of colon cancer [85]. In colon cancer cells, activation of the Wnt/beta-catenin pathway decreases PPAR gamma activity [86]. Beta-catenin can also interact with RXR alpha. In *APC*- and *p53*-mutated colorectal cancer cells, RXR agonists inactivate beta-catenin via RXR alpha. RXR alpha-mediated inactivation of oncogenic beta-catenin occurs in parallel with a reduction in cell proliferation [87]. Mutations in PPAR gamma are linked with human colon cancer [88]. In normal untransformed cells, PPAR gamma induces CPD through both the CBD of PPAR gamma and the TCF binding domain of beta-catenin (Figure 1). In transformed cells, there is no oncogenic beta-catenin degradation. In colon carcinogenesis, PPAR gamma can suppress tumorigenesis by downregulating the oncogene beta-catenin [89]. An early treatment by means of PPAR gamma agonists, and before the onset of carcinogenesis, might prevent tumor development. In many cell types, PPAR gamma agonists induce antitumorigenic effects, probably due to their antiproliferative and prodifferentiation effects. Troglitazone inhibits development of tumors that are derived from colon cancer cells [90]. In transplantable tumors derived from human colon cancer cells, troglitazone induces a significant reduction of growth. Troglitazone fed to rodents decreases the formation of aberrant crypt foci, which is an early stage in the development of colon carcinoma [91]. Activation of PPAR gamma induces CPD in cells that express an APC-containing destruction complex although the oncogenic beta-catenin inhibits the expression of PPAR gamma target genes [6]. Mutations in the TCF/LEF binding domain of an oncogenic beta-catenin leads to both decreased interaction with PPAR gamma and inhibition of PPAR gamma activity [6]. Conversely, in some cases, PPAR gamma activation induces deleterious procarcinogenic effects. Thus, in APC *Min* mice, used as a model for human familial adenomatous polyposis, TZDs increase the number of colon tumors [92, 93]. Numerous studies on cancer and PPAR gamma have focused on the potential for employing PPAR gamma agonists in cancer treatment. As a monotherapy, PPAR gamma agonists have induced little success in clinical trials. Results have been shown promise with combined treatments in culture and animal models. A role for PPAR gamma as a tumor suppressor and inducer of differentiation of cancer stem cells has also been investigated. Various conclusions concerning the prevalence of PPAR gamma mutations in cancer have been observed [94].

6.5. Inactivation of PPAR Gamma and Activation of the Wnt/Beta-Catenin Pathway in Type 2 Diabetes. TZDs are potent insulin-sensitizers and certain TZDs represent a therapeutic target for the treatment of type 2 diabetes. However, the involvement of PPAR gamma in numerous pathways generates negative side-effects after PPAR gamma activation by TZDs in tissues or cells not concerned by the disease [95]. PPAR gamma enables activation of GLUT2 and GK in liver and beta-cells and contributes to the beneficial effects induced by TZDs, which improve glucose homeostasis in type 2 diabetic patients. Moreover, dominant-negative mutation in the *PPAR gamma* gene is associated with severe hyperglycemia in patients. This provides a genetic link between PPAR gamma and type 2 diabetes [96]. Humans with dominant-negative mutations in PPAR gamma manifest partial lipodystrophy and severe peripheral and hepatic insulin resistance [97]. Expression of TNF-alpha, which induces insulin resistance, is reduced by PPAR gamma ligands, suggesting that the insulin-sensitizing effect of TZDs is related to its anti-inflammatory properties [98]. PPAR gamma has a significantly lower expression in obese type 2 diabetics than in nondiabetic obese subjects [99].

The Wnt/beta-catenin signaling pathway is involved in diabetes mellitus [100]. Wnt signaling and TCF7L2 are negative regulators of hepatic gluconeogenesis, and TCF7L2

belongs to the downstream effectors of insulin in hepatocytes [101]. Wnt/beta-catenin may represent a link between diabetes and cancer, due to the strong genetic association between specific polymorphisms in the TCF7L2 (TCF4) gene and diabetes [102, 103]. TCF7L2 polymorphisms enhance the risk of developing type 2 diabetes [104–106]. Mutations in LRP5 lead to the development of diabetes and obesity [107]. The Wnt pathway is involved in glucose-induced insulin secretion [108] and production of the incretin hormone glucagon-like peptide-1 [109–111]. Polymorphisms in Wnt5B are associated with a higher risk of developing type 2 diabetes [112]. Otherwise, the human LRP5 gene maps within the IDDM4 region on chromosome 11q13 [113, 114]. Conversely, TCF7L2 knockdown increases human pancreatic beta-cell apoptosis and reduces beta-cell proliferation and glucose-stimulated insulin secretion [115].

7. Conclusions

PPAR gamma is downregulated while the canonical Wnt/beta-catenin pathway is upregulated in both type 2 diabetes and colon cancer. Wnt activates some crucial metabolic key enzymes, such as PDKs in the two pathologies. In colon cancer, this leads to aerobic glycolysis or the Warburg effect. Decreased PDH activity by upregulated PDK modifies metabolic flexibility that is, the capacity of the cell to adjust glucose and fatty acid oxidation. Competition between glucose and fatty acids for oxidation occurs at the level of the PDH complex, whose activity is decreased by PDKs. In colon cancer, partial deviation of pyruvate toward lactate contributes to protein synthesis, which are required for cell growth and proliferation. These major metabolic alterations induced by upregulated Wnt/beta-catenin signaling and downregulated PPAR gamma may partly account for the frequently encountered association between type 2 diabetes and colon cancer.

Abbreviations

APC: Adenomatous polyposis coli
ARVC: Arrhythmogenic right ventricular
              dysplasia/cardiomyopathy
CPD: Beta-catenin proteasomal
              degradation
CBD: Catenin binding domain
Dsh: Dishevelled
EMT: Epithelial-mesenchymal transition
Fzd: Frizzled
GK: Glucokinase
GLUT: Glucose transporter
GSK-3beta: Glycogen synthase kinase-3beta
IGF-1:   Insulin growth factor
LDH-A: Lactate dehydrogenase-A
LRP5/6:   LDL receptor-related protein 5/6
              coreceptors
LRP5/6:   Low-density lipoprotein
              receptor-related protein 5/6
MCT-1:   Monocarboxylate lactate
              transporter-1

PPAR gamma: Peroxisome proliferator-activated receptor gamma
PGC-1 alpha: Peroxisome proliferator-activated receptor-gamma coactivator-1 alpha
PDH: Pyruvate dehydrogenase
PDK: Pyruvate dehydrogenase kinase
RXR Alpha: Retinoid X receptor alpha
TCF/LEF: T-cell factor/lymphoid enhancer factor
TZD: Thiazolidinedione
TCA: Tricarboxylic acid.

Competing Interests

The authors declare no conflict of interests.

Authors' Contributions

Yves Lecarpentier, Victor Claes, Alexandre Vallée, and Jean-Louis Hébert have equally contributed to this review.

Acknowledgments

The authors would like to thank Dr Christophe Locher, Director of the Clinical Research Center, Meaux Hospital, and Mr Vincent Gobert, Administrative Manager of the Clinical Research Center, Meaux Hospital, Meaux, France, for their valuable support in making the necessary research facilities available for this study. The manuscript has been revised by Brian Keogh, PhD.

References

[1] D. L. Gerhold, F. Liu, G. Jiang et al., "Gene expression profile of adipocyte differentiation and its regulation by peroxisome proliferator-activated receptor-γ agonists," *Endocrinology*, vol. 143, no. 6, pp. 2106–2118, 2002.

[2] G. D. Girnun, F. E. Domann, S. A. Moore, and M. E. C. Robbins, "Identification of a functional peroxisome proliferator-activated receptor response element in the rat catalase promoter," *Molecular Endocrinology*, vol. 16, no. 12, pp. 2793–2801, 2002.

[3] C. Sharma, A. Pradeep, L. Wong, A. Rana, and B. Rana, "Peroxisome proliferator-activated receptor γ activation can regulate β-catenin levels via a proteasome-mediated and adenomatous polyposis coli-independent pathway," *The Journal of Biological Chemistry*, vol. 279, no. 34, pp. 35583–35594, 2004.

[4] I. Takada, A. P. Kouzmenko, and S. Kato, "Wnt and PPARγ signaling in osteoblastogenesis and adipogenesis," *Nature Reviews Rheumatology*, vol. 5, no. 8, pp. 442–447, 2009.

[5] D. Lu and D. A. Carson, "Repression of β catenin signaling by PPARγ ligands," *European Journal of Pharmacology*, vol. 636, no. 1–3, pp. 198–202, 2010.

[6] J. Liu, H. Wang, Y. Zuo, and S. R. Farmer, "Functional interaction between peroxisome proliferator-activated receptor γ and β-catenin," *Molecular and Cellular Biology*, vol. 26, no. 15, pp. 5827–5837, 2006.

[7] Y. Lecarpentier, V. Claes, G. Duthoit, and J.-L. Hébert, "Circadian rhythms, Wnt/beta-catenin pathway and PPAR alpha/gamma profiles in diseases with primary or secondary cardiac dysfunction," *Frontiers in Physiology*, vol. 5, article 429, 2014.

[8] A. Vallee and Y. Lecarpentier, "Alzheimer disease: crosstalk between the canonical Wnt/beta-catenin pathway and PPARs alpha and gamma," *Frontiers in Neuroscience*, vol. 10, article 459, 2016.

[9] Y. Lecarpentier and A. Vallée, "Opposite interplay between PPAR gamma and canonical Wnt/beta-catenin pathway in amyotrophic lateral sclerosis," *Frontiers in Neurology*, vol. 7, article no. 100, 2016.

[10] M. Moldes, Y. Zuo, R. F. Morrison et al., "Peroxisome-proliferator-activated receptor γ suppresses Wnt/β-catenin signalling during adipogenesis," *Biochemical Journal*, vol. 376, no. 3, pp. 607–613, 2003.

[11] D. Corrado, C. Basso, G. Thiene et al., "Spectrum of clinico-pathologic manifestations of arrhythmogenic right ventricular cardiomyopathy/dysplasia: a multicenter study," *Journal of the American College of Cardiology*, vol. 30, no. 6, pp. 1512–1520, 1997.

[12] E. Garcia-Gras, R. Lombardi, M. J. Giocondo et al., "Suppression of canonical Wnt/β-catenin signaling by nuclear plakoglobin recapitulates phenotype of arrhythmogenic right ventricular cardiomyopathy," *The Journal of Clinical Investigation*, vol. 116, no. 7, pp. 2012–2021, 2006.

[13] F. Djouadi, Y. Lecarpentier, J.-L. Hébert, P. Charron, J. Bastin, and C. Coirault, "A potential link between peroxisome proliferator-activated receptor signalling and the pathogenesis of arrhythmogenic right ventricular cardiomyopathy," *Cardiovascular Research*, vol. 84, no. 1, pp. 83–90, 2009.

[14] D. Lu, H. B. Cottam, M. Corr, and D. A. Carson, "Repression of β-catenin function in malignant cells by nonsteroidal anti-inflammatory drugs," *Proceedings of the National Academy of Sciences of the United States of America*, vol. 102, no. 51, pp. 18567–18571, 2005.

[15] E. L. Abbot, J. G. McCormack, C. Reynet, D. G. Hassall, K. W. Buchan, and S. J. Yeaman, "Diverging regulation of pyruvate dehydrogenase kinase isoform gene expression in cultured human muscle cells," *FEBS Journal*, vol. 272, no. 12, pp. 3004–3014, 2005.

[16] C. Gao and S.-K. Yao, "Diabetes mellitus: a 'true' independent risk factor for hepatocellular carcinoma?" *Hepatobiliary and Pancreatic Diseases International*, vol. 8, no. 5, pp. 465–473, 2009.

[17] M. Gerber, "Background review paper on total fat, fatty acid intake and cancers," *Annals of Nutrition and Metabolism*, vol. 55, no. 1–3, pp. 140–161, 2009.

[18] P. Hillon, B. Guiu, J. Vincent, and J.-M. Petit, "Obesity, type 2 diabetes and risk of digestive cancer," *Gastroentérologie Clinique et Biologique*, vol. 34, no. 10, pp. 529–533, 2010.

[19] M. J. Khandekar, P. Cohen, and B. M. Spiegelman, "Molecular mechanisms of cancer development in obesity," *Nature Reviews Cancer*, vol. 11, no. 12, pp. 886–895, 2011.

[20] A. G. Renehan, M. Tyson, M. Egger, R. F. Heller, and M. Zwahlen, "Body-mass index and incidence of cancer: a systematic review and meta-analysis of prospective observational studies," *The Lancet*, vol. 371, no. 9612, pp. 569–578, 2008.

[21] P. Vigneri, F. Frasca, L. Sciacca, G. Pandini, and R. Vigneri, "Diabetes and cancer," *Endocrine-Related Cancer*, vol. 16, no. 4, pp. 1103–1123, 2009.

[22] R. Vigneri, "Diabetes: diabetes therapy and cancer risk," *Nature Reviews Endocrinology*, vol. 5, no. 12, pp. 651–652, 2009.

[23] E. Giovannucci, D. M. Harlan, M. C. Archer et al., "Diabetes and cancer: a consensus report," *CA: A Cancer Journal for Clinicians*, vol. 60, no. 4, pp. 207–221, 2010.

[24] P. J. H. L. Peeters, M. T. Bazelier, H. G. M. Leufkens, F. De Vries, and M. L. De Bruin, "The risk of colorectal cancer in patients with type 2 diabetes: associations with treatment stage and obesity," *Diabetes Care*, vol. 38, no. 3, pp. 495–502, 2015.

[25] I. Cheng, C. P. Caberto, A. Lum-Jones et al., "Type 2 diabetes risk variants and colorectal cancer risk: the multiethnic Cohort and PAGE studies," *Gut*, vol. 60, no. 12, pp. 1703–1711, 2011.

[26] R. J. O. Dowling, M. Zakikhani, I. G. Fantus, M. Pollak, and N. Sonenberg, "Metformin inhibits mammalian target of rapamycin-dependent translation initiation in breast cancer cells," *Cancer Research*, vol. 67, no. 22, pp. 10804–10812, 2007.

[27] E. Giovannucci, D. M. Harlan, M. C. Archer et al., "Diabetes and cancer: a consensus report," *Diabetes Care*, vol. 33, no. 7, pp. 1674–1685, 2010.

[28] P. Pisani, "Hyper-insulinaemia and cancer, meta-analyses of epidemiological studies," *Archives of Physiology and Biochemistry*, vol. 114, no. 1, pp. 63–70, 2008.

[29] J. M. Berster and B. Göke, "Type 2 diabetes mellitus as risk factor for colorectal cancer," *Archives of Physiology and Biochemistry*, vol. 114, no. 1, pp. 84–98, 2008.

[30] J. A. Johnson, B. Carstensen, D. Witte, S. L. Bowker, L. Lipscombe, and A. G. Renehan, "Diabetes and cancer (1): evaluating the temporal relationship between type 2 diabetes and cancer incidence," *Diabetologia*, vol. 55, no. 6, pp. 1607–1618, 2012.

[31] R. T. Moon, B. Bowerman, M. Boutros, and N. Perrimon, "The promise and perils of Wnt signaling through β-catenin," *Science*, vol. 296, no. 5573, pp. 1644–1646, 2002.

[32] R. T. Moon, A. D. Kohn, G. V. De Ferrari, and A. Kaykas, "WNT and β-catenin signalling: diseases and therapies," *Nature Reviews Genetics*, vol. 5, no. 9, pp. 691–701, 2004.

[33] R. Nusse, "Wnt signaling in disease and in development," *Cell Research*, vol. 15, no. 1, pp. 28–32, 2005.

[34] H. Clevers, "Wnt/β-catenin signaling in development and disease," *Cell*, vol. 127, no. 3, pp. 469–480, 2006.

[35] T.-C. He, A. B. Sparks, C. Rago et al., "Identification of c-MYC as a target of the APC pathway," *Science*, vol. 281, no. 5382, pp. 1509–1512, 1998.

[36] M. Shtutman, J. Zhurinsky, I. Simcha et al., "The cyclin D1 gene is a target of the β-catenin/LEF-1 pathway," *Proceedings of the National Academy of Sciences of the United States of America*, vol. 96, no. 10, pp. 5522–5527, 1999.

[37] S. Angers and R. T. Moon, "Proximal events in Wnt signal transduction," *Nature Reviews Molecular Cell Biology*, vol. 10, no. 7, pp. 468–477, 2009.

[38] K. T. Pate, C. Stringari, S. Sprowl-Tanio et al., "Wnt signaling directs a metabolic program of glycolysis and angiogenesis in colon cancer," *The EMBO Journal*, vol. 33, no. 13, pp. 1454–1473, 2014.

[39] A. Chocarro-Calvo, J. M. García-Martínez, S. Ardila-González, A. De la Vieja, and C. García-Jiménez, "Glucose-induced β-catenin acetylation enhances Wnt signaling in cancer," *Molecular Cell*, vol. 49, no. 3, pp. 474–486, 2013.

[40] M. Bienz and H. Clevers, "Linking colorectal cancer to Wnt signaling," *Cell*, vol. 103, no. 2, pp. 311–320, 2000.

[41] T. Brabletz, F. Hlubek, S. Spaderna et al., "Invasion and metastasis in colorectal cancer: epithelial-mesenchymal transition, mesenchymal-epithelial transition, stem cells and β-catenin," *Cells Tissues Organs*, vol. 179, no. 1-2, pp. 56–65, 2005.

[42] A. Klaus and W. Birchmeier, "Wnt signalling and its impact on development and cancer," *Nature Reviews Cancer*, vol. 8, no. 5, pp. 387–398, 2008.

[43] H. Clevers and R. Nusse, "Wnt/β-catenin signaling and disease," *Cell*, vol. 149, no. 6, pp. 1192–1205, 2012.

[44] C. B. Thompson, "Wnt meets Warburg: another piece in the puzzle?" *EMBO Journal*, vol. 33, no. 13, pp. 1420–1422, 2014.

[45] O. Warburg, "On the origin of cancer cells," *Science*, vol. 123, no. 3191, pp. 309–314, 1956.

[46] R. J. DeBerardinis, J. J. Lum, G. Hatzivassiliou, and C. B. Thompson, "The biology of cancer: metabolic reprogramming fuels cell growth and proliferation," *Cell Metabolism*, vol. 7, no. 1, pp. 11–20, 2008.

[47] M. G. Vander Heiden, L. C. Cantley, and C. B. Thompson, "Understanding the warburg effect: the metabolic requirements of cell proliferation," *Science*, vol. 324, no. 5930, pp. 1029–1033, 2009.

[48] T. E. Roche, J. C. Baker, X. Yan et al., "Distinct regulatory properties of pyruvate dehydrogenase kinase and phosphatase isoforms," *Progress in Nucleic Acid Research and Molecular Biology*, vol. 70, pp. 33–75, 2001.

[49] T. K. Hunt, R. S. Aslam, S. Beckert et al., "Aerobically derived lactate stimulates revascularization and tissue repair via redox mechanisms," *Antioxidants and Redox Signaling*, vol. 9, no. 8, pp. 1115–1124, 2007.

[50] M. van de Wetering, E. Sancho, C. Verweij et al., "The β-catenin/TCF-4 complex imposes a crypt progenitor phenotype on colorectal cancer cells," *Cell*, vol. 111, no. 2, pp. 241–250, 2002.

[51] P. Chafey, L. Finzi, R. Boisgard et al., "Proteomic analysis of β-catenin activation in mouse liver by DIGE analysis identifies glucose metabolism as a new target of the Wnt pathway," *Proteomics*, vol. 9, no. 15, pp. 3889–3900, 2009.

[52] D. R. Wise, R. J. Deberardinis, A. Mancuso et al., "Myc regulates a transcriptional program that stimulates mitochondrial glutaminolysis and leads to glutamine addiction," *Proceedings of the National Academy of Sciences of the United States of America*, vol. 105, no. 48, pp. 18782–18787, 2008.

[53] R. Nusse, "Wnt signaling and stem cell control," *Cell Research*, vol. 18, no. 5, pp. 523–527, 2008.

[54] C. V. Dang, "Rethinking the warburg effect with Myc micro-managing glutamine metabolism," *Cancer Research*, vol. 70, no. 3, pp. 859–862, 2010.

[55] C. Niehrs and S. P. Acebron, "Mitotic and mitogenic Wnt signalling," *EMBO Journal*, vol. 31, no. 12, pp. 2705–2713, 2012.

[56] R. C. Osthus, H. Shim, S. Kim et al., "Deregulation of glucose transporter 1 and glycolytic gene expression by c-Myc," *Journal of Biological Chemistry*, vol. 275, no. 29, pp. 21797–21800, 2000.

[57] J.-W. Kim, P. Gao, Y.-C. Liu, G. L. Semenza, and C. V. Dang, "Hypoxia-inducible factor 1 and dysregulated c-Myc cooperatively induce vascular endothelial growth factor and metabolic switches hexokinase 2 and pyruvate dehydrogenase kinase 1," *Molecular and Cellular Biology*, vol. 27, no. 21, pp. 7381–7393, 2007.

[58] M. I. Koukourakis, A. Giatromanolaki, A. L. Harris, and E. Sivridis, "Comparison of metabolic pathways between cancer cells and stromal cells in colorectal carcinomas: a metabolic survival role for tumor-associated stroma," *Cancer Research*, vol. 66, no. 2, pp. 632–637, 2006.

[59] S. M. Wigfield, S. C. Winter, A. Giatromanolaki, J. Taylor, M. L. Koukourakis, and A. L. Harris, "PDK-1 regulates lactate production in hypoxia and is associated with poor prognosis in

head and neck squamous cancer," *British Journal of Cancer*, vol. 98, no. 12, pp. 1975–1984, 2008.

[60] D. Baumunk, U. Reichelt, J. Hildebrandt et al., "Expression parameters of the metabolic pathway genes pyruvate dehydrogenase kinase-1 (PDK-1) and DJ-1/PARK7 in renal cell carcinoma (RCC)," *World Journal of Urology*, vol. 31, no. 5, pp. 1191–1196, 2013.

[61] T. McFate, A. Mohyeldin, H. Lu et al., "Pyruvate dehydrogenase complex activity controls metabolic and malignant phenotype in cancer cells," *The Journal of Biological Chemistry*, vol. 283, no. 33, pp. 22700–22708, 2008.

[62] G. Sutendra, P. Dromparis, A. Kinnaird et al., "Mitochondrial activation by inhibition of PDKII suppresses HIF1a signaling and angiogenesis in cancer," *Oncogene*, vol. 32, no. 13, pp. 1638–1650, 2013.

[63] H. Lu, R. A. Forbes, and A. Verma, "Hypoxia-inducible factor 1 activation by aerobic glycolysis implicates the Warburg effect in carcinogenesis," *Journal of Biological Chemistry*, vol. 277, no. 26, pp. 23111–23115, 2002.

[64] C. Pinheiro, A. Longatto-Filho, C. Scapulatempo et al., "Increased expression of monocarboxylate transporters 1, 2, and 4 in colorectal carcinomas," *Virchows Archiv*, vol. 452, no. 2, pp. 139–146, 2008.

[65] S. Zhang, M. W. Hulver, R. P. McMillan, M. A. Cline, and E. R. Gilbert, "The pivotal role of pyruvate dehydrogenase kinases in metabolic flexibility," *Nutrition and Metabolism*, vol. 11, article 10, 2014.

[66] I.-K. Lee, "The role of pyruvate dehydrogenase kinase in diabetes and obesity," *Diabetes and Metabolism Journal*, vol. 38, no. 3, pp. 181–186, 2014.

[67] B. Huang, P. Wu, M. M. Bowker-Kinley, and R. A. Harris, "Regulation of pyruvate dehydrogenase kinase expression by peroxisome proliferator-activated receptor-α ligands, glucocorticoids, and insulin," *Diabetes*, vol. 51, no. 2, pp. 276–283, 2002.

[68] H.-S. Kwon, B. Huang, T. G. Unterman, and R. A. Harris, "Protein kinase B-α inhibits human pyruvate dehydrogenase kinase-4 gene induction by dexamethasone through inactivation of FOXO transcription factors," *Diabetes*, vol. 53, no. 4, pp. 899–910, 2004.

[69] R. R. Attia, P. Sharma, R. C. Janssen et al., "Regulation of pyruvate dehydrogenase kinase 4 (PDK4) by CCAAT/enhancer-binding protein β (C/EBPβ)," *Journal of Biological Chemistry*, vol. 286, no. 27, pp. 23799–23807, 2011.

[70] Y. I. Kim, F. N. Lee, W. S. Choi, S. Lee, and J. H. Youn, "Insulin regulation of skeletal muscle PDK4 mRNA expression is impaired in acute insulin-resistant states," *Diabetes*, vol. 55, no. 8, pp. 2311–2317, 2006.

[71] T. L. Pehleman, S. J. Peters, G. J. F. Heigenhauser, and L. L. Spriet, "Enzymatic regulation of glucose disposal in human skeletal muscle after a high-fat, low-carbohydrate diet," *Journal of Applied Physiology*, vol. 98, no. 1, pp. 100–107, 2005.

[72] S. J. Peters, R. A. Harris, P. Wu, T. L. Pehleman, G. J. F. Heigenhauser, and L. L. Spriet, "Human skeletal muscle PDH kinase activity and isoform expression during a 3-day high-fat/low-carbohydrate diet," *American Journal of Physiology—Endocrinology and Metabolism*, vol. 281, no. 6, pp. E1151–E1158, 2001.

[73] A. Elbrecht, Y. Chen, C. A. Cullinan et al., "Molecular cloning, expression and characterization of human peroxisome proliferator activated receptors γ1 and γ2," *Biochemical and Biophysical Research Communications*, vol. 224, no. 2, pp. 431–437, 1996.

[74] L. Fajas, D. Auboeuf, E. Raspé et al., "The organization, promoter analysis, and expression of the human PPARγ gene," *The Journal of Biological Chemistry*, vol. 272, no. 30, pp. 18779–18789, 1997.

[75] B. Desvergne and W. Wahli, "Peroxisome proliferator-activated receptors: nuclear control of metabolism," *Endocrine Reviews*, vol. 20, no. 5, pp. 649–688, 1999.

[76] S. M. Rangwala and M. A. Lazar, "Peroxisome proliferator-activated receptor γ in diabetes and metabolism," *Trends in Pharmacological Sciences*, vol. 25, no. 6, pp. 331–336, 2004.

[77] F. Picard and J. Auwerx, "PPARγ and glucose homeostasis," *Annual Review of Nutrition*, vol. 22, pp. 167–197, 2002.

[78] H.-I. Kim and Y.-H. Ahn, "Role of peroxisome proliferator-activated receptor-γ in the glucose-sensing apparatus of liver and β-cells," *Diabetes*, vol. 53, supplement 1, pp. S60–S65, 2004.

[79] N. Wang, G. Yang, Z. Jia et al., "Vascular PPARγ controls circadian variation in blood pressure and heart rate through Bmal1," *Cell Metabolism*, vol. 8, no. 6, pp. 482–491, 2008.

[80] Y. Lecarpentier, V. Claes, and J.-L. Hébert, "PPARs, cardiovascular metabolism, and function: near- or far-from-equilibrium pathways," *PPAR Research*, vol. 2010, Article ID 783273, 10 pages, 2010.

[81] B. N. Finck, C. Bernal-Mizrachi, D. H. Han et al., "A potential link between muscle peroxisome proliferator-activated receptor-α signaling and obesity-related diabetes," *Cell Metabolism*, vol. 1, no. 2, pp. 133–144, 2005.

[82] A. Ben-Ze'ev and B. Geiger, "Differential molecular interactions of β-catenin and plakoglobin in adhesion, signaling and cancer," *Current Opinion in Cell Biology*, vol. 10, no. 5, pp. 629–639, 1998.

[83] J. Zhurinsky, M. Shtutman, and A. Ben-Ze'ev, "Differential mechanisms of LEF/TCF family-dependent transcriptional activation by β-catenin and plakoglobin," *Molecular and Cellular Biology*, vol. 20, no. 12, pp. 4238–4252, 2000.

[84] P. J. Morin, A. B. Sparks, V. Korinek et al., "Activation of β-catenin-Tcf signaling in colon cancer by mutations in β-catenin or APC," *Science*, vol. 275, no. 5307, pp. 1787–1790, 1997.

[85] R. Najdi, R. Holcombe, and M. Waterman, "Wnt signaling and colon carcinogenesis: beyond APC," *Journal of Carcinogenesis*, vol. 10, article no. 5, 2011.

[86] E. Å. Jansson, A. Are, G. Greicius et al., "The Wnt/β-catenin signaling pathway targets PPARγ activity in colon cancer cells," *Proceedings of the National Academy of Sciences of the United States of America*, vol. 102, no. 5, pp. 1460–1465, 2005.

[87] J.-H. Xiao, C. Ghosn, C. Hinchman et al., "Adenomatous polyposis coli (APC)-independent regulation of β-catenin degradation via a retinoid X receptor-mediated pathway," *Journal of Biological Chemistry*, vol. 278, no. 32, pp. 29954–29962, 2003.

[88] P. Sarraf, E. Mueller, W. M. Smith et al., "Loss-of-function mutations in PPARγ associated with human colon cancer," *Molecular Cell*, vol. 3, no. 6, pp. 799–804, 1999.

[89] G. D. Girnun, W. M. Smith, S. Drori et al., "APC-dependent suppression of colon carcinogenesis by PPARγ," *Proceedings of the National Academy of Sciences of the United States of America*, vol. 99, no. 21, pp. 13771–13776, 2002.

[90] P. Sarraf, E. Mueller, D. Jones et al., "Differentiation and reversal of malignant changes in colon cancer through PPARγ," *Nature Medicine*, vol. 4, no. 9, pp. 1046–1052, 1998.

[91] E. Osawa, A. Nakajima, K. Wada et al., "Peroxisome proliferator-activated receptor γ ligands suppress colon carcinogenesis induced by azoxymethane in mice," *Gastroenterology*, vol. 124, no. 2, pp. 361–367, 2003.

[92] E. Saez, P. Tontonoz, M. C. Nelson et al., "Activators of the nuclear receptor PPARγ enhance colon polyp formation," *Nature Medicine*, vol. 4, no. 9, pp. 1058–1061, 1998.

[93] A. M. Lefebvre, I. Chen, P. Desreumaux et al., "Activation of the peroxisome proliferator-activated receptor gamma promotes the development of colon tumors in C57BL/6J-APCMin/+ mice," *Nature Medicine*, vol. 4, pp. 1053–1057, 1998.

[94] G. T. Robbins and D. Nie, "PPAR gamma, bioactive lipids, and cancer progression," *Frontiers in Bioscience*, vol. 17, no. 5, pp. 1816–1834, 2012.

[95] L. Gelman, J. N. Feige, and B. Desvergne, "Molecular basis of selective PPARγ modulation for the treatment of Type 2 diabetes," *Biochimica et Biophysica Acta*, vol. 1771, no. 8, pp. 1094–1107, 2007.

[96] I. Barroso, M. Gurnell, V. E. F. Crowley et al., "Dominant negative mutations in human PPARγ associated with severe insulin resistance, diabetes mellitus and hypertension," *Nature*, vol. 402, no. 6764, pp. 880–883, 1999.

[97] D. B. Savage, G. D. Tan, C. L. Acerini et al., "Human metabolic syndrome resulting from dominant-negative mutations in the nuclear receptor peroxisome proliferator-activated receptor-γ," *Diabetes*, vol. 52, no. 4, pp. 910–917, 2003.

[98] N. Marx, J. Froehlich, L. Siam et al., "Antidiabetic PPARγ-activator rosiglitazone reduces MMP-9 serum levels in type 2 diabetic patients with coronary artery disease," *Arteriosclerosis, Thrombosis, and Vascular Biology*, vol. 23, no. 2, pp. 283–288, 2003.

[99] S. G. Dubois, L. K. Heilbronn, S. R. Smith, J. B. Albu, D. E. Kelley, and E. Ravussin, "Decreased expression of adipogenic genes in obese subjects with type 2 diabetes," *Obesity*, vol. 14, no. 9, pp. 1543–1552, 2006.

[100] W. Ip, Y.-T. A. Chiang, and T. Jin, "The involvement of the wnt signaling pathway and TCF7L2 in diabetes mellitus: the current understanding, dispute, and perspective," *Cell and Bioscience*, vol. 2, no. 1, article 28, 2012.

[101] W. Ip, W. Shao, Y.-T. A. Chiang, and T. Jin, "The Wnt signaling pathway effector TCF7L2 is upregulated by insulin and represses hepatic gluconeogenesis," *American Journal of Physiology—Endocrinology and Metabolism*, vol. 303, no. 9, pp. E1166–E1176, 2012.

[102] R. Saxena, L. Gianniny, N. P. Burtt et al., "Common single nucleotide polymorphisms in TCF7L2 are reproducibly associated with type 2 diabetes and reduce the insulin response to glucose in nondiabetic individuals," *Diabetes*, vol. 55, no. 10, pp. 2890–2895, 2006.

[103] V. Lyssenko, "The transcription factor 7-like 2 gene and increased risk of type 2 diabetes: an update," *Current Opinion in Clinical Nutrition and Metabolic Care*, vol. 11, no. 4, pp. 385–392, 2008.

[104] J. C. Florez, "The new type 2 diabetes gene TCF7L2," *Current Opinion in Clinical Nutrition and Metabolic Care*, vol. 10, no. 4, pp. 391–396, 2007.

[105] K. R. Owen and M. I. McCarthy, "Genetics of type 2 diabetes," *Current Opinion in Genetics and Development*, vol. 17, no. 3, pp. 239–244, 2007.

[106] M. N. Weedon, "The importance of TCF7L2," *Diabetic Medicine*, vol. 24, no. 10, pp. 1062–1066, 2007.

[107] T. Jin, "The WNT signalling pathway and diabetes mellitus," *Diabetologia*, vol. 51, no. 10, pp. 1771–1780, 2008.

[108] T. Fujino, H. Asaba, M.-J. Kang et al., "Low-density lipoprotein receptor-related protein 5 (LRP5) is essential for normal cholesterol metabolism and glucose-induced insulin secretion," *Proceedings of the National Academy of Sciences of the United States of America*, vol. 100, no. 1, pp. 229–234, 2003.

[109] Z. Ni, Y. Anini, X. Fang, G. Mills, P. L. Brubaker, and T. Jin, "Transcriptional activation of the proglucagon gene by lithium and β-catenin in intestinal endocrine L cells," *The Journal of Biological Chemistry*, vol. 278, no. 2, pp. 1380–1387, 2003.

[110] F. Yi, P. L. Brubaker, and T. Jin, "TCF-4 mediates cell type-specific regulation of proglucagon gene expression by β-catenin and glycogen synthase kinase-3β," *Journal of Biological Chemistry*, vol. 280, no. 2, pp. 1457–1464, 2005.

[111] F. Yi, J. Sun, G. E. Lim, I. G. Fantus, P. L. Brubaker, and T. Jin, "Cross talk between the insulin and Wnt signaling pathways: evidence from intestinal endocrine L cells," *Endocrinology*, vol. 149, no. 5, pp. 2341–2351, 2008.

[112] A. Kanazawa, S. Tsukada, A. Sekine et al., "Association of the gene encoding wingless-type mammary tumor virus integration-site family member 5B (WNT5B) with type 2 diabetes," *American Journal of Human Genetics*, vol. 75, no. 5, pp. 832–843, 2004.

[113] P. J. Hey, R. C. J. Twells, M. S. Phillips et al., "Cloning of a novel member of the low-density lipoprotein receptor family," *Gene*, vol. 216, no. 1, pp. 103–111, 1998.

[114] R. C. J. Twells, C. A. Mein, F. Payne et al., "Linkage and association mapping of the LRP5 locus on chromosome 11q13 in type 1 diabetes," *Human Genetics*, vol. 113, no. 2, pp. 99–105, 2003.

[115] L. Shu, N. S. Sauter, F. T. Schulthess, A. V. Matveyenko, J. Oberholzer, and K. Maedler, "Transcription factor 7-like 2 regulates β-cell survival and function in human pancreatic islets," *Diabetes*, vol. 57, no. 3, pp. 645–653, 2008.

14

Cellular and Biophysical Pipeline for the Screening of Peroxisome Proliferator-Activated Receptor Beta/Delta Agonists: Avoiding False Positives

Natália Bernardi Videira (ID),[1,2] **Fernanda Aparecida Heleno Batista,**[1]
Artur Torres Cordeiro (ID),[1] **and Ana Carolina Migliorini Figueira** (ID)[1]

[1]*Brazilian Biosciences National Laboratory (LNBio), Brazilian Center for Research in Energy and Materials (CNPEM),*
13083-970 Campinas, SP, Brazil
[2]*Graduate Program in Biosciences and Technology of Bioactive Products, Institute of Biology, State University of Campinas (Unicamp),*
Campinas, SP, Brazil

Correspondence should be addressed to Ana Carolina Migliorini Figueira; ana.figueira@lnbio.cnpem.br

Academic Editor: Stéphane Mandard

Peroxisome proliferator-activated receptor beta/delta (PPARß/δ) is considered a therapeutic target for metabolic disorders, cancer, and cardiovascular diseases. Here, we developed one pipeline for the screening of PPARß/δ agonists, which reduces the cost, time, and false-positive hits. The first step is an optimized 3-day long cellular transactivation assay based on reporter-gene technology, which is supported by automated liquid-handlers. This primary screening is followed by a confirmatory transactivation assay and by two biophysical validation methods (thermal shift assay (TSA) and (ANS) fluorescence quenching), which allow the calculation of the affinity constant, giving more information about the selected hits. All of the assays were validated using well-known commercial agonists providing trustworthy data. Furthermore, to validate and test this pipeline, we screened a natural extract library (560 extracts), and we found one plant extract that might be interesting for PPARß/δ modulation. In conclusion, our results suggested that we developed a cheaper and more robust pipeline that goes beyond the single activation screening, as it also evaluates PPARß/δ tertiary structure stabilization and the ligand affinity constant, selecting only molecules that directly bind to the receptor. Moreover, this approach might improve the effectiveness of the screening for agonists that target PPARß/δ for drug development.

1. Introduction

Peroxisome proliferator-activated receptor beta/delta (PPARß/δ) is a lipid-activated transcription factor, which is a member of the nuclear receptors (NR) superfamily that regulates the activation or silencing of several target genes. PPARß/δ is ubiquitously expressed in humans, although it is mainly found in the skin, placenta, brain, liver, kidneys, spleen, fat skeletal muscle, and digestive tube [1–3].

PPARß/δ is involved in some metabolic pathways such as energy metabolism, homeostasis, adipogenesis, and lipid metabolism [4–6]. Several studies have suggested that PPARß/δ modulation by agonists regulates food intake, body weight, insulin sensitivity, adiposity, and body mass [5, 7]. It has also been associated with diverse physiopathological processes, such as inflammation, obesity, dyslipidemia, diabetes, cancer, and cardiovascular diseases [6, 8–10]. PPARß/δ also has described extra-metabolic roles including neuroprotective effects against brain diseases, such as multiple sclerosis, strokes, Alzheimer's disease, and Parkinson's disease, and acts in cell differentiation and proliferation, immune regulation, oxidative stress, and skin biology [2, 3, 11].

The diversity in PPARß/δ function has been related to its ability to accommodate and bind different ligands in its ligand binding domain (LBD), with a wide range of natural and synthetic ligands. Among the natural ligands, there are fatty acids, prostaglandins, and leukotrienes [12, 13]. Several high affinity and subtype-specific PPARß/δ agonists have been developed and submitted for clinical trials for the treatment of metabolic diseases [1, 14]; however no ligand has been made available for clinical use.

Due to the high number of people affected by PPARß/δ-related disorders, the development of specific ligands to modulate the receptor activity becomes of great importance. Here, we developed and set up a suitable, cheaper, and robust screening pipeline for the better identification of PPARß/δ agonists. In the first step of this pipeline, we optimized the cell-based transactivation assay to be 1 to 2 days shorter and with the use of less reagents than the previously described ones, significantly reducing the costs in time and money for big screening campaigns. Additionally, we introduced two validation methods to avoid false positives: a thermal shift assay (TSA) to check PPARß/δ tertiary structure stabilization by the hit candidates, indicating direct binding to the protein, followed by an ANS fluorescence quenching assay to determine the compound/extract affinity for the PPARß/δ hydrophobic pocket.

To date, most of the screening methods for PPARs were based only on transactivation assays, which is the most common and well-established protocol to measure the activity of nuclear receptors [15–19]. However, this method may allow the selection of false-positive compounds that may activate PPARß/δ in an indirect way without agonist properties. To overcome this gap, we propose a pipeline in which the transactivation assay is followed by biophysical assays to confirm that the compound directly bound to the PPARß/δ ligand pocket.

Particularly, the major differences in our pipeline in comparison to other proposed PPARß/δ transactivation methods are the reduction of the assay length and volume; the cell carrier; automation; and the addition of biophysical validation methods [15–18]. Moreover, this pipeline was assessed by specific PPARß/δ agonists (GW0742, GW501516, and L-165,041) and the Z'-factor. In summary, we propose that this pipeline is a stable, cheaper, faster, and more robust tool to identify PPARß/δ agonists, and moreover, we tested a natural product library against the developed pipeline.

2. Material and Methods

2.1. Reagents. The materials for cell culture: Dulbecco's modified Eagle's medium (DMEM) was purchased from GIBCO Corporation (Carlsbad, CA, USA), fetal bovine serum (FBS) was obtained from CULTILAB (Campinas, SP, Brazil), and charcoal-stripped FBS and Penicillin/Streptomycin was obtained from GIBCO Corporation (Grand Island, NE, USA). Lipofectamine 2000® transfection reagent was obtained from Life Technologies (Indianapolis, IN, USA). The Dual Luciferase® Assay Reporter System was obtained from Promega Corporation (Madison, WI, USA). GW0742 (CAS 317318-84-6), GW501516 (CAS 317318-70-0), Bezafibrate (CAS41859-67-0), and L-165,041 (CAS 79558-09-1) were purchased from Sigma Corporation (St Louis, MO, USA).

2.2. Plasmids. The cell culture assays were performed after transfection of (i) pBIND-PPARß/δ, expressing Gal4-DBD

and PPARß/δ-LBD fusion protein, and (ii) pGRE-LUC, which contains a Gal4 response element followed by firefly luciferase reporter gene. The PPARß/δ:GAL4 protein, when activated by a ligand, can induce the transcription of the luciferase reporter gene from pGRE-LUC. The pBIND-PPARß/δ modified vector and pGRE-LUC were a gift from Dr. Paul Webb (the Methodist Hospital Research Institute, Houston, EUA) [15, 17]. For transfection efficiency control (vector normalization), we used pRL-TK vector, which constitutively expresses *Renilla reniformis* luciferase [20, 21]. For *in vitro* protein assays, we used pET28a-His-LBD-PPARδ, which contains the LBD gene of human PPARß/δ (aa 171-441) fused with His-tag [5].

2.3. Cell Culture. 293T (ATCC® CRL-3216™) cells were maintained in DMEM supplemented with 10% (v/v) fetal bovine serum (FBS) and antibiotics (100 units/mL penicillin and 100 mg/mL streptomycin). Cells were grown in a 5% CO_2, 95% air-humidified atmosphere, at 37°C.

2.4. PPARß/δ Transactivation Assay. The rationale of the primary screening assay is described in Figure 1. First, 293T cells at 70–90% confluence were transiently cotransfected with the plasmids pBIND-PPARß/δ, pGRE-LUC, and pRL in 100 × 20 mm plates with Lipofectamine 2000® transfection reagent, following the manufacturer's protocol. The transfected cells were incubated for 6 hours in a 5% CO_2, 95% air-humidified atmosphere at 37°C.

In the meantime, the screening compounds (plant extracts) were reformatted to a 96-well plate (screening plates, white microplates, Perkin Elmer) containing 50 μL of DMEM supplemented with 10% charcoal-stripped FBS at final concentration of 10 μg/mL with Thermo Scientific™ Versette™ Automated Liquid Handler equipped with a 96-tip head. In each assay plate, column 1 was set up as negative control (vehicle, 1% dimethyl sulfoxide (DMSO)) and column 12 was set up as positive control (1 μM GW0742, ~0.00047 μg/mL).

After transfection, cells were seeded in 96-well white microplates (4×10^4 cells per well), which already contained the controls or test compounds/extracts, in a final volume of 100 μL per well of DMEM supplemented with 10% charcoal-stripped FBS and antibiotics (100 units/mL penicillin and 100 mg/mL streptomycin). Experimental conditions were adjusted to ensure linearity during the entire assay.

After 24 hours, the medium was aspirated with Thermo Scientific Versette Automated Liquid Handler, and luciferase activity was measured in each well with the Dual Luciferase Assay Reporter System (Promega). The reading solutions were added with Thermo Scientific Multidrop Combi Reagent Dispenser as follows: first, 20 μL of lysis solution, followed by 20 min of plate incubation; then 25 μL of LAR II substrate, followed by luminescence measurements in CLARIOstar® (BMG Labtech) plate reader; finally, 25 μL of Stop&Glo® substrate was added and luminescence was measured.

We performed vector normalization with the raw luminescence data to control for differences in transfection efficiency between samples. For vector normalization we

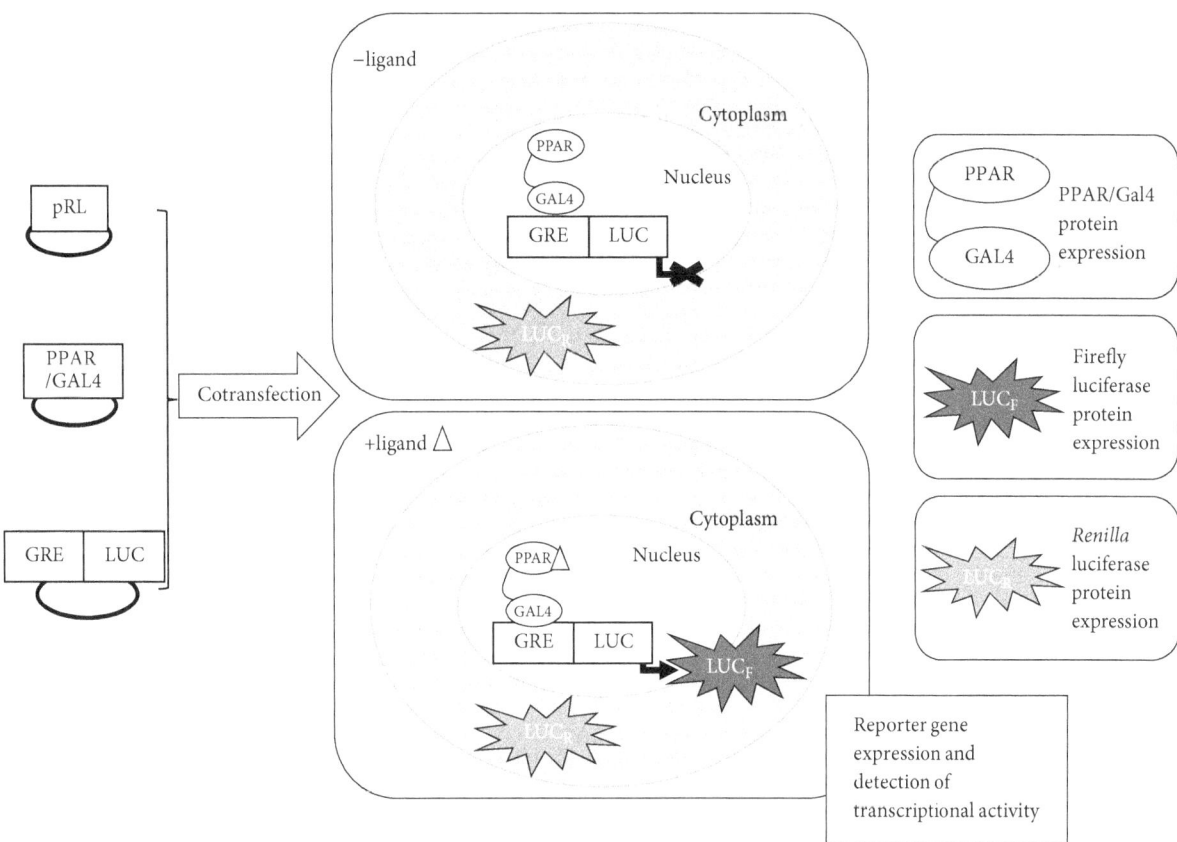

FIGURE 1: Principle of the *in vitro* PPARß/δ transactivation assay. This assay is based on the transient transfection of the 293T cell line with three plasmids: pBIND-PPARß/δ encoding a chimera of Gal4-DBD and PPARß/δ-LBD genes (PPAR/GAL4); pGRE-LUC, which owns one GAL4 response element upstream of a firefly luciferase reporter gene (LUC$_F$); and the pRL vector, which constitutively express *Renilla* luciferase (LUC$_R$). The transfected cells express both PPARß/δ and *Renilla* luciferase constitutively. When the transfected cell is exposed to a molecule that works as a ligand (+ligand), such as GW0742, PPARß/δ moves into the nucleus, binds to GRE-LUC, and triggers the expression of LUC$_F$, which is the expected PPARß/δ activation effect in this assay. The reporter-gene expression correlates with the bioactivity of PPARß/δ in the sample. *Note.* For simplicity, only PPARß/δ monomer binding to GRE has been depicted.

calculate luciferase signal/*Renilla* signal. The assay performance was assessed by plate statistics (signal-to-background ratio, Z'-factor, coefficient of variation) [22] and apparent cytotoxicity was a measure of *Renilla* luciferase parameters. For Z'-factor calculation, we consider, after vector normalization, the positive controls (GW0742) as signal, and negative controls (DMSO) as background. For cytotoxicity, wells with expression of *Renilla* reporter five standard deviations (5 × SD) below the mean value of the controls treatment were considered cytotoxic and consequently were disregarded. We considered as hit candidates compounds/extracts with luminescence *firefly/Renilla* ratio 7 times above the standard deviation of negative controls (DMSO) from the same plate. This last criterion takes in account the intrinsic variation of the negative controls signals by plate. In the screening graphics, the ratio *firefly/Renilla* for all the wells was normalized, positive control mean indicates 100% activation, and negative control mean was considered 0% activation. To confirm the hit candidates, all the selected extracts were retested in triplicate.

2.5. MTT Cytotoxicity Assay. Additionally, we related the 3-(4,5-dimethyl-2-thia-zoyl)-2,5-diphenyl-2H-tetrazolium bromide (MTT) results with *Renilla* reporter expression to assess when a test compound/extract might be toxic to the cells, only based on *Renilla* reporter expression. Then, 4×10^4 293T cells per well were seeded in a 96-well transparent microplates (Sarstedt) in 0.1%, 1%, 3%, 5%, 10%, and 50% DMSO and 1 µM GW0742 and the general viability of the cells was determined by reduction of MTT to formazan [23]. After 20 hours of DMSO incubation, cell media were changed to phosphate buffer saline (PBS), and 10% MTT (5 mg/mL in PBS) was added to each well. Cells were incubated at 37°C, for 3 h, PBS was removed, and 100 µL DMSO was added to dissolve the formazan crystals. The absorbance was measured at 562 nm using an EnSpire® Multimode Plate Reader (Perkin Elmer). The experiment was performed in 4 independent experiments. Data were analyzed by 2-way ANOVA followed by Sidak's multiple comparison test in GraphPad Prism software.

2.6. Protein Expression. The human PPARß/δ ligand binding domain (hPPARß/δ LBD) cDNA (amino acids 171–441) inserted into pET28a vector (Novagen, USA) was heterologous expressed in *Escherichia coli* BL21(DE3) strain. The protein was purified in buffer A (20 mM HEPES pH 7.5, 300 mM NaCl, 5% glycerol) onto a Talon Superflow Metal Affinity Resin (BD Biosciences Clontech, Palo Alto, CA), according to the previously described protocol [5].

2.7. Thermal Shift Assay (TSA). This assay was performed following qualitative and quantitative approaches. Qualitative TSA used 10 μM of hPPARß/δ LBD, 5x SYPRO® Orange (Sigma Aldrich) in buffer containing 20 mM HEPES pH 7.5, 200 mM NaCl, and 5% glycerol, and 30 μM (~0.01 μg/mL) of commercial agonists (1 protein : 3 ligand) or 140 μg/mL of extracts from the tested library were added in a Microamp 96-well plate (Applied Biosystems). Quantitative TSA was performed in same conditions, varying ligand/extract concentrations (ligand concentrations were 0.3, 0.5, 1, 3, 5, 10, 30, and 50 μM; extract concentration were 5, 10, 30, 50, 100, 300, and 500 μg/mL). The experiment was performed at 7500 PCR Real Time System (Applied Biosystems), and measurements were taken from 9°C to 89°C, with a gradient of 1°C per minute, totalizing 80 measurements [23]. The assay was performed in triplicate and data were analyzed at OriginPro8.1. For Kd determination data were fitted using Hill1 model (OriginPro 8.1).

2.8. ANS Fluorescence Quenching. The conditions for 8-anilinonaphthalene-1-sulfonic acid (ANS) assay was optimized in terms of protein and ANS concentrations (Supplementary Material Figure 1), in order to define if ANS quenching was really promoted by PPARß/δ ligand binding. In a 96-well black microplate (Greiner Bio-One), 2 μM hPPARß/δ LBD and 20 μM ANS were incubated in 20 mM HEPES pH 7.5, 200 mM NaCl, and 5% glycerol, at 4°C. After 1 hour, the compounds or extracts were added to the mixture. For the commercial agonist test, 0.3 μM (0.0001 μg/mL), 0.5 μM (0.0002 μg/mL), 1 μM (0.0004 μg/mL), 3 μM (0.001 μg/mL), 5 μM (0.002 μg/mL), 10 μM (0.004 μg/mL), 30 μM (0.01 μg/mL), and 50 μM (0.02 μg/mL) concentrations were used; for the extracts, 5 μg/mL, 10 μg/mL, 30 μg/mL, 50 μg/mL, 100 μg/mL, 300 μg/mL, 500 μg/mL, and 1 mg/mL concentrations were used. The assay was read on EnSpire Multimode Plate Reader (Perkin Elmer) with 380 nm excitation and emission scanning between 400 and 600 nm, at 25°C. The maximum fluorescence emission intensities (480 nm) were plotted versus each compound/extract concentration for affinity constant calculation, at OriginPro 8.0, through Hill1 sigmoidal adjust.

2.9. Natural Extract Library. PPARß/δ primary screening was performed against 560 hydroalcoholic extracts from the Phytobios library. The Phytobios library was kindly provided by Chemistry of Natural Products Library (LQPN) from the Brazilian National Bioscience Laboratory (LNBio/CNPEM) in partnership with Phytobios Ltda, which planned and assembled the library. The Phytobios/LNBio library regularly has extracted plant samples from Amazonian forest, Atlantic

forest, Cerrado, and Caatinga. Each sample is accompanied by precise collecting location by GPS; plant identification by a qualified botanical taxonomist; and a deposit of testimony exsiccate in a certified herbarium. Each collection gets at least 5 kg of leaves (and/or roots and or barks). After processing, each sample gives about 20 g of dry extract, enough for many test repetitions and each sample is fractionated in 9 (nine) chromatographic fractions and immediately plated in 384 wells plates and frozen for further assays. Therefore 10 (ten) samples = 9 fractions + the crude extract are available for testing. This processing allows access to low concentration and yet unknown bioactive substances that are generally hidden by the majoritarian substances. All samples were submitted to analysis by mass spectrometry + molecular networking technique (data not shown). The tested library contained 560 hydroalcoholic extracts from Brazilian plants assembled in two 384 microplates. The compounds were preplated in 384 well microplates at the stock concentration of 10 mg/mL, in 100% DMSO. Before screening, compounds were transferred to daughter plates and diluted to 1 mg/mL, in 100% DMSO. Columns 1, 2, 23, and 24 from daughter plates were empty, and the positive and negative controls were filled in the screening plates.

3. Results

3.1. Optimizing the Screening Conditions. Here we measured the PPARß/δ activity in transactivation assays under different circumstances with the goal of determining the best screening conditions. This screening setup included the evaluation of luciferase substrate volumes, the medium for drug-incubation, and the cell number per well (Figure 2).

First, we tested different volumes of the Dual Luciferase Assay Reporter System components to define the best signal-to-noise ratio without harming the assay quality. The solution volumes recommended by the manufacturer are 100 μL of luciferase substrate per well. However, we verified that 25 μL of each substrate is sufficient to provide a high signal with good discrimination between the activated and nonactivated PPARß/δ (Figure 2(a)). In this way, we reduced the cost and reagent usage by 75% without losing signal information. This reduction represents a major decrease in the cost of high- and medium-throughput assays, as these campaigns usually screen hundreds and thousands of compounds at the same time.

Another important verification was related to the definition of the best medium composition used in the assay that improved the data quality. Since natural fatty acids work as PPARß/δ natural ligands and FBS contains many of these natural fatty acids, 10% FBS-supplemented DMEM may not be suitable for PPARß/δ agonist screening [15, 16, 18]. To overcome this limitation, we tested different medium compositions during compound/extract incubation. Our results showed that serum-free DMEM was considered inadequate since GW0742 activation was low, and the calculated Z'-factor of tested plate was below the reliability limit (Z'-factor = 0.21) [22] (Figure 2(b)). On the other hand, the assay performed with 10% FBS charcoal-stripped-supplemented DMEM showed a higher agonist-activation fold and better

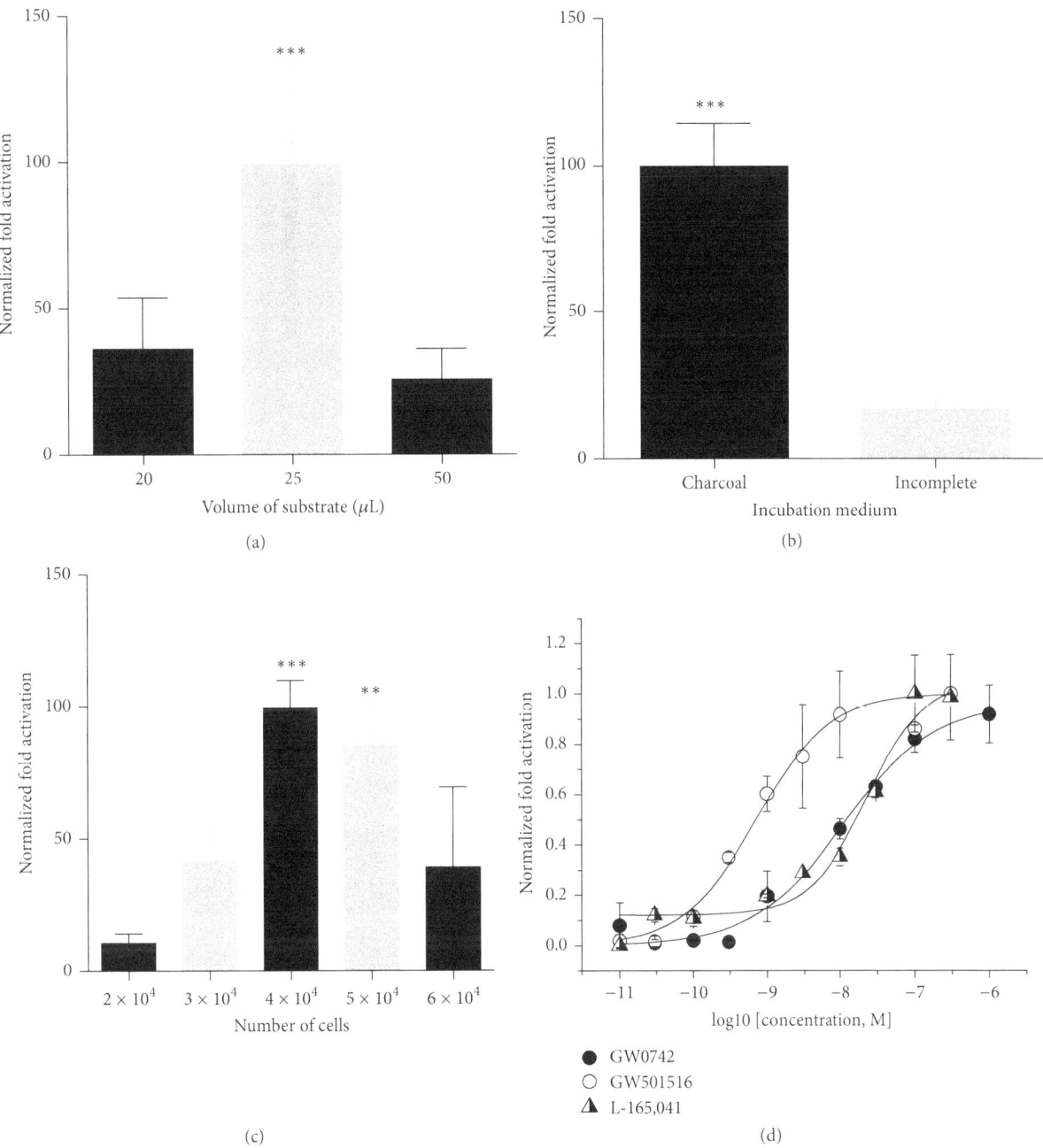

FIGURE 2: Optimization of the screening protocols. When not specified, the positive control was 1 μM of GW0742 and the number of cells was 4×10^4 cell/well. Bar graphs represent the specific fold activation normalized by the highest activation presented as the mean ± SD. p values were calculated by the unpaired t-test (**$p < 0.01$ and ***$p < 0.001$). All bar graphs and calculations were performed with GraphPad Prism. (a) Evaluation of substrate volumes. Cell lysis was performed in 20 μL of passive lysis buffer, and the volumes of LAR II and Stop & Glo substrates were varied (50, 25, and 20 μL). The results show that the best signal of PPARß/δ activation was measured with 25 μL of each substrate. The data is from one experiment with 6 technical replicates. (b) Evaluation of the best ligand incubation medium. In this test, 293T cells were incubated with GW0742 in 10% charcoal-stripped FBS DMEM (charcoal) or in DMEM (incomplete), and the activation fold of PPARß/δ was measured in each condition. Z'-factor charcoal = 0.62; Z'-factor incomplete = 0.21. Charcoal-supplemented medium was chosen as the best option for our assays, and this medium composition was used in the ligand screening for PPARß/δ. One representative experiment is shown out of three independent replicates. (c) Evaluation of the number of cells per well. Cells were seeded at 2×10^4, 3×10^4, 4×10^4, 5×10^4, and 6×10^4 cells per well, and the activation fold of PPARß/δ was measured in each condition to determine the best quantity of cells in each assay. Based on these results, we chose 4×10^4 cells per well to perform PPARß/δ ligand screening. One representative experiment is shown out of four independent replicates. (d) PPARß/δ dose-response activation in the presence of the commercial agonists (GW0742, GW501516, and L-165,041). Concentrations varied from 10^{-11} to 10^{-6} M. Data are expressed as the normalized activation fold as 1 (maximum activation) and 0 (vehicle-treated cells) and represent the mean of 2 independent experiments with 3 technical triplicates. Graphs and dose-response calculations were performed in OriginPro 8.0. GW0742: $R^2 = 0.98549$ and $EC_{50} = 1.08708E - 8$; GW601516: $R^2 = 0.98028$ and $EC_{50} = 7.10385E - 10$; L-165,041: $R^2 = 0.9725$ and $EC_{50} = 2.23969E - 8$.

Z'-factor (0.56). Due to these results, the 10% FBS charcoal-stripped-supplemented DMEM was selected as the incubation medium for PPARß/δ agonist screening assays.

Interestingly, instead of HeLa or Cos-1, we chose the 293T cell lineage, which had not yet been described for PPARß/δ screening assays. This lineage is easy to cultivate, grow, and transfect as well as being one of the most industrially relevant cell lines due to the fact that it is cGMP compliant [24]. Additionally, we checked different concentrations of cells per well in the range (10,000–40,000) previously described for other cellular types [15, 17, 19]. Our results showed PPARß/δ activation of 199-fold when 40,000 cells were seeded per well (Figure 2(c)). Therefore, this quantity was selected due to its higher activation and small deviation.

In summary, we standardized that the best conditions for running our PPARβ/δ-screening assay use 40,000 transfected cells per well and incubation in 10% FBS charcoal-stripped-supplemented DMEM and with a 75% reduction of luciferase substrates (25 μL of both the luciferase substrates LAR II and Stop & Glo®).

3.2. Sensitivity of the Assay against Known Agonists.

To verify the sensitivity of our assay, we measured the PPARß/δ activation under treatment with its commercial agonists GW0742, GW501516, and L-165,041 in dose-response curves (10^{-11}–10^{-6} M) (Figure 2(d)). These ligands are pure compounds known to induce high cellular transactivation of PPARß/δ [5, 7, 25]. By our results, we calculated the following EC_{50} for each tested compound: $EC_{50\ GW501516} = 0.71$ nM, $EC_{50\ GW0742} = 10.87$ nM, and $EC_{50\ L-165,041} = 26.40$ nM on the same nanomolar scale found in the literature ($EC_{50\ GW501516} = 1.8$ nM [7], $EC_{50\ GW0742} = 1$–3.5 nM [5], and $EC_{50\ L-165,041} = 125$ nM [25]). These results confirm that the proposed transactivation assay is robust enough to discriminate low activation signals from possible hit candidates, as it is capable of identifying signals from commercial agonists in concentrations lower than 1 nM.

3.3. Renilla Reporter Expression as an Indicator of Cytotoxicity.

Renilla reporter expression is commonly used as a control for the transfection efficiency [20, 21]. Here, we propose using *Renilla* reporter expression as a parameter for indirect cytotoxicity. Since cells were transfected in a batch prior to plating in the screening plates, *Renilla* reporter expression among wells should be on the same order of magnitude among wells and decreases in this signal should indicate cytotoxicity [21]. The concentration of GW0742 (1 μM, 1% DMSO as vehicle), used as a positive control in the screening, had no statistical difference in comparison with 0.1% or 1% DMSO (concentration used in our negative control), showing that GW0742 has no cytotoxicity. Using toxic concentrations of DMSO (3–50%), we demonstrated that analyses of the *Renilla* reporter expression had the same outcome as the MTT cytotoxicity experiment (Figure 3); that is, we can imply, with statistical significance ($p < 0.0001$), that compounds or extracts that led to low *Renilla* reporter expressions also resulted in high cellular toxicity. Therefore, we defined low *Renilla* reporter expression as an indirect cytotoxicity parameter of

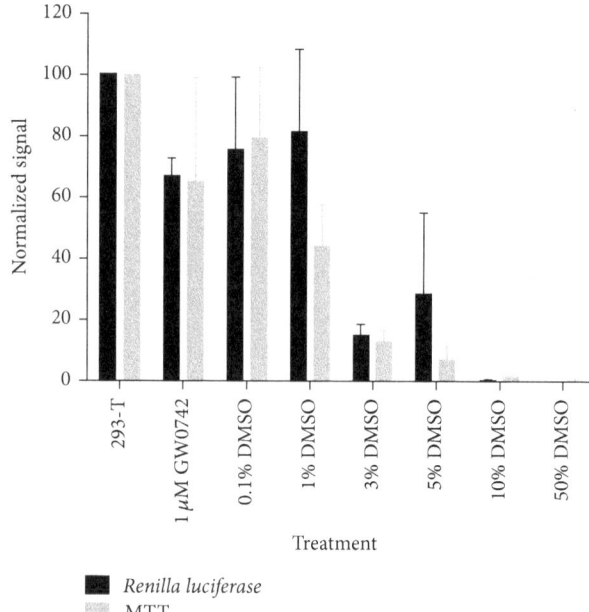

FIGURE 3: Development of a cytotoxic parameter. Comparison between the *Renilla* reporter expression with the MTT cytotoxicity signal in different DMSO concentrations (0.1%, 1%, 3%, 5%, 10%, and 50%) in order to validate the *Renilla* reporter expression as an indirect cytotoxicity parameter. One micromolar GW0742 diluted in DMSO, with a final concentration of 1% DMSO, was used as the positive control in the screening. Statistical analyses proved that our indirect cytotoxic parameter (*Renilla* reporter expression) can be used to identify cytotoxic compounds as well as the MTT cytotoxicity assay. Through analyzing the 2-way ANOVA statistics, there is no statistical difference (ns) between the two types of experiments, and the effect of the DMSO concentration was considered extremely significant according to GraphPad Prism. Followed by Sidak's multiple comparison test, the toxicity increases in concentrations above 3% of DMSO with statistical significance. Data are the mean ± SD ($n = 4$ independent replicates).

our assay, and in further screenings, compounds/extracts that led to low transfection signals were disregarded. In this manner, in one transactivation assay, we obtained two types of different results: the primary firefly reporter, which indicated PPARß/δ activation, and a second control with *Renilla* luciferase to detect the cytotoxicity.

3.4. Transactivation Screening with a Real Library.

After optimization of the cell-based transactivation assay with well-known commercial agonists, we submitted this assay to one natural extract library (Phytobios library). Our results showed that most of the extracts/fractions and negative controls presented low firefly luciferase expression and, therefore, a low *firefly/Renilla* ratio (Figure 4(a)). On the other hand, treatment with the positive controls presented high firefly luciferase expression and a high *firefly/Renilla* ratio, as expected.

After our data analysis, we found 31 possible hit candidates for PPARß/δ agonists (extracts 1–31), which showed activation rates from 1.3- to 2.1-fold. However, the obtained

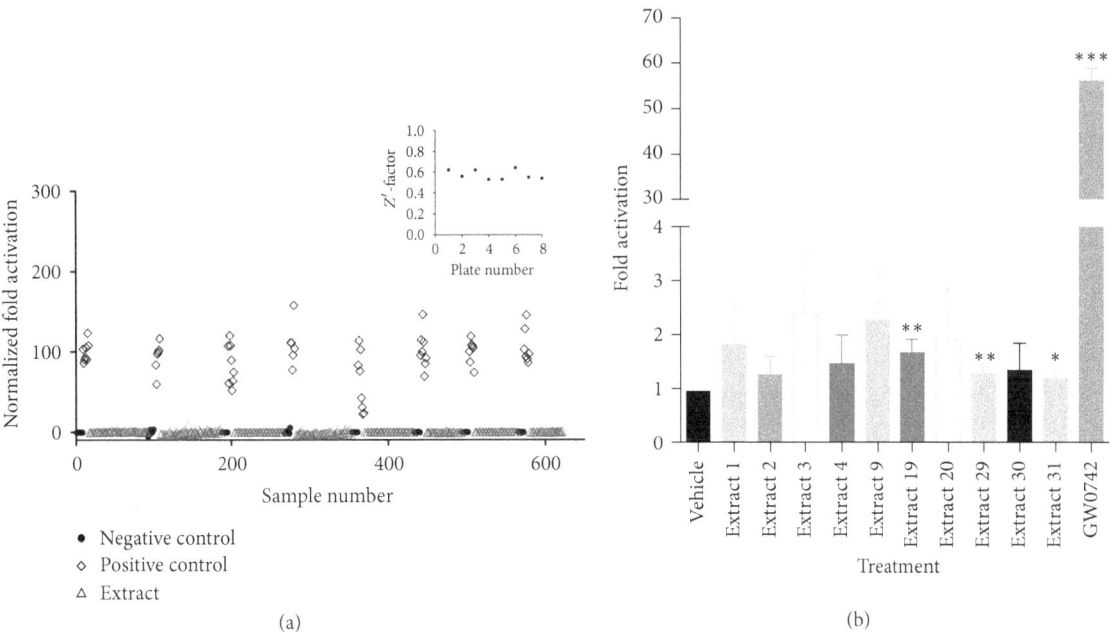

FIGURE 4: High-throughput screening assay and statistics. (a) HTS results are expressed by the *firefly/Renilla* ratio of each compound normalized by positive and negative controls, which were set as 100% and 0%, respectively, for each plate. It is possible to observe that the positive control varied among different plates and wells. Despite the fact that the searched extracts presented low PPARß/δ activation, they still presented significant differences in comparison to the negative controls (signal 7 times higher than the negative control standard deviation). Insert: Z' values for each screened plate presented the high reliability of the data. (b) Confirmatory transactivation assay in triplicate using the possible hit candidates from the previously screened Phytobios library with 1 μM GW0742 as the positive control, 1% DMSO as the negative control (vehicle), and 0.01 mg/mL of the tested extracts. We considered confirmed hit candidate extracts that showed *firefly/Renilla* ratios seven times higher than the standard deviation (>7 × DP) for the negative control treatment for at least two of the three replicates. Data are the mean ± SD. p values were calculated by the unpaired t-test ($^{*}p < 0.05$, $^{**}p < 0.01$, and $^{***}p < 0.001$) with GraphPad Prism.

signal was much lower than the ones obtained in positive control treatment. These results could be explained by the fact that GW0742 is a commercial agonist with high specificity and affinity for PPARß/δ [5]. This means that this ligand has already been submitted to optimization steps through lead generation, while the Phytobios library is composed of raw plant extracts, which are a mixture of different compounds in different concentrations that need further fractionation and improvement. For all screening plates, we obtained an appropriate Z'-factor higher than the 0.5 limit (0.53–0.64) [26], indicating that our assay is reliable and suitable enough for PPARß/δ agonist screening (Figure 4(b)). The variability of PPARß/δ activation by the positive control (GW0742), even though the same batch of transfected cells, culture medium, agonist aliquot, and reading solutions was used, did not interfere in the Z'-factor assessment and was considered intrinsic to the experiment.

Next, to confirm the selected hit candidates, we performed a secondary transactivation screening. After this confirmatory screening, our results presented 10 possible hit candidates (extract 1, extract 2, extract 3, extract 4, extract 9, extract 19, extract 20, extract 29, extract 30, and extract 31), with activation rates from 1.2- to 2.4-fold (Figure 4(b)). When compared with GW0742 PPARß/δ-activation (56-fold), all fractions showed a much lower signal, but the signals were still above our selection criteria based on the standard

deviation of negative controls. Moreover, as was mentioned above, the library contains raw plant extracts, which are a mix of diverse compounds in different concentrations, and probably, the compounds that activate PPARß/δ are present in very low amounts. In this context, the low PPARß/δ activation rates found with the extracts should be considered to be very significant.

3.5. Qualitative TSA Worked as a Confirmatory Assay for PPARß/δ Structure Stabilization by the Hit Candidate. The qualitative TSA was one additional validation methodology of our screening, measuring the tertiary structure stabilization of the PPARß/δ before and after ligand binding. As it was reported, NR ligands increase NR structural stability mainly because the ligand binding organizes specific interactions in their LBD pocket, which raises the degree of solvent protection and therefore, makes their structure more rigid [27–30].

Here, we first tested commercial agonists; our results showed that this technique is able to discriminate among specific agonists, not-specific agonists, and apo-PPARß/δ (Figures 5(a)-5(b)). The specific agonists (GW0742, GW501516, and L-165,041) lead to an increase in the protein melting temperatures (T_m) in comparison to the apo-PPARß/δ T_m, indicating tertiary structure stabilization (Figure 5(a)). In particular, the GW0742 agonist stabilizes the tertiary structure

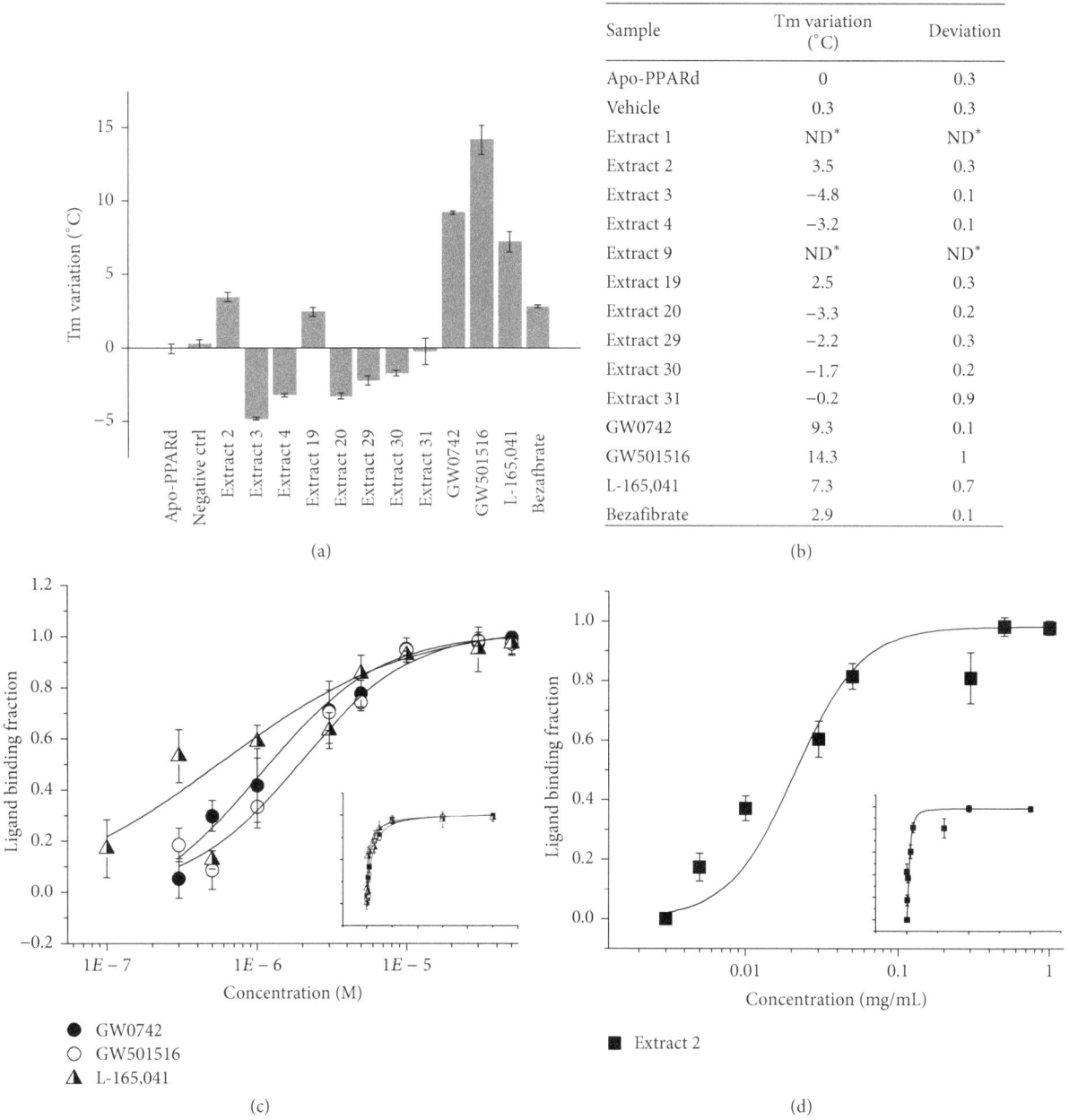

FIGURE 5: Validation assays of PPARß/δ ligand screening. (a) Thermal shift assay of hit candidates. Ten micromolar PPARß/δ with commercial agonists (GW0742, GW501516, L-165,041, and Bezafibrate) at 30 μM or extracts at 0.14 mg/mL. The vehicle is DMSO. Experiments were performed in triplicate. Data are the mean ± SD. (b) Table with T_m variation and standard deviation for the extracts/compounds from the thermal shift. The experiment was performed in triplicate. ND*: not defined. It is possible to verify that two possible hit candidates stabilized the receptor structure by more than 2.5°C, indicating direct binding to the receptor. (c)-(d) Dissociation curves for PPARß/δ ligands and hit candidates. Normalized fluorescence intensity at the emission maximum (480 nm) versus the ligand/fraction concentration, adjusted by the Hill1 approach with OriginPro 8.0. Dissociation curves for the commercial agonists varied from 10^{-7} to 10^{-5} μM. In the dissociation curve, the concentration varied from 0.003 to 1 mg/mL. Data are the mean ± SD (n = 3 independent replicates).

of PPARß/δ, as was previously reported [5], increasing its T_m by 9.3 ± 0.1°C. The other specific agonists, GW501516 and L-165,041, also increased the T_m values of PPARß/δ by 14.3 ± 1°C and 7.3 ± 0.7°C, respectively. Bezafibrate, a PPAR pan-agonist with very low specificity to PPARß/δ that provides low activation [31], presented a T_m increase of only 2.9 ± 0.1°C,

suggesting that the assay is sensitive to evaluate low-specificity hit candidates that might appear during compound screening.

In parallel, the TSA results of the hit candidates showed that 2 selected fractions (extract 1 and extract 9) did not shown the expected melting curves, indicating that these

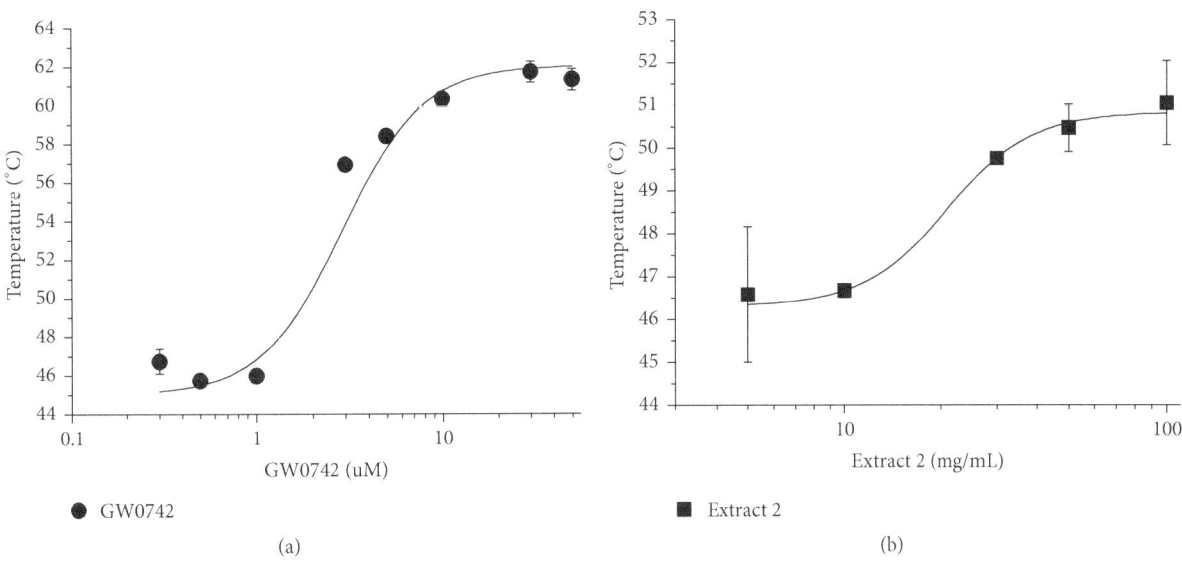

FIGURE 6: Quantitative TSA of PPARß/δ in different concentrations of GW0742 (a) and extract 2 (b). The curves were made using $10\,\mu M$ PPARß/δ. The GW0742 concentrations were 0.3, 0.5, 1, 3, 5, 10, 30, and $50\,\mu M$, and the extract 2 concentrations were 5, 10, 30, 50, and 100 $\mu g/mL$ (higher concentrations of the extract were discarded since they absorb in the used wavelengths). The temperature was varied from 20°C to 90°C in a ramp of 1°C/minute. The T_m variations in the entire curves were approximately 16°C for GW0742 and 5°C for extract 2. Data are the mean ± SD ($n = 3$ independent replicates).

extracts somehow might destabilize the tertiary structure of PPARß/δ or even not directly bind to this receptor. On the other hand, 2 fractions (extract 2 and extract 19) increased the PPARß/δ T_m by 3.5 ± 0.3°C and 2.5 ± 0.3°C, respectively, in comparison with the T_m of apo-PPARß/δ (Figure 5(a)). This result suggests that these extracts may have components that physically bind to the receptor and promote the stabilization of the protein structure.

3.6. ANS Fluorescence Quenching Determines the Affinity of the Hits in the Ligand Binding Pocket of PPARß/δ.

The third experiment of this pipeline is the ANS fluorescence quenching assay, which determines the affinity of the selected hit candidate in the PPARß/δ hydrophobic binding site. In this assay, the ANS probe binds to the hydrophobic ligand binding pocket (LBP) of PPARß/δ, and it can be displaced by PPARß/δ ligands, causing fluorescence quenching (Supplementary Figure 1). As the agonist concentration increases, the fluorescence quenching becomes higher. Several tests were performed to evaluate the best probe: protein ratio for the best assay performance (Supplementary Figure 1). We also made PPARß/δ-ligand/extract binding curves with a 1 : 1 (probe : protein) stoichiometry, which showed that these molecule/extract ratios were effective in dissociating ANS from the PPARß/δ binding site, even in unsaturated ANS concentrations (Supplementary Figure 2). Finally, after all of the performed tests, we standardized the experiments with a 5-fold excess of ANS (Figures 5(c)-5(d)) to guarantee that all of the PPARß/δ is saturated by ANS and all of the conformational modifications caused by ligands/extracts in the receptor's LBP will provoke ANS probe displacement. After that, we measured and calculated the apparent dissociation

constants (Kd_{app}) of PPARß/δ bound to commercial agonists GW0742 ($1.2 ± 0.3\,\mu M$), GW501516 ($1.8 ± 0.1\,\mu M$), and L-165,041 ($1.09 ± 0.08\,\mu M$) (Figure 5(c)). Bezafibrate did not dislocate the ANS probe, with a behavior similar to the negative control (vehicle, DMSO) (Supplementary Figure 2), which is explained by its low specificity and affinity for PPARß/δ [31]. This result means that our pipeline is sensitive enough to evaluate low-specificity hit candidates. However, it is not possible to determine the Kd of this type of candidate. Finally, our results showed an apparent dissociation constant (Kd_{app}) of 0.022 ± 0.008 mg/mL for the hit candidate extract 2 (Figure 5(d)), which is very close to the concentration used in the cellular transactivation assay (0.01 mg/mL).

3.7. Quantitative TSA Also Allows the Calculation of the Dissociation Constant.

To confirm the apparent dissociation constant calculated by the ANS quenching assay, we conducted a quantitative thermal shift assay using increasing concentrations of GW0742 (positive control) and extract 2. To our knowledge, this is the first time that an ANS quenching assay was performed to characterize the binding affinities between the PPARß/δ binding pocket and ligands. Therefore, we submitted the extract and the commercial ligand to a more established protocol for the calculation of the dissociation constant [32]. By our results, we obtained a Kd_{app} of 20 ± 3.7 $\mu g/mL$ for extract 2 and a Kd_{app} of 2.6 ± 0.2 μM for GW0742, which are very close and on the same order of magnitude as the ones obtained by the ANS quenching assay. In this way, we confirm that both the ANS quenching assay and TSA can be used for PPARß/δ dissociation constant evaluation, which present reliable results (Figure 6).

4. Discussion

The purpose of our study was to delineate a pipeline to search and characterize PPARß/δ agonists through a faster and cheaper transactivation primary screening, followed by two biophysical methods, aiming to exclude false positives and select molecules or extracts that directly bind and activate PPARß/δ.

The choice of the cellular transactivation reporter-gene assay as the first step in this pipeline enables the screening to start from a more physiological point of view [33, 34]. In this case, the selected molecules or extracts must permeate the cellular membranes, find and bind to the receptor, and promote its activation. Although other methods, such as TSA, ANS, and FRET, have been proposed to evaluate NR ligand binding [35–37], we consider that the transactivation assay produces quantitative and functional information in a short period of time, which makes it one of the most relevant and important assays for compound screening and drug discovery applied to NRs [33, 34]. Meanwhile, although *in vitro* FRET is the easiest to set up with commercial kits, it does not correlate with cellular conditions [37, 38]. ANS fluorescence quenching is also cheaper; nevertheless, it is laborious and time-demanding for HTS screening, beyond the fact that it is an *in vitro* approach [36, 39]. Moreover, even though TSA is designed to be applied in ligand screening [35, 40], it does not consider the intrinsic fluorescence of natural extracts or the high hydrophobicity of PPARß/δ LBD, which may interfere with the fluorescence signal. In summary, TSA, ANS, and FRET share the disadvantages of biophysical assays as they do not always correlate well with in vivo studies [34].

In summary, we suggest that transactivation reporter-gene assays in cell culture are the most verisimilar assays, as they exploit the natural signaling pathway of NRs; when ligands are added to the system, the receptor is activated and there is the consequent production of reporter protein, which can be measured [33]. Therefore, biophysical methods can and should be used as additional steps of screening pipelines, as they give important information for hit characterization like direct binding confirmation (TSA) and dissociation constant evaluation (ANS and TSA). In comparison with FRET and Lantha-Screen, which may be considered cheaper than commercial kits, these chosen validation methods present the disadvantage of providing indirect results with coactivator measurements [41–43].

After extensive investigation, we established a 3-day transactivation assay, which is a reduction of 1 to 2 days in length in comparison with other transiently transfected cell assays [15–17]. We also optimized the incubation medium (10% charcoal-stripped FBS-supplemented DMEM) and cellular concentration (40,000 cells/well) for our experiment. The major improvement was the 75% reduction in the luciferase substrate volume, which represents a 75% reduction in the kit usage as well as cost, and it brings innovation and advantages when compared with the other transactivation assays in 96-well plates [15–17, 19].

Several reporter-gene screenings for NRs in general have been described as efficient and fast ways to obtain NR physiological responses in high-throughput screening [18, 44–47].

Regarding PPARß/δ assays, most of them use transient transfection taking one or two days longer than our proposed method [15–17], with just one exception, which is based on permanent gene reporter transfect cells [19]. Our reduction in the assay length represents decreased costs for screening campaigns. Furthermore, we found in some reports individually made transfections in each well of the microplate [16], and we consider that this approach cannot confirm if all of the wells were equally transfected and received the same amount of DNA. Following other HTS screening assays [15, 17, 18], we chose to perform transfection in a batch prior to plating the cells, as we considered that the cells would be more homogenously transfected, with all cells contained in the well submitted to the same treatment.

Another special detail in our screening assay is the fact that we chose a $1\,\mu M$ concentration for the positive controls. Although the EC_{50} values for most agonists used (GW0742, GW501516, and L-165,041) are in the nanomolar range, the majority of transactivation assays and screenings for PPARß/δ use a range between 0.1 and 40 μM of commercial agonists as a positive control [16, 17, 19, 48]. In addition, as we showed, the proposed transactivation assay is sensitive enough to detect PPARß/δ agonists in concentrations varying from 10^{-11} to 10^{-6} M, as we obtained the following EC_{50} values for the commercial agonists: $EC_{50\;GW501516} = 0.71\,nM$, $EC_{50\;GW0742} = 10.87\,nM$, and $EC_{50\;L-165,041} = 26.40\,nM$. In this way, our results indicate that our assay can be used to detect, at a low level, an agonist that activates PPARß/δ.

Following the sequence of our pipeline, two biophysical methods (TSA and ANS fluorescence quenching) were employed to characterize PPARß/δ ligand binding along with Kd evaluation. Several studies had shown that a ligand-NR complex has an increased structural stability in comparison to its apo form [27–30]. Qualitative TSA results provided measurement of the PPARß/δ LBD structural stability in the absence or presence of commercial ligands, and the results were able to discriminate between high affinity (GW0742, GW501516, and L-165,041) and low affinity (as the pan-PPAR agonist Bezafibrate) PPARß/δ ligands [5, 7, 25, 31]. Furthermore, the ANS quenching assay and quantitative TSA evaluated the selected compounds/extracts bound to hPPARß/δ LBD, providing dissociation constant values. Few studies show affinity constants between the NRs and their ligands, and most of them are based on cellular dose-response assays, which calculate indirect constant affinities [7, 25]. Here, we show an improvement in ligand binding characterization methods, using an ANS fluorescence quenching assay and quantitative TSA, which are able to evaluate the affinities of compounds/extracts that bind to the PPARß/δ LBD pocket. These approaches for PPARß/δ ligand characterization were compared themselves, and the apparent dissociation constants found in both methodologies were in the same range, increasing the data reliability of our Kd evaluations. Finally, application of these methodologies also has the advantage of measuring the relative activity of a compound (or a mixture of substances) without the requirement of prior information about the chemical structure of the ligand [36]. Therefore, we proposed that these methodologies are useful as additional steps in the screening of natural extract libraries.

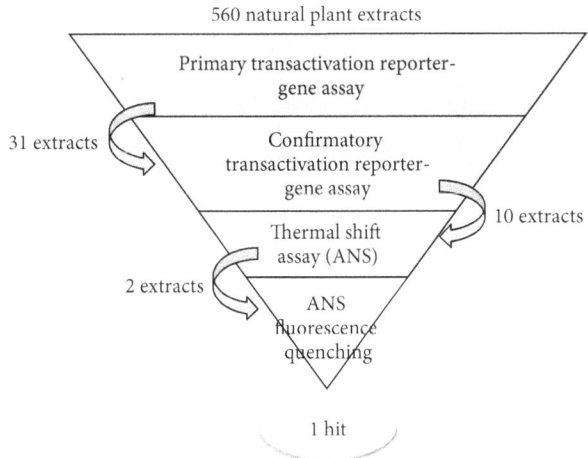

FIGURE 7: Screening pipeline for PPARß/δ agonists. Our proposed screening pipeline for PPARß/δ agonists is composed of 3 complementary assays. The primary transactivation reporter-gene assay screening and the confirmatory transactivation reporter-gene assay utilize a cellular transactivation reporter-gene assay that has been optimized to a 3-day long experiment with 40,000 cells and only 25 μL of the luciferases substrates per well, reducing the time and cost of the screening assay. The two following validation assays are the thermal shift (TSA) to check if the compounds/extracts previously selected stabilize the PPARß/δ tertiary structure and the ANS fluorescence quenching to determine the compound affinity to the hydrophobic pocket of PPARß/δ. We submitted a 560-natural extract library to the proposed pipeline and found 31 possible hit candidates in the primary transactivation screening. Ten hit candidates were selected in the confirmatory cellular transactivation. The TSA selected 2 extracts, and one of them showed a 0.02 mg/mL affinity constant in the ANS quenching assay.

As it has been extensively reported, natural extracts are good starting points to select compounds that may play important roles in treating or preventing human metabolic diseases or regulating physiological functions [49]. In addition, natural plant extracts could improve the chemical diversity of compounds, increasing the choices of finding new molecules with biological activity [50], especially in the case of libraries that explore particular biomes of Brazilian diversity. Studies have shown that one new focus in the treatment of metabolic syndromes is searching for novel agonists for PPARs from natural products, which present low toxicity and high efficiency [49, 50]. However, it is important to mention that the screening of natural extract libraries could result in low activity signals since each tested fraction/extract is composed of different compounds, and only one of them might present activity against a specific target. In this context, the measured activities tend to be smaller than the ones obtained from the positive controls, which are generally composed of one isolated compound [15, 17].

To test and best characterize our developed pipeline, we performed a validation screening with 560 natural extracts from the Phytobios library and found 31 possible hit candidates (Figure 7). All of the screening plates presented the statistical parameter Z'-factor values higher than the 0.5 limit

(0.53–0.64) [22], indicating the robustness and reliability of this assay. The observed variation of the positive control activation fold among different plates was considered to be an intrinsic variability of the cellular assay, as it has been reported previously [5, 15, 17, 19, 48].

After confirming 10 hit candidates in a secondary transactivation assay, we started the selection of these extracts through the TSA and ANS assays, avoiding possible indirect and allosteric interactions. From the qualitative TSA results, two extracts have increased the receptor melting temperature, which means that they contain chemical components that bind and stabilize the tertiary structure of the receptor [27, 28]. However, qualitative TSA allows the selection of extracts with components that interact with other hydrophobic sites in the protein structure (besides LBD) [40]. To overcome this limitation, the ANS fluorescence quenching assay was applied to confirm the physical interaction between the compounds/extracts and PPARß/δ LBD, and it allows the evaluation of the apparent dissociation constants (Kd_{app}). We selected the best extract from the library (extract 2), which binds PPARß/δ with a Kd_{app} of 22 ± 8 μg/mL. Moreover, we performed an additional Kd_{app} evaluation, employing quantitative TSA. By using this technique, we obtained a Kd_{app} of 20.9 ± 3.7 μg/mL for extract 2, showing the reliability of our Kd evaluations.

In addition, it is important to mention that the found apparent affinity constant (Kd_{app}) for extract 2 is close to the concentration used in the cellular assay (0.01 mg/mL), which may explain the low-fold of activation (1.31-fold) found in the transactivation assay. Since extract 2 is a mixture of diverse chemical compounds, we suggest that at least one of its components provides PPARß/δ activation, binding to the receptor with a higher affinity. Thus, the use of higher extract concentrations would probably increase the degree of PPARß/δ activation. However, we observed that higher extract 2 concentrations were cytotoxic to cells (data not shown), and therefore, it would be interesting to fractionate this extract to concentrate and separate its bioactive compounds in order to decrease the cytotoxicity and possibly increase PPARß/δ activation.

5. Conclusion

In summary, we developed and validated a pipeline to screening for new PPARß/δ agonists in libraries of compounds or natural extracts. The first living cell screening gives information about the ability of the hit candidates to activate PPARß/δ. We optimized this assay in length (3 days long) and in the volume of reading reagents (75% reduction), which represents a real decrease in cost for screening campaigns. We also obtained information about the compound cytotoxicity, which adds an improvement in the obtained information from the primary screening. To exclude indirect activators of PPARß/δ, we joined two *in vitro* biophysics assays, creating a pipeline that searches for compounds/extracts that can activate, stabilize the tertiary structure, and bind to the hydrophobic pocket of PPARß/δ, allowing calculation of the apparent affinity constant. We screened a 560-natural extract library to test our pipeline and found 31 possible hit candidates in the primary cellular transactivation screening; from these, 10 hit candidates were selected in the confirmatory cellular transactivation, where 2 were selected by qualitative TSA, but only one was selected as a hit since it presented a real capacity to bind and activate PPARß/δ with a relatively high affinity. To date, our proposed pipeline presents more information than just a cellular activation screening, as it ranges from the cellular to the biophysical point of view, allowing the calculation of apparent affinity constants besides the traditional EC_{50} calculation. Moreover, we reduced the reagent use and time of the assay, which is relevant for big screening campaigns. Finally, this approach may improve the effectiveness of screening for agonists targeting PPARß/δ for drug development, with a significant reduction in the time and cost for the transactivation assay.

Conflicts of Interest

The authors declare that there are no conflicts of interest regarding the publication of this article.

Acknowledgments

The authors acknowledge the LNBio facilities, LPP, LEC, and LDEE for the protein purification, spectroscopy, and screening devices. They acknowledge LQPN and Phytobios Pesquisa, Desenvolvimento e Inovação Ltda for kindly providing the Phytobios library. This work was supported by Fundação de Amparo à Pesquisa do Estado de São Paulo (FAPESP) (Grant nos. 2013/22648-3 and 2016/16476-2) and Conselho Nacional de Desenvolvimento Científico e Tecnológico (CNPq) (Grant no. 403433/2016-9).

Supplementary Materials

Supplementary 1. Supplementary Figure 1: tests of probe : protein concentrations for ANS fluorescence quenching assay. ANS quenching tests of probe and protein concentrations. hPPARß/δ LBD concentrations varied from 0.25 to 2 μM; ANS concentrations varied from 5 to 20 μM. Protein-ANS mixtures were incubated for 1 hour at 4°C. After, GW0742 was added at 0.3 μM, 0.5 μM, 1 μM, 3 μM, and 5 μM. DMSO was used as vehicle. The assay was read on the EnSpire Multimode Plate Reader (Perkin Elmer) with 380 nm excitation and emission scanning between 400 and 600 nm, at 25°C. The fluorescence emission intensities were plotted for each combination of protein and probe 9 10 11 12 13 14 15 16 concentrations in all emission wavelengths (400–600 nm). The chosen protein and ANS concentrations were 2 uM and 10 uM, which presented best signal-to-ratio noise without much reagent usage. In graphs 1–4 hPPARß/δ concentration varied in the presence of 5 μM ANS; 5–8, hPPARß/δ concentration varied in the presence of 10 μM ANS; 9–12, hPPARß/δ concentration varied in the presence of 15 μM ANS; and 13–16 hPPARß/δ concentration varied in the presence of 20 μM ANS.

Supplementary 2. Supplementary Figure 2: ANS quenching curves of PPARß/δ submitted to GW0742 (left) or extract 02

(right) titration. 10 μM of hPPARß/δ LBD and 10 μM of ANS were used. The found Kds (6.3 ± 1.3 μM fo GW0742 and 113.9 ± 75 μg/mL for extract 2) are probably overestimated, due to the fact that there are more than one possible ANS binding site in hPPARß/δ LBD, which are not necessary located into the LBP, but it is still possible to observe that both GW0742 and extract 02 dislocated ANS from PPARß/δ LBP. Data are the mean $\pm$ SD ($n = 3$ independent replicates).

Supplementary 3. Supplementary Figure 3: ANS fluorescence quenching assay for PPARδ commercial agonist and hit candidate. 2 μM hPPARß/δ LBD and 20 μM ANS were incubated for 1 hour at 4°C. After, compounds or extracts were added to the mixture at 0.3 μM, 0.5 μM, 1 μM, 3 μM, 5 μM, 10 μM, 30 μM, and 50 μM (commercial compounds), or at 0.005 mg/mL, 0.01 mg/mL, 0.03 mg/mL, 0.05 mg/mL, 0.1 mg/mL, 0.3 mg/mL, 0.5 mg/mL, and 1 mg/mL (extracts). DMSO was used as vehicle (negative control). The assay was read on the EnSpire Multimode Plate Reader (Perkin Elmer) with 380 nm excitation and emission scanning between 400 and 600 nm, at 25°C. The fluorescence emission intensities were plotted for each compound/extract concentration in all emission wavelengths (400–600 nm). GW0742, GW501516, L-165,041, and the hit candidate extract 2 showed quenching in the ANS fluorescence. Bezafibrate had the same pattern as the vehicle (DMSO) and did not show a fluorescence quenching, meaning that the compound could not dislocate the ANS from PPARß/δ binding pocket.

References

[1] L. Michalik, J. Auwerx, J. P. Berger et al., "International union of pharmacology. LXI. Peroxisome proliferator-activated receptors," *Pharmacological Reviews*, vol. 58, no. 4, pp. 726–741, 2006.

[2] S. Aleshin, M. Strokin, M. Sergeeva, and G. Reiser, "Peroxisome proliferator-activated receptor (PPAR)β/δ, a possible nexus of PPARα- and PPARγ-dependent molecular pathways in neurodegenerative diseases: review and novel hypotheses," *Neurochemistry International*, vol. 63, no. 4, pp. 322–330, 2013.

[3] A. Iwashita, Y. Muramatsu, T. Yamazaki et al., "Neuroprotective efficacy of the peroxisome proliferator-activated receptor δ-selective agonists in vitro and in vivo," *The Journal of Pharmacology and Experimental Therapeutics*, vol. 320, no. 3, pp. 1087–1096, 2007.

[4] L. Michalik and W. Wahli, "Involvement of PPAR nuclear receptors in tissue injury and wound repair," *The Journal of Clinical Investigation*, vol. 116, no. 3, pp. 598–606, 2006.

[5] F. A. H. Batista, D. B. B. Trivella, A. Bernardes et al., "Structural insights into human peroxisome proliferator activated receptor delta (PPAR-delta) selective ligand binding," *PLoS ONE*, vol. 7, no. 5, Article ID e33643, 2012.

[6] N. S. Tan, M. Vázquez-Carrera, A. Montagner, M. K. Sng, H. Guillou, and W. Wahli, "Transcriptional control of physiological and pathological processes by the nuclear receptor PPARβ/δ," *Progress in Lipid Research*, vol. 64, pp. 98–122, 2016.

[7] W. R. Oliver Jr., J. L. Shenk, M. R. Snaith et al., "A selective peroxisome proliferator-activated receptor δ agonist promotes reverse cholesterol transport," *Proceedings of the National Acadamy of Sciences of the United States of America*, vol. 98, no. 9, pp. 5306–5311, 2001.

[8] R. Müller, "PPARβ/δ in human cancer," *Biochimie*, vol. 136, pp. 90–99, 2017.

[9] T. A. Ajith and T. G. Jayakumar, "Peroxisome proliferator-activated receptors in cardiac energy metabolism and cardiovascular disease," *Clinical and Experimental Pharmacology and Physiology*, vol. 43, no. 7, pp. 649–658, 2016.

[10] A. S. Grewal, M. Beniwal, D. Pandita, B. S. Sekhon, and V. Lather, "Recent Updates on peroxisome proliferator-activated receptor δ agonists for the treatment of metabolic syndrome," *Medicinal Chemistry*, vol. 12, no. 1, pp. 3–21, 2016.

[11] A. Montagner, W. Wahli, and N. S. Tan, "Nuclear receptor peroxisome proliferator activated receptor (PPAR) β/δ in skin wound healing and cancer," in *European Journal of Dermatology*, vol. 25, pp. 4–11, 1 edition, 2015.

[12] F. Biscetti, G. Straface, D. Pitocco, F. Zaccardi, G. Ghirlanda, and A. Flex, "Peroxisome proliferator-activated receptors and angiogenesis," *Nutrition, Metabolism & Cardiovascular Diseases*, vol. 19, no. 11, pp. 751–759, 2009.

[13] T. Varga, Z. Czimmerer, and L. Nagy, "PPARs are a unique set of fatty acid regulated transcription factors controlling both lipid metabolism and inflammation," *Biochimica et Biophysica Acta*, vol. 1812, no. 8, pp. 1007–1022, 2011.

[14] J. Zhang, X. Liu, X.-B. Xie, X.-C. Cheng, and R.-L. Wang, "Multitargeted bioactive ligands for PPARs discovered in the last decade," *Chemical Biology & Drug Design*, pp. 635–663, 2016.

[15] N. Matsuura, K. Gamo, H. Miyachi et al., "γ-Mangostin from garcinia mangostana pericarps as a dual agonist that activates both PPARα and PPARδ," *Bioscience, Biotechnology, and Biochemistry*, vol. 77, no. 12, pp. 2430–2435, 2013.

[16] M. L. Takacs and B. D. Abbott, "Activation of mouse and human peroxisome proliferator-activated receptors (α, β/δ, γ) by perfluorooctanoic acid and perfluorooctane sulfonate," *Toxicological Sciences*, vol. 95, no. 1, pp. 108–117, 2007.

[17] Z.-N. Xia, Y.-X. Lin, L.-X. Guo et al., "Development of a cell-based high-throughput peroxisome proliferator- activated receptors (PPARs) screening model and its application for evaluation of the extracts from Rhizoma Coptis," *Journal of Asian Natural Products Research*, vol. 15, no. 3, pp. 225–234, 2013.

[18] G. S. Grover, B. A. Turner, C. N. Parker, J. Meier, D. S. Lala, and P. H. Lee, "Multiplexing nuclear receptors for agonist identification in a cell-based reporter gene high-throughput screen," *Journal of Biomolecular Screening*, vol. 8, no. 3, pp. 239–246, 2003.

[19] M. Seimandi, G. Lemaire, A. Pillon et al., "Differential responses of PPARα, PPARδ, and PPARγ reporter cell lines to selective PPAR synthetic ligands," *Analytical Biochemistry*, vol. 344, no. 1, pp. 8–15, 2005.

[20] F. Fan and K. V. Wood, "Bioluminescent assays for high-throughput screening," *ASSAY and Drug Development Technologies*, vol. 5, no. 1, pp. 127–136, 2007.

[21] A. Paguio, P. Stecha, K. V. Wood, and F. Fan, "Improved dual-luciferase reporter assays for nuclear receptors," *Current Chemical Genomics*, vol. 4, no. 1, pp. 13–19, 2010.

[22] J.-H. Zhang, T. D. Y. Chung, and K. R. Oldenburg, "A simple statistical parameter for use in evaluation and validation of high throughput screening assays," *Journal of Biomolecular Screening*, vol. 4, no. 2, pp. 67–73, 1999.

[23] F. H. Niesen, H. Berglund, and M. Vedadi, "The use of differential scanning fluorimetry to detect ligand interactions that promote protein stability," *Nature Protocols*, vol. 2, no. 9, pp. 2212–2221, 2007.

[24] L. Cervera, S. Gutiérrez, F. Gòdia, and M. M. Segura, "Optimization of HEK 293 cell growth by addition of non-animal derived components using design of experiments," *BMC Proceedings*, vol. 5, no. Suppl 8, p. P126, 2011.

[25] C. Ekambomé Bassène, F. Suzenet, N. Hennuyer et al., "Studies towards the conception of new selective PPARβ/δ ligands," *Bioorganic & Medicinal Chemistry Letters*, vol. 16, no. 17, pp. 4528–4532, 2006.

[26] T. Mosmann, "Rapid colorimetric assay for cellular growth and survival: application to proliferation and cytotoxicity assays," *Journal of Immunological Methods*, vol. 65, no. 1-2, pp. 55–63, 1983.

[27] A. C. M. Figueira, D. M. Saidemberg, P. C. T. Souza et al., "Analysis of agonist and antagonist effects on thyroid hormone receptor conformation by hydrogen/deuterium exchange," *Molecular Endocrinology*, vol. 25, no. 1, pp. 15–31, 2011.

[28] Y. Hamuro, S. J. Coales, J. A. Morrow et al., "Hydrogen/deuterium-exchange (H/D-Ex) of PPARγ LBD in the presence of various modulators," *Protein Science*, vol. 15, no. 8, pp. 1883–1892, 2006.

[29] P. Pissios, I. Tzameli, P. J. Kushner, and D. D. Moore, "Dynamic stabilization of nuclear receptor ligand binding domains by hormone or corepressor binding," *Molecular Cell*, vol. 6, no. 2, pp. 245–253, 2000.

[30] F. Rastinejad, P. Huang, V. Chandra, and S. Khorasanizadeh, "Understanding nuclear receptor form and function using structural biology," *Molecular Endocrinology*, vol. 51, no. 3, pp. T1–T21, 2013.

[31] T. M. Willson, P. J. Brown, D. D. Sternbach, and B. R. Henke, "The PPARs: from orphan receptors to drug discovery," *Journal of Medicinal Chemistry*, vol. 43, no. 4, pp. 527–550, 2000.

[32] P. Cimmperman, L. Baranauskiene, S. Jachimovičiute et al., "A quantitative model of thermal stabilization and destabilization of proteins by ligands," *Biophysical Journal*, vol. 95, no. 7, pp. 3222–3231, 2008.

[33] G. Bagchi Bhattacharjee and S. M. Paul Khurana, "In vitro reporter assays for screening of chemicals that disrupt androgen signaling," *Journal of Toxicology*, vol. 2014, Article ID 701752, 7 pages, 2014.

[34] C. Lai, X. Jiang, and X. Li, "Development of luciferase reporter-based cell assays," *ASSAY and Drug Development Technologies*, vol. 4, no. 3, pp. 307–315, 2006.

[35] K. DeSantis, A. Reed, R. Rahhal, and J. Reinking, "Use of differential scanning fluorimetry as a high-throughput assay to identify nuclear receptor ligands," *Nuclear Receptor Signaling*, vol. 10, p. e002, 2012.

[36] S. Zorrilla, B. Garzón, and D. Pérez-Sala, "Selective binding of the fluorescent dye 1-anilinonaphthalene-8-sulfonic acid to peroxisome proliferator-activated receptor γ allows ligand identification and characterization," *Analytical Biochemistry*, vol. 399, no. 1, pp. 84–92, 2010.

[37] T. Hilal, V. Puetter, C. Otto, K. Parczyk, and B. Bader, "A dual estrogen receptor TR-FRET assay for simultaneous measurement of steroid site binding and coactivator recruitment," *Journal of Biomolecular Screening*, vol. 15, no. 3, pp. 268–278, 2010.

[38] J. R. Gunther, Y. Du, E. Rhoden et al., "A set of time-resolved fluorescence resonance energy transfer assays for the discovery of inhibitors of estrogen receptor-coactivator binding," *Journal of Biomolecular Screening*, vol. 14, no. 2, pp. 181–193, 2009.

[39] R. Jasuja, J. Ulloor, C. M. Yengo et al., "Kinetic and thermodynamic characterization of dihydrotestosterone-induced

conformational perturbations in androgen receptor ligand-binding domain," *Molecular Endocrinology*, vol. 23, no. 8, pp. 1231–1241, 2009.

[40] M. Vivoli, H. R. Novak, J. A. Littlechild, and N. J. Harmer, "Determination of protein-ligand interactions using differential scanning fluorimetry," *Journal of Visualized Experiments*, no. 91, Article ID e51809, 2014.

[41] J. F. Glickman, X. Wu, R. Mercuri et al., "A comparison of ALPHAscreen, TR-FRET, and TRF as assay methods for FXR nuclear receptors," *Journal of Biomolecular Screening*, vol. 7, no. 1, pp. 3–10, 2002.

[42] J. Liu, K. S. Knappenberger, H. Käck et al., "A homogeneous in vitro functional assay for estrogen receptors: Coactivator recruitment," *Molecular Endocrinology*, vol. 17, no. 3, pp. 346–355, 2003.

[43] M. S. Ozers, K. M. Ervin, C. L. Steffen et al., "Analysis of ligand-dependent recruitment of coactivator peptides to estrogen receptor using fluorescence polarization," *Molecular Endocrinology*, vol. 19, no. 1, pp. 25–34, 2005.

[44] E. Sonneveld, J. A. C. Riteco, H. J. Jansen et al., "Comparison of in vitro and in vivo screening models for androgenic and estrogenic activities," *Toxicological Sciences*, vol. 89, no. 1, pp. 173–187, 2006.

[45] D. Sedlák, A. Paguio, and P. Bartůněk, "Two panels of steroid receptor luciferase reporter cell lines for compound profiling," *Combinatorial Chemistry & High Throughput Screening*, vol. 14, no. 4, pp. 248–266, 2011.

[46] N. Andruska, C. Mao, M. Cherian, C. Zhang, and D. J. Shapiro, "Evaluation of a luciferase-based reporter assay as a screen for inhibitors of estrogen-ERα-induced proliferation of breast cancer cells," *Journal of Biomolecular Screening*, vol. 17, no. 7, pp. 921–932, 2012.

[47] C.-W. Hsu, J. Zhao, R. Huang et al., "Quantitative high-throughput profiling of environmental chemicals and drugs that modulate farnesoid X receptor," *Scientific Reports*, vol. 4, article no. 6437, 2014.

[48] A.-M. Krogsdam, C. A. F. Nielsen, S. Neve et al., "Nuclear receptor corepressor-dependent repression of peroxisome-proliferator-activated receptor δ-mediated transactivation," *Biochemical Journal*, vol. 363, part 1, pp. 157–165, 2002.

[49] T. H.-W. Huang, A. W. Teoh, B.-L. Lin, D. S.-H. Lin, and B. Roufogalis, "The role of herbal PPAR modulators in the treatment of cardiometabolic syndrome," *Pharmacological Research*, vol. 60, no. 3, pp. 195–206, 2009.

[50] D. Rigano, C. Sirignano, and O. Taglialatela-Scafati, "The potential of natural products for targeting PPARα," *Acta Pharmaceutica Sinica B (APSB)*, vol. 7, no. 4, pp. 427–438, 2017.

15

MicroRNAs-Dependent Regulation of PPARs in Metabolic Diseases and Cancers

Dorothea Portius, Cyril Sobolewski, and Michelangelo Foti

Department of Cell Physiology and Metabolism and Diabetes Center, Faculty of Medicine, University of Geneva, Geneva, Switzerland

Correspondence should be addressed to Michelangelo Foti; michelangelo.foti@unige.ch

Academic Editor: Valeria Amodeo

Peroxisome proliferator-activated receptors (PPARs) are a family of ligand-dependent nuclear receptors, which control the transcription of genes involved in energy homeostasis and inflammation and cell proliferation/differentiation. Alterations of PPARs' expression and/or activity are commonly associated with metabolic disorders occurring with obesity, type 2 diabetes, and fatty liver disease, as well as with inflammation and cancer. Emerging evidence now indicates that microRNAs (miRNAs), a family of small noncoding RNAs, which fine-tune gene expression, play a significant role in the pathophysiological mechanisms regulating the expression and activity of PPARs. Herein, the regulation of PPARs by miRNAs is reviewed in the context of metabolic disorders, inflammation, and cancer. The reciprocal control of miRNAs expression by PPARs, as well as the therapeutic potential of modulating PPAR expression/activity by pharmacological compounds targeting miRNA, is also discussed.

1. Introduction

Peroxisome proliferator-activated receptors (PPARs) are a family of nuclear receptors involved in various biological functions but with a prominent role in metabolic homeostasis of carbohydrates and lipids [1]. The three PPAR isoforms, PPARα (NR1C1), PPARβ/δ (NR1C2), and PPARγ (NR1C3), share 60% to 80% of structural homology [2, 3] and exhibit a distinct tissue expression pattern but can exert similar or different physiological functions [3]. In the canonical model, PPARs are activated in the cytoplasm by specific ligands [1–6] and then translocate into the nucleus, where they form a complex predominantly with the nuclear receptor Retinoid-X-Receptor (RXR), to transactivate gene expression by binding to PPAR response elements (PPREs) on gene promoters [6, 7]. In contrast, noncanonical PPAR activity suppresses gene transcription through direct protein-protein interactions with other transcription factors, for example, the nuclear factor-kB (NFkB) or activated protein-1 (AP-1) [1, 3]. PPARs activity is also tightly dependent on the binding of other cofactors such as PGC1α (peroxisome proliferator-activated receptor coactivator-1α) and p300 or CREB binding protein—or on the contrary on the binding of corepressor proteins, for example, NCOR (nuclear receptor corepressor) or SMRT (silencing mediator for retinoid and thyroid hormone receptor), which hamper PPARs interactions with PPRE [3].

Through complex regulatory mechanisms, PPARs exert a tight control on energy homeostasis by modulating the expression of key genes involved in lipid metabolism [5, 6], adipocytes differentiation [5], and carbohydrate metabolism [5, 6]. The implication of PPARs in inflammatory processes and specific cancers is further suggested by recent studies (reviewed in [3, 8, 9]). These key and pleiotropic roles of PPARs in cellular processes have led to the development of pharmacologic agonists, for example, thiazolidinediones and fibrates [10, 11], to treat metabolic disorders or other diseases such as atherosclerosis [2, 5, 12]. However, long-term treatment with PPARs agonists triggers uncontrolled side effects in patients (e.g., oedema, weight gain, heart failure, and bone fractures) and in some cases they may even promote tumorigenesis [6, 8, 13]. Alternative therapeutic options to control distinct PPARs activities in specific tissues are therefore desirable but require that we deepen our understanding of the molecular mechanisms controlling PPARs expression/activity in diseases.

Recently, a wealth of studies has suggested that epigenetic mechanisms, for example, DNA methylation, histone modifications, or small noncoding RNA (i.e., microRNAs), importantly affect physiological or pathological mechanisms involved in a wide variety of diseases and cancers. In the case of PPARs, methylation of their promoters [14, 15], or histone acetylation [16], has been reported to affect PPARs expression and physiological processes under their control. More recently, other epigenetic alterations, in particular those leading to abnormal microRNAs (miRNAs) expression, have also been implicated in the regulation of PPARs expression or activity [17]. Indeed several miRNAs were reported to either directly target PPARs mRNA or to indirectly affect their expression/activities by targeting PPARs-associated cofactors and repressors, thus providing a further level of complexity in these regulatory mechanisms [18–20].

In this review, we discuss the current knowledge about miRNAs-dependent regulation of PPARs and their cofactors in physiological and pathological processes. Most of available studies dealing with this topic are restrained to metabolic diseases (e.g., diabetes, fatty liver diseases, and cardiovascular diseases) and associated cancers (e.g., liver cancers) in tissues where the role of PPARs is well characterized (e.g., liver, adipose tissue, muscles, and heart). Other rare studies investigating PPARs regulation by miRNAs in different tissues (e.g., bone marrow, neurons, and cartilage) or type of cancers (e.g., neuroblastoma, prostate cancer), unrelated to metabolic disorders, are also considered. Finally, the reciprocal regulation of specific miRNAs by PPARs, as well as potential miRNA-based pharmacological approaches to therapeutically modulate PPARs expression and/or activity, was also examined.

2. miRNAs

MicroRNAs (miRNAs) are endogenous small noncoding RNAs of approximately 16–22 nucleotides, which bind to complementary sequences (seed sequences) in the $3'$UTR of target mRNAs and mediate either their decay or translation inhibition [21, 22]. miRNAs are encoded within intronic, intergenic regions or in polycistronic clusters [19, 23], and their biogenesis starts with a RNA polymerase II-dependent transcription of a primary transcript (pri-miRNA), which is then matured by a nuclear microprocessor complex (RNase III Drosha and its mammalian double-stranded RNA-binding partner DGCR8). This leads to the release of a pre-miRNA, which is then exported into the cytoplasm by Exportin-5, where the RNase III Dicer1, together with its binding partner TARP2 (T-cell receptor gamma-chain constant region), removes the pre-miRNA hairpin loop and generates a miRNA duplex of mature miRNA (guide strand) and of a complementary strand (passenger strand or miRNA*). The guide strand and the miRNA* are then associated with Argonaute proteins and incorporated into the RNA-induced silencing complex (RISC). A second maturation step is initiated within the RISC to separate both strands and the mature miRNA binds to the $3'$UTR of target mRNAs. Recent evidence also indicates a pathophysiological role of the passenger strand of miRNA (miRNA*) in specific conditions,

although it frequently appears to be degraded and devoid of any functions [19, 21, 23, 24].

More than 2000 miRNAs have been identified and it is considered that 60% of human genes are regulated by miRNAs with around 45 000 miRNA targets within the transcriptome [21–23, 25]. miRNAs act within an intricate regulatory network, where one specific miRNA can control the expression of several hundred mRNAs and conversely one mRNA can be targeted by several miRNAs [19, 23]. Through their wide action, miRNAs are involved in the control of almost all cellular functions and alterations of their expression/activity are observed in various pathological conditions including metabolic diseases and associated cancers [2, 21, 22, 25–29]. The bulk of the studies investigating PPARs and associated cofactors/repressors (e.g., RXR, NCOR) regulation by miRNAs has been performed in the frame of metabolic diseases, where the role of PPARs is the best characterized. Indeed, bioinformatics analyses using the miRWalk 2.0 platform (http://zmf.umm.uni-heidelberg.de/apps/zmf/mirwalk2/index.html), which integrates different prediction software programs for miRNA-mRNA interactions, point to multiple candidate miRNAs potentially targeting directly PPAR isoforms. However, only a restricted number of these candidates have been validated by experimental approaches (see Table 1). Combining MetaCore™ and miRWalk 2.0 based analyses in human studies exclusively revealed that 606 miRNAs were implicated in human cancers, and among those 34 are in metabolic disorders (e.g., obesity, diabetes, hepatomegaly, fatty liver diseases, hypertension, dyslipidemia, and other diabetic complications). Among the 606 cancer-related miRNAs, eight were targeting PPARα, four were targeting PPARβ/δ, and eight were targeting PPARγ. Interestingly, two miRNAs targeting PPARα (miR-21 and miR-519d) and two miRNAs targeting PPARγ (miR-27 and miR-20) were also previously associated with metabolic diseases (Figure 1). Although such predictive analyses using available software programs are subject to multiple biases and should be considered with extreme caution, they suggest that fine-tuning of PPARs signaling by miRNAs may sit at the crossroad between metabolic diseases and cancers in human.

3. miRNAs-Dependent Regulation of PPARs in Metabolic Diseases and Cancer

3.1. miRNAs-Dependent Regulation of PPARα. PPARα is a nutritional sensor adapting metabolic homeostasis to energy deprivation [3]. It is mostly expressed in the liver, where it regulates lipid catabolism (i.e., β-oxidation) and critical genes (e.g., fatty acid transport protein 1, CD36, Acyl-CoA oxidase 1, and Carnitine palmitoyltransferase 1) involved in fatty acid transport [68] and in ketogenesis (e.g., Hmgcs2, Hmgcl) [68]. PPARα exerts also an anti-inflammatory function, as evidenced in mouse models of acute inflammation [68]. This effect results from an attenuation of proinflammatory cytokines (e.g., Il-6, Il-1β) expression as well as an upregulation of anti-inflammatory factors such as Il-1ra (Il-1 receptor antagonist) or IκBα [68]. PPARα is also expressed in other organs such as adipose tissues, heart, skeletal muscles, and kidneys, where it controls also some aspects of the glucose

TABLE 1: Experimentally validated miRNAs targeting PPAR isoforms in specific tissues and pathophysiological processes.

(a) PPARα

miRNA	Biological process	Cell/tissue	Reference
Human studies			
miR-9	Cancer cell invasion and proliferation	HCC tissue Hepatic cell lines	Drakaki et al., 2015 [30]
	Lipid metabolism	HCC tissue Hepatic cell lines	Cui et al., 2015 [31]
miR-10b	Hepatic steatosis	Hepatic cell lines	Zheng et al., 2010 [32]
miR-21	Vascular inflammation	Endothelial cell lines	Zhou et al., 2011 [33]
	Liver cell injury Inflammation Fibrosis	Liver tissue Primary biliary and hepatic inflammatory cells	Loyer et al., 2015 [34]
miR-33	Liver fibrosis	Hepatic stellate cell line	Li et al., 2014 [35]
miR-141-3p	HBV replication	Hepatic cell line	Hu et al., 2012 [36]
miR-199a-5p	Hepatic steatosis	Liver tissue Hepatic cell lines	Li et al., 2014 [37]
miR-506	Drug resistance	Colon cancer cell line	Tong et al., 2011 [38]
miR-519d	Adipocyte differentiation	White adipose tissue Primary preadipocytes	Martinelli et al., 2010 [39]
Rodent studies			
miR-21	Liver cell injury Inflammation Fibrosis	Liver tissue Primary biliary and hepatic inflammatory cells	Loyer et al., 2015 [34]
miR-22	Cardiac hypertrophy Cardiac contractility	Heart tissue Primary neonatal cardiomyocytes	Gurha et al., 2013 [40]
miR-27	Adipocyte differentiation	Brown/white adipose tissue, primary adipose derived stromal cells, brown preadipocyte cell line	Sun et al., 2014 [41]
miR-124-3p	Protein secretion	Isolated neutrophils	Baek et al., 2008 [42]
miR-199a-5p	Hepatic steatosis	Liver tissue Hepatic cell lines	Li et al., 2014 [37]

(b) PPARβ/δ

miRNA	Biological process	Cell/tissue	Reference
Human studies			
miR-199a miR-214	Mitochondrial metabolism	Myocardium Primary cardiomyocytes	El Azzouzi et al., 2013 [43]
miR-9	Inflammation	Isolated monocytes	Thulin et al., 2013 [44]
miR-138	Wound healing, Proliferation, migration	Skin tissue Hypertrophic scar fibroblasts	Xiao et al., 2015 [45]
Rodent studies			
miR-199a miR-214	Mitochondrial metabolism	Myocardium Primary cardiomyocytes	El Azzouzi et al., 2013 [43]

(c) PPARγ

miRNA	Biological process	Cell/tissue	Reference
Human studies			
miR-20	Osteogenic differentiation	Bone marrow derived stromal cell line	Zhang et al., 2011 [46]

(c) Continued.

miRNA	Biological process	Cell/tissue	Reference
miR-27a	Proliferation	HCC tissue Hepatic cell lines	Li et al., 2015 [47]
	Proliferation	Lung tissue Pulmonary endothelial cell lines	Kang et al., 2013 [48]
miR-27b	Inflammation	Isolated monocytes Monocyte cell line	Jennewein et al., 2010 [49]
	Adipocyte differentiation	Adipose derived stromal cell line	Karbiener et al., 2009 [50]
	Tumor growth and progression	Neuroblastoma cell line	Lee et al., 2012 [51]
miR-34a miR-34c	Liver fibrosis	Primary hepatic stellate cells Hepatic stellate cell line	Li et al., 2015 [52]
miR-128-3p	Liver fibrosis	Primary hepatic stellate cells Hepatic stellate cell line	Povero et al., 2015 [53]
miR-130	Adipocyte differentiation	Primary preadipocytes	Lee et al., 2011 [54]
	Epithelial-mesenchymal transition Cancer cell migration and invasion	HCC tissue Hepatic cell lines	Tu et al., 2014 [55]
miR-130a	Type 2 diabetes mellitus	White adipose tissue Adipocyte cell line	Jiao et al., 2015 [56]
miR-138	Adipocyte differentiation	Primary adipose derived stromal cells	Yang et al., 2011 [57]
miR-548d-5p	Adipocyte differentiation	Bone marrow derived stromal cells	Sun et al., 2014 [58]
Rodent studies			
miR-27	Adipocyte differentiation	White adipose tissue, Primary white adipocytes Primary adipose derived stromal cells Preadipocyte cell line	Kim et al., 2010 [59]
	Adipocyte differentiation	Brown/white adipose tissue Primary adipose derived stromal cells Brown pre-adipocyte cell line	Sun et al., 2014 [41]
miR-27a	Proliferation	Lung tissue Pulmonary endothelial cell lines	Kang et al., 2013 [48]
	Renal fibrosis	Kidney tissue Kidney tubular epithelial cells	Hou et al., 2016 [60]
miR-27b	Cardiac hypertrophy Heart failure	Myocardium Primary cardiomyocytes	Wang et al., 2012 [61]
miR-34a miR-34c	Liver fibrosis	Primary hepatic stellate cells Hepatic stellate cell line	Li et al., 2015 [52]
miR-128-3p	Liver fibrosis	Primary hepatic stellate cells Hepatic stellate cell line	Povero et al., 2015 [53]

(c) Continued.

miRNA	Biological process	Cell/tissue	Reference
miR-130	Adipocyte inflammation	Preadipocyte cell line	Kim et al., 2013 [62]
	Liver fibrosis	Primary hepatic stellate cells Hepatic stellate cell line	Lu et al., 2015 [63]
miR-130a	Type 2 diabetes mellitus	White adipose tissue Adipocyte cell line	Jiao et al., 2015 [56]
miR-210	Osteoporosis	Primary bone marrow derived stromal cells	Liu et al., 2015 [64]
miR-301a	Adipocyte inflammation	White adipose tissue Preadipocyte cell line	Li et al., 2016 [65]
miR-302a	Adipocyte differentiation	White adipose tissue Pre-adipocyte cell line	Jeong et al., 2014 [66]
miR-540	Adipocyte differentiation	Primary adipose derived stromal cells	Chen et al., 2015 [67]

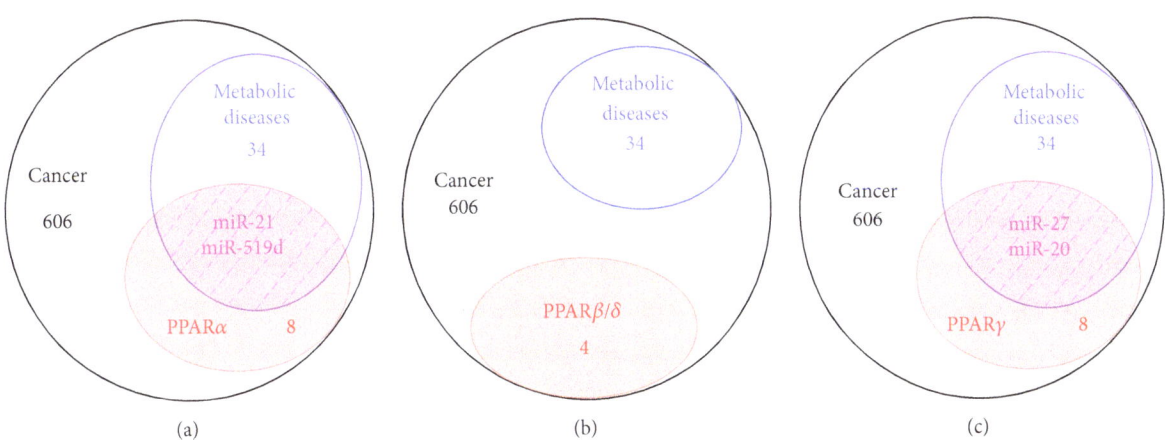

(a)   (b)   (c)

FIGURE 1: Human miRNAs targeting PPAR isoforms and involved in metabolic diseases and cancer. MetaCore pathway analysis software from Thomson Reuters was used to identify experimentally the number of validated human miRNAs involved in cancer (grey circle). Among those, the numbers of miRNAs involved in metabolic diseases, also identified by MetaCore pathway analysis, are indicated in blue circles. In red circles are the number of miRNAs identified using miRWalk 2.0 atlas and targeting PPARα (Panel (a)), PPARβ/δ (Panel (b)), and PPARγ (Panel (c)). The identities of miRNAs targeting specific PPAR isoforms and involved in both cancer and metabolic diseases are indicated in violet. miRWalk 2.0 atlas is a software integrating 12 different prediction algorithms (miRWalk 2.0, MicroT4, miRanda, miRBridge, miRDB, miRMap, miRNAMap, PICTAR2, PITA, RNA22, RNAhybrid, and TargetScan) for identification of miRNAs target mRNAs.

and lipid homeostasis (i.e., β-oxidation) [6, 68, 69]. PPARα is usually activated through the binding of specific ligands, in particular unsaturated fatty acids (ω-3 fatty acids), eicosanoid derivatives (e.g., 8-hydroxy-eicosatetraenoic acid, prostacyclin), or metabolized fatty acids (e.g., oxidized fatty acids) [6]. Alterations of PPARα expression or activity were associated with a variety of human pathologies such as obesity, liver diseases, inflammation, and cancers [3, 68, 69]. It is now clear that deregulations of specific miRNA can significantly contribute to PPARα abnormal signaling in these pathophysiological conditions (see experimentally validated miRNAs targeting PPARα in Table 1 and Figure 2). Such alterations have been investigated only in specific tissues, such as the liver or adipose tissue, as well as in inflammatory cells and cartilage and specific tumors (e.g., in the colon). Whether PPARα expression/activity is affected by miRNAs in other metabolically active tissues, for example, skeletal muscles or pancreas, remains to be established.

3.1.1. miRNAs-Dependent Regulation of PPARα in the Liver.
In the liver, PPARα is implicated in the lipid catabolism and inflammatory processes [68]. miRNAs-dependent alterations of PPARα signaling are reported by numerous studies to contribute to the onset of liver diseases such as nonalcoholic fatty liver disease (NAFLD) [19, 21, 29], chronic diseases associated with viral infections (HBV, HCV) [70], or hepatic cancers [30, 71].

Hepatic Steatosis. Two miRNAs were shown to alter PPARα expression in hepatocytes and to lead to steatosis development (Table 1) [19, 69]. Upregulation of miR-199a-5p was observed in various in vivo mouse models of obesity (ob/ob

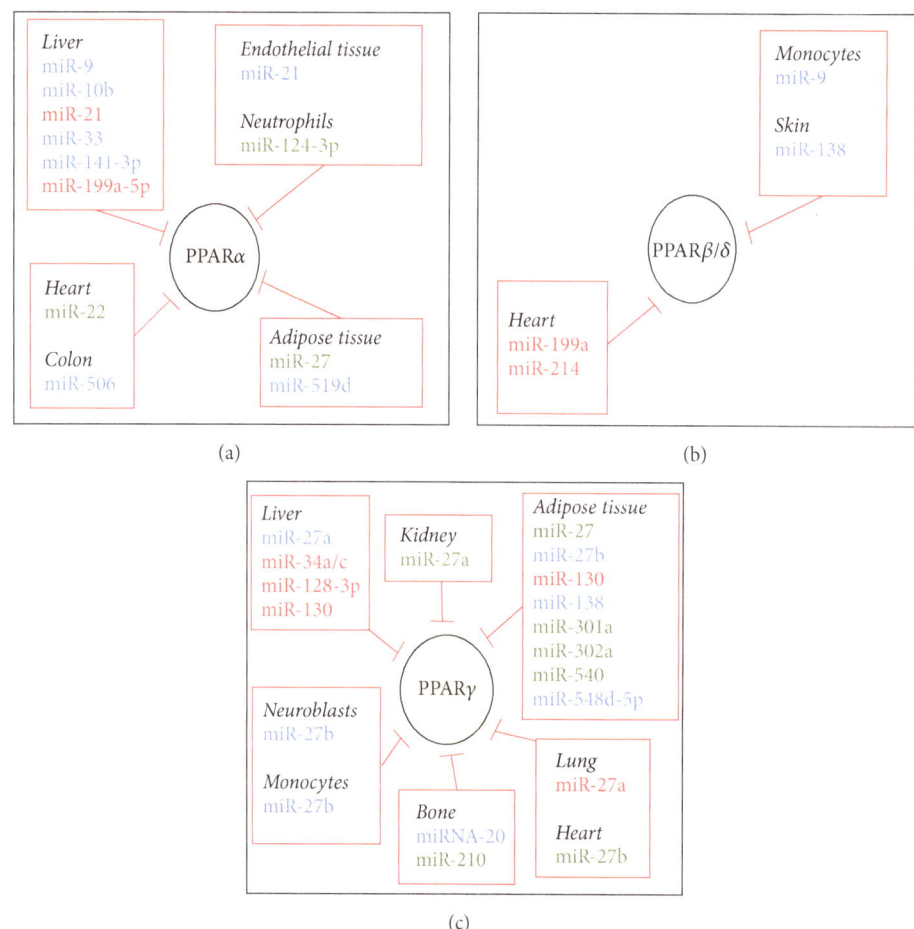

FIGURE 2: miRNAs targeting PPAR isoforms in specific tissues. miRNAs (also referred to in Table 1) that have been experimentally demonstrated to specifically target PPARα (Panel (a)), PPARβ/δ (Panel (b)), and PPARγ (Panel (c)) in different tissues are illustrated. miRNAs identified in human studies are in blue, those identified in mouse/rat studies are in green, and those identified in both human and rodents studies are in red.

and db/db mice, mice fed a high-fat diet), as well as in liver samples from patients with NAFLD. In vitro analyses of hepatoma cell lines (HepG2 and murine AML12 cells) exposed to fatty acids as a surrogate model of steatosis further confirm an upregulation of miR-199a-5p, which in turn downregulates PPARα and caveolin-1 thereby promoting abnormal cellular redox equilibrium and fatty acids intracellular accumulation [37]. In human hepatic LO2 cells, Zheng et al. uncover another miRNA, miR-10b, upregulated following exposure to fatty acids and having a unique binding site in the PPARα 3′UTR sequence [32]. However, the relevance of miR-10b alterations in human liver metabolic disorders was not evaluated.

Hepatic Inflammation and Fibrosis. PPARα downregulation by miRNAs was recently suggested to trigger hepatic inflammation and fibrosis. Indeed, Loyer et al. [34] reported an upregulation of miR-21 in biliary and inflammatory cells of mice and patients with nonalcoholic steatohepatitis (NASH). They further discover that miR-21 was promoting hepatic inflammation and fibrosis by suppressing PPARα expression

in these cells. Interestingly, in mice knockout, specifically for miR-21 in hepatocytes, PPARα expression was not altered, even when mice were challenged with an obesogenic diet, therefore suggesting that, in different cell types, miR-21 may have different activities and/or cellular targets [34, 72]. In hepatic stellate cells (HSCs), which are the main non-parenchymal liver cells contributing to the abnormal extracellular matrix deposition in liver fibrosis, miR-33 and miR-27a/-27b were also found upregulated and to target PPARα and the PPARα cofactor RXR, respectively. Inhibition of these miRNAs with synthetic nucleotides in rat primary and immortalized human HSCs (LX-2 cells) increased PPARα expression concomitantly with a decreased activation of the cells, thus suggesting a tight link between HSC activation and PPARα expression [35, 73].

Hepatic Carcinogenesis. The role of PPARα in cancer is still debated but few studies suggested that miRNAs-dependent alterations of PPARα expression/activity are relevant for the development of hepatocellular carcinoma (HCC). In particular, high-throughput screening of human HCC samples revealed 28 miRNAs differentially expressed with top hits for miR-9, miR-21, and miR-224 [30]. In addition to miR-21, which is discussed in the previous section, prediction software programs identified conserved miR-9 binding sites within the 3'UTR of PPARα. miR-9 upregulation correlated with tumor invasiveness, cell growth, and tumor stage, but whether this was related to a decreased PPARα expression remains unclear. Indeed, whereas the direct regulation of PPARα by miR-9 in human HCC cells was confirmed by luciferase reporter assay [31], molecular analysis of human Snu-449 and HepG2 cancer cell lines indicated an indirect role for miR-9 overexpression in PPARα downregulation [30].

3.1.2. miRNAs-Dependent Regulation of PPARα in the Adipose Tissue.

PPARα assumes important functions in brown adipose tissue and adaptive thermogenesis and browning of white adipose tissue [41]. Although experimental evidence in human showing miRNAs-dependent PPARα regulation in brown/white adipose tissue is scarce, several animal models have suggested such regulatory mechanisms. For example, miR-27a and miR-27b, which are downregulated in mouse brown/white adipose tissue after cold exposure, directly modulate components of the adipocyte transcriptional network including PPARα [41]. MiR-519d, which is increased in subcutaneous white adipose tissue of obese subjects as compared to nonobese individuals, decreases fatty acid catabolism, and increases intracellular lipid accumulation by directly repressing PPARα [39]. Finally, other miRNAs upregulated in brown adipose tissue and/or white adipose tissue of diet-induced obese mice, or during human white and beige adipose differentiation, for example, miR-106b/miR-93 [74, 75] and miR-26a and miR-26b [50], have been correlated with alterations of PPARα expression. However, whether PPARα is a direct target of these miRNAs was not investigated.

3.1.3. miRNAs-Dependent Regulation of PPARα in Other Cell Types/Organs

Inflammatory Cells and Cartilage. Functional miRNAs-dependent PPARα alteration in inflammatory processes was suggested by two studies. First, miR-21, which is upregulated in cultured human endothelial cells from umbilical vein exposed to oscillatory shear stress, was shown to directly inhibit PPARα translation [33]. The decreased expression of PPARα in turn promotes AP1-dependent upregulation of VCAM-1 (vascular cell adhesion molecule-1) and MCP-1 (monocyte chemotactic protein-1), which favor the adhesion of inflammatory cells [33]. In a second study, bioinformatics and molecular analyses combined with clinical data identified an increased expression of miR-22 in osteoarthritic cartilage, which was correlated with PPARα downregulation and an increased body-mass-index (BMI) of patients [76]. However, this study did not provide any direct molecular link between miR-22 upregulation and PPARα downregulation.

Nonhepatic Cancers. The only evidence that PPARα may potentially behave as a tumor suppressor downregulated by aberrantly expressed miRNAs in transformed cells comes from a study performed in a drug-resistant colon cancer cell line (SW1116) showing that miR-506 overexpression in this cancer cell model directly affects PPARα expression [38]. In another study, the growth inhibitory properties of 1.25-dihydroxyvitamin D3 in human prostate adenocarcinoma cells (LNCaP) were associated with an increased expression of the miR-17/92 cluster, which correlated with PPARα downregulation, but whether miR-17/92 directly target PPARα was not investigated [77].

3.2. miRNAs-Dependent Regulation of PPARβ/δ.

PPARβ/δ is ubiquitously expressed with the highest levels in liver, intestine, kidneys, and skeletal muscles [6, 78]. Major PPARβ/δ activators are natural ligands such as polyunsaturated fatty acids, prostaglandin derivatives (e.g., prostacyclin), or components of VLDL (Very Low Density Lipoproteins) particles [6]. This PPAR isoform regulates multiple cellular processes including developmental aspects, the lipid metabolism, insulin sensitivity, vascular function, and anti-inflammatory responses [4, 6, 44, 79]. The best-characterized role of PPARβ/δ has been described in metabolically active tissues. In the liver, PPARβ/δ appears to increase glucose utilization through the pentose-phosphate pathway and to promote lipogenesis [80]. However, in mice fed an obesogenic diet, activation of PPARβ/δ surprisingly prevents the development of steatosis [81]. In muscles and white adipose tissue, PPARβ/δ exerts an adaptive response to fasting and exercise by favoring fatty acids oxidation [82], through the direct induction of key genes involved in this process (e.g., mitochondrial CPT-1 (Carnitine palmitoyltransferase-1) and FoxO1 (Forkhead box protein O1)) [82, 83]. In brown adipose tissue, PPARβ/δ contributes to adaptive thermogenesis by inducing the expression of UCP-1 and UCP-3 [81, 82] and to β-oxidation, by upregulating several genes involved in this process (e.g., long chain acyl-CoA synthetase, Acyl-CoA oxidase). In addition to these well established roles of PPARβ/δ, this isoform was further implicated in the regulation of multiple other cellular processes including developmental aspects, vascular function, and anti-inflammatory responses [4, 6, 44, 79]. Finally, in cancer, the role of PPARβ/δ is controversial with evidence pointing at PPARβ/δ as an oncogene (e.g., in breast and prostate tumors) [84] or as a tumor suppressor (e.g., in colon cancer) [4, 6, 85]. Despite the key functions of PPARβ/δ, solid experimental evidence indicating miRNAs-dependent regulation of this isoform is very limited and restricted to studies described below (see Table 1 and Figure 2).

3.2.1. miRNAs-Dependent Regulation of PPARβ/δ in the Liver.

Based on Affymetrix microarrays, in vivo inhibition of miR-122 by antisense oligonucleotides (ASO) in mice affected hundreds of hepatic mRNAs including PPARβ/δ [86]. Whether miR-122 directly targets PPARβ/δ is still undetermined; however its downregulation following injection of miR-122 inhibitors in mice was suggested to affect circadian clock-dependent energy homeostasis and in particular regulation of lipid transport and catabolism [86].

3.2.2. miRNAs-Dependent Regulation of PPARβ/δ in the Heart.

By stimulating fatty acid utilization in the myocardium, PPARβ/δ exerts a protective vascular function. In a mouse model of heart failure, an impaired fatty acid oxidation and a metabolic switch towards glycolysis were attributed to the direct repression of PPARβ/δ by two miRNAs, miR-199a and miR-214, which are upregulated following aortic pressure overload and subsequent heart failure [43].

3.2.3. miRNAs-Dependent Regulation of PPARβ/δ in Monocytes/Macrophages.

PPARβ/δ exerts an anti-inflammatory function, by promoting the switch from proinflammatory M1 macrophages to the anti-inflammatory M2 macrophages in the liver and in adipose tissue [44]. Bioinformatics and luciferase reporter assays revealed the presence of a functional miR-9 binding site within PPARβ/δ 3′UTR in human monocytes. Downregulation of PPARβ/δ and its targets genes was further observed in proinflammatory M1 macrophages treated with lipopolysaccharide (LPS) and correlated with an upregulation of miR-9 in these cells, thus suggesting a potential functional regulation of PPARβ/δ by miR-9 in monocytes and macrophages [44].

3.2.4. miRNAs-Dependent Regulation of PPARβ/δ in Other Cell Types/Organs.

MiRNAs-dependent PPARβ/δ regulation was finally reported in hypertrophic scar formation, where PPARβ/δ promotes proliferation of fibroblasts. A decrease in miR-138 expression was noted in scar tissue as compared to paired normal skin tissues and inversely correlated with the level of PPARβ/δ. Further analyses using luciferase reporter assays and synthetic miR-138 mimics and inhibitor nucleotides in human hypertrophic scar fibroblasts (hHSFs) confirmed that PPARβ/δ is a direct target of miR-138 and the functional relevance of this regulatory mechanism in hHSFs proliferation [45].

3.3. miRNAs-Dependent Regulation of PPARγ.

There are two PPARγ isoforms (PPARγ1 and PPARγ2). PPARγ1 is broadly expressed in adipose tissue, liver, intestine, kidneys, small intestine, immune cells, and endothelium, while PPARγ2 is predominantly expressed in the adipose tissue [2, 3, 6]. Activation of PPARγ is induced mostly by unsaturated fatty acids and endogenous arachidonic acid-derived metabolites (e.g., leukotriene B4 and eicosatetraenoic acid). The best-described functions of PPARγ are to transcriptionally promote adipocyte differentiation and lipogenesis as well as *de novo* lipogenesis in the liver [5, 87]. In addition, PPARγ controls also the expression of various adipocyte genes involved in glucose homeostasis (e.g., Glut4 expression) and endocrine signaling (e.g., adiponectin, resistin, and TNFα) affecting insulin sensitivity in other peripheral organs such as liver and muscles [2, 3, 5, 12]. Finally, several other cellular processes including cholesterol transport, kidney function, food intake, and inflammation have been suggested to be modulated by PPARγ isoforms [2, 3, 5, 12]. Consistent with the role of PPARγ in glucose and lipid homeostasis, an abnormal activity of PPARγ is often associated with the development of metabolic disorders (e.g., obesity, type 2 diabetes, and fatty liver disease) [5]. In contrast, in cancer, increasing evidence indicates a beneficial tumor suppressive role for PPARγ (e.g., gastric, pancreatic, and hepatic cancers) [2, 6,

88]. As illustrated in Table 1 and Figure 2, posttranscriptional regulation of PPARγ by miRNAs has been reported in many pathophysiological situations.

3.3.1. miRNAs-Dependent Regulation of PPARγ in the Liver

Hepatic Fibrosis. PPARγ is a negative regulator of hepatic stellate cells (HSCs) activation [89]. The induction of various miRNAs expressed in nonalcoholic steatohepatitis (NASH) and fibrosis correlated with PPARγ downregulation and overexpression of profibrogenic markers like α-SMA. Among those miRNAs, upregulation of miR-34a/-34c [52], miR-128-3p [53], and miR-130a/miR-130b [63] in activated human or rat HSCs was reported to directly bind the 3′UTR of PPARγ and to repress its expression. miRNAs-dependent PPARγ downregulation in hepatic fibrosis can also occur through indirect mechanisms. For example, in HSCs from mice treated with CCL4 to induce fibrosis, miR-132 is downregulated thereby leading to an increase of one of its targets, MeCP2 (Methyl CpG binding protein 2), and repression of PPARγ transcription *via* different epigenetic mechanisms [90].

Hepatitis C Virus (HCV) Infection. Infection of Huh-7.5 hepatoma cells with a HCV-derived JFH1 strain induces expression of miR-27a. This miRNA directly targets PPARγ thereby reducing lipid synthesis and increasing lipid secretion [91], two processes likely promoting HCV replication and virions egress.

Hepatic Carcinogenesis. PPARγ has a tumor suppressive function in hepatocarcinogenesis [7, 51, 92–95]. PPARγ downregulation in HCC correlated with upregulation of specific miRNAs [3, 93, 96], among which the best characterized ones are miR-130b and miR-27a. These two miRNAs directly target PPARγ and decrease its expression thus promoting cancer cells growth and aggressiveness [47, 55].

3.3.2. miRNAs-Dependent Regulation of PPARγ in Adipose Tissue

Adipocyte Differentiation. Regulation of PPARγ activity/ expression by miRNAs represents an important posttranscriptional mechanism controlling adipocyte differentiation. Several miRNAs in murine and human preadipocytes, including miR-540, miR-302a, miR-138, miR-548d-5p, miR-130, and miR-27, were described to bind the 3′UTR of PPARγ and to decrease its expression thus preventing differentiation towards mature adipocytes [54, 57–59, 67, 97, 98]. In particular, miR-130 was reported to be downregulated in mice fed an obesogenic diet and in adipocytes of obese and type 2 diabetic patients, who also have high levels of PPARγ in adipose tissues and a low abundance of preadipocytes [54, 56, 62]. Further in vitro analyses using embryonic fibroblasts-derived preadipocytes (3T3-L1) indicated that synthetic nucleotides mimicking or inhibiting miR-130a were able to modulate PPARγ expression and its downstream target genes involved in glucose and lipid metabolism [56]. miR-27a and miR-27b are other key miRNAs regulating adipocyte differentiation, and both are downregulated during adipocyte differentiation, thus leading to an induction of PPARγ [59]. Consistent with this role, expression of miR-27a/-27b is lower in obese ob/ob mice as compared to lean animals and decreases during adipogenic differentiation of 3T3-L1 cells and mouse bone marrow derived mesenchymal stem cells (OP9 cell line). In the same study, miR-27a/miR-27b mimic nucleotides decreased PPARγ expression and prevented adipocyte differentiation. However, experimental evidence indicated that the mechanisms by which miR-27 affect PPARγ expression are indirect [98].

Inflammation. The role of PPARγ in adipose tissue inflammation is still poorly characterized, but downregulation of miR-301a, which directly targets PPARγ, was correlated with the production of proinflammatory cytokines in obese mice and in 3T3L1 preadipocytes [65].

3.3.3. miRNAs-Dependent Regulation of PPARγ in Bone Marrow.
The commitment of mesenchymal stem cells (MSCs) in the bone marrow towards osteogenic or adipogenic differentiation might be also tightly dependent on PPARγ regulation by miRNAs. Indeed, miR-548d-5p, which is downregulated during adipogenic differentiation of human bone marrow derived MSCs, targets the 3$'$UTR of PPARγ. Overexpression of this miRNA abrogates adipogenic differentiation and increases the osteogenic potential of MSCs by downregulating PPARγ and C/EBPα [58]. Induction of other miRNAs such as miR-20 during osteogenic differentiation leads also to a direct downregulation of PPARγ [46]. In addition, miR-17-5p and miR-106a also promote adipogenesis and inhibit osteogenic differentiation in human adipose derived MSCs by indirect mechanisms, which increase C/EBPα and PPARγ expressions [99]. Finally, alterations of the osteogenic/adipogenic differentiation balance is an important component of specific osteogenic-related disorders such as osteoporosis and deregulation of the expression of miRNAs targeting PPARγ, for example, miR-210, have been involved in these diseases [64, 100].

3.3.4. miRNAs-Dependent Regulation of PPARγ in the Heart.
Upregulation of miR-27b expression was shown in heart-specific smad4 knockout mice, which develop cardiac hypertrophy [61]. Overexpression of this miRNA specifically in cardiomyocytes using transgenic mice was sufficient to induce cardiac hypertrophy through PPARγ downregulation [61]. Conversely, treatment of a mouse model of heart failure with miR-27b inhibitors (antagomirs) improved cardiovascular functions by increasing PPARγ expression [61]. Similarly, in vivo inhibition of miR-128 by antagomirs protected cardiomyocytes from apoptosis in a model of myocardial ischemia/reperfusion injury and increased PPARγ expression in neonatal rat ventricular myocytes (NRVM) [101]. However, whether miR-128 modulates PPARγ through direct or indirect mechanisms was not assessed in this study.

3.3.5. miRNAs-Dependent Regulation of PPARγ in Other Cell Types/Organs.
In addition to its role in hepatocytes, adipocytes, and cardiomyocytes, the relevance of miR-27b

targeting of PPARγ was also highlighted in several other tissues (inflammatory cells, renal tubular cells, and pulmonary endothelial cells as well as neuroblastoma).

Inflammatory Cells. PPARγ is a potent inhibitor of M1 macrophage activation (Th1 proinflammatory macrophages) and promoter of M2 macrophage activation (Th2 anti-inflammatory macrophages) [102]. Upregulation of miR-27b in human macrophages upon LPS exposure was demonstrated to directly target PPARγ and to elicit a Th1 differentiation [49]. Although these findings suggest that miR-27b-dependent downregulation of PPARγ may represent a key process in macrophage polarization, whether miR-27b controls M2 macrophage activation *via* PPARγ was however not investigated.

Kidneys. Upregulation of miR-27a occurs in glucose-stimulated rat renal proximal tubular cell line (NRK-52E cells) and renal tubular epithelial cells of streptozotocin-induced diabetic rats. In these cellular contexts, the increased miR-27a expression was shown to trigger PPARγ downregulation, which in turn promoted renal fibrosis [60].

Lung. In mice and human pulmonary artery endothelial cells (HPAECs), hypoxia upregulates miR-27a expression and decreases PPARγ expression [103]. Given the important antiproliferative, and antithrombotic and vasodilatory effects of PPARγ on the lung vasculature [104], upregulation of miR-27a may thus represent an important contributor to the development of pulmonary hypertension.

Neuroblastoma Cells. Although miR-27b-dependent downregulation of PPARγ promotes cell proliferation in HCC, it may lead to opposite effects in other cancers [7, 51, 92–95]. This is the case in the SK-N-AS neuroblastoma cells and derived mouse xenografts, where miR-27b was shown to repress PPARγ expression resulting in a decreased inflammatory response and tumor growth [51, 105, 106].

4. Indirect Regulation of PPARs by miRNAs

The activity of PPARs is tightly linked to the binding of transcriptional partners (i.e., RXR, Prdm16), cofactors/repressors (e.g., PGC1α, NCOR), or other regulators (e.g., Sirt1) [3]. Most of the PPARs binding partners and cofactors are also finely tuned by specific miRNAs, which thereby indirectly regulate the expression/activity of PPARs isoforms [18, 107–112]. A brief overview of miRNAs targeting PPARs binding partners and cofactors is provided in the next section (see Figure 3).

4.1. miRNAs-Dependent Regulation of PPARs Binding/Heterodimerization Partners

4.1.1. miRNAs Dependent Regulation of RXRs.
RXR isoforms (RXRα/β/γ) are the obligate binding partners for PPARs. Together they form heterodimeric complexes and induce gene transactivation by binding to PPAR response elements (PPREs) [3]. As illustrated in Figure 3, several miRNAs have

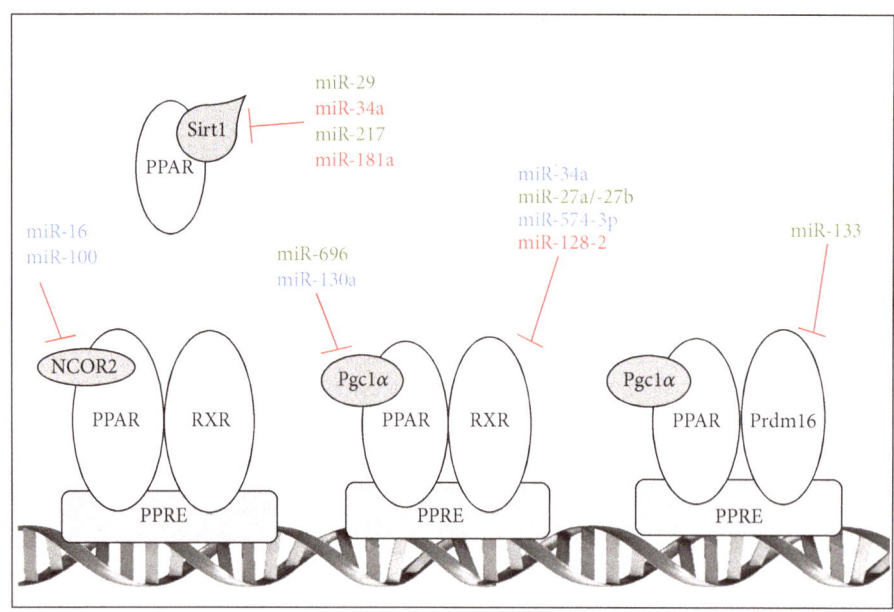

FIGURE 3: miRNAs targeting PPAR transcriptional partners, cofactors/repressors, and other regulators. miRNAs that have been experimentally demonstrated to specifically target PPAR transcriptional partners (RXR and Prdm16), PPAR cofactors (Pgc1α), PPAR repressors (NCOR2), and other PPAR regulators (Sirt1) are illustrated. miRNAs identified in human studies are in blue, those identified in mouse/rat studies are in green, and those identified in both human and rodents studies are in red. *PPAR: peroxisome proliferator-activated receptor α, β/δ, or γ; RXR: Retinoid-X-Receptor; Prdm16: PR domain-containing 16; Sirt1: Sirtuin-1; NCOR2: nuclear receptor corepressor 2 (SMRT); Pgc1α: peroxisome proliferator-activated receptor gamma coactivator 1; PPRE: peroxisome proliferator response element.*

been reported to directly target RXR isoforms thus affecting indirectly PPARs activities [108, 109, 113, 114]. For example, miR-128-2 was shown to suppress cholesterol efflux in HepG2 cells and in the liver of diet-induced obese mice by binding to the 3′UTR of RXRα and of ATP-binding cassette transporters (ABCA1 and ABCG1) and repressing their expressions [114]. Chondrogenesis, which is inhibited by RXRα, was also promoted in mesenchymal stem cells by miR-574-3p, which downregulates specifically RXRα expression [113]. Interestingly, specific miRNAs targeting PPARγ, that is, miR-34a and miR-27a/b, also control RXRα expression in liver cells [73, 98, 109]. Indeed upregulation of miR-34a, which was correlated with fibrosis development, downregulates RXRα by binding within the coding region and not the 3′UTR of this isoform in hepatocytes [109]. In the case of miR-27a and miR-27b, these two miRNAs were upregulated in rat activated HSCs and decrease RXRα expression through 3′UTR-dependent mechanisms [73, 98]. It thus appears that abnormal miRNAs-dependent inhibition of RXRα in distinct liver cells contributes to the development of hepatic fibrogenesis. Finally, inhibition of RXRα by upregulation of miR-27a was also reported in aggressive rhabdomyosarcoma (RMS) [108]. Altogether, these studies suggest that particular miRNAs, such as miR-34a and the miR-27 family, may affect PPARs signaling by simultaneously targeting different key players in this pathway.

4.1.2. miRNAs-Dependent Regulation of Prdm16. During brown adipogenesis, Prdm16 (PR domain-containing 16)

instead of RXRα heterodimerizes with PPARγ2 and mediates brown adipocyte differentiation [115]. MiR-133a was demonstrated to regulate directly Prdm16 expression in immortalized brown preadipocytes [18] and inhibition of miR-133a and miR-133b led to an increased expression of adipogenic markers including PPARγ as well as differentiation towards mature brown adipocytes [18, 116, 117].

4.1.3. miRNAs-Dependent Regulation of PGC1α. PGC1α is a critical transcriptional coactivator of PPARγ in brown preadipocytes and of PPARα in white preadipocytes (3T3-L1 cells) [118]. To date only two miRNAs have been described in hepatocytes to directly target PGC1α mRNA: (i) miR-696, which is upregulated with obesity, decreases PGC1α expression in the liver of ob/ob mice [119] and (ii) miR-130a, which is downregulated in HBV-infected human hepatocytes, increases PGC1α and PPARγ expression thus favoring HBV replication [120].

4.1.4. miRNAs-Dependent Regulation of NCOR. In the absence of PPARs ligands, the transcriptional activity of PPARs is inhibited by the binding of corepressors such NCOR proteins [12]. miRNAs-dependent regulation of NCOR proteins is supported by two studies showing that (i) miR-16 in LPS-activated human monocytes (U937) and biliary epithelial cells (H69) targets SMRT (NCOR2), which leads to NF-κB-mediated transactivation of the IL-8 gene [107], and (ii) miR-100 targets SMRT (NCOR2) in glioblastoma cells thereby inhibiting their proliferation [112].

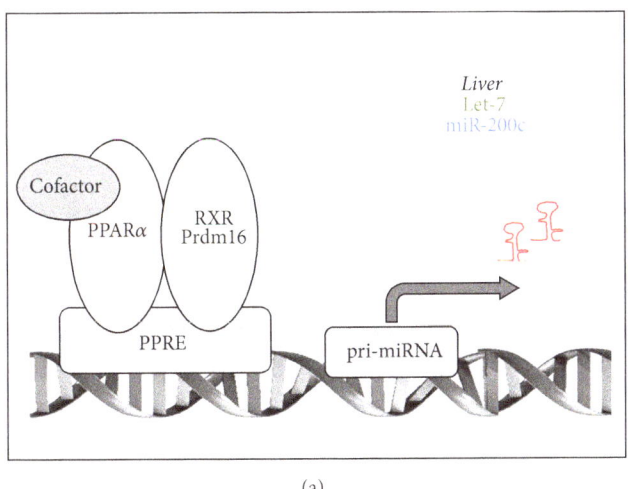
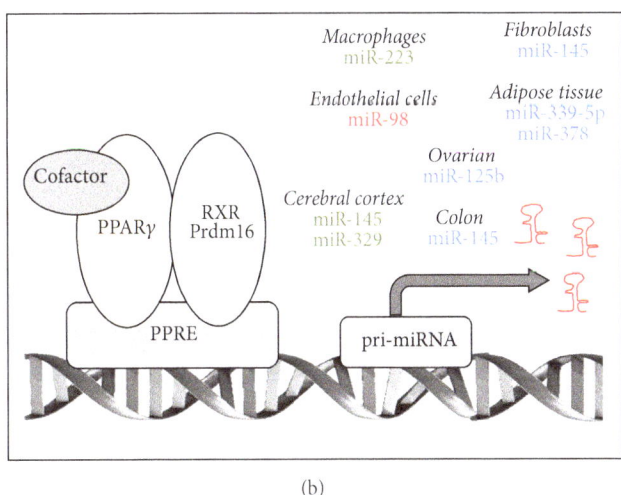

(a)   (b)

FIGURE 4: miRNAs expression induced by PPARα and PPARγ. Induction of miRNAs by PPARα (Panel (a)) and PPARγ (Panel (b)) binding to PPRE in pri-miRNA promoters in specific tissues is indicated. miRNAs identified in human studies are in blue, those identified in mouse/rat studies are in green, and those identified in both human and rodents studies are in red. *RXR: Retinoid-X-Receptor; Prdm16: PR domain-containing 16; PPRE: peroxisome proliferator response element.*

4.1.5. miRNAs-Dependent Regulation of Sirtuin-1. The NAD-dependent deacetylase Sirtuin-1 (Sirt1) is a critical regulator of PPAR signaling and of energy homeostasis [121]. Posttranscriptional control of SIRT1 and other sirtuins by miRNAs represents important regulatory mechanism for this protein family and has been extensively reviewed elsewhere [111]. Among the various miRNAs directly targeting SIRT1, miR-217 [122], miR-181a [123], miR-29 [124], and miR-34a [125] in particular were shown to affect hepatic lipid metabolism, insulin sensitivity, or carcinogenesis by modulating SIRT1 expression. Of note, miR-34a is also a direct regulator of PPARγ and RXRα expression [111, 125–128] therefore supporting again the biological relevance of fine-tuning PPARs signaling by modulating several factors involved in this transcriptional pathway.

5. miRNAs Regulated by PPARs

Recent evidence indicates that the expression of particular miRNAs can also be under the transcriptional control of PPARs [129] (see Figure 4). Most of the studies reviewed here rely on the identification of PPAR response elements (PPREs) within the promoter of genes encoding pri-miRNAs or on the effects of PPARs agonists [17, 96, 130, 131]. miRNAs described to date to be regulated by PPARs are short-listed in Table 2.

5.1. PPARα- and PPARβ/δ-Dependent Regulation of miRNAs Expression. Limited information is available on PPARα- and PPARβ/δ-dependent regulation of miRNAs expression. PPARα was suggested to promote the expression of let-7 and miR-200c in hepatic cancer cells. Indeed, expression of let-7, which targets c-myc in hepatocytes, was decreased in mice treated with the PPARα agonist Wy-14,643, which in turn fostered myc-dependent liver oncogenesis [71]. In Huh-7 hepatoma cells, PPARα in synergy with another nuclear receptor,

that is, LRH-1 (liver receptor homolog-1), was proposed also to drive miR-200c transcription through a direct binding to its promoter [132]. Although the role of miR-200c in HCC was not investigated in this study, miR-200 was previously shown to have tumor suppressive activities by inhibiting cell migration [135]. Regarding PPARβ/δ, treatment of HUVEC endothelial cells with a PPARβ/δ agonist (GW501516) led to an increase of miR-100 expression, which improved lipidemia and vascular function [136]. However, as for the study using PPARα agonists, a direct binding of PPARβ/δ to the miR-100 promoter was not investigated and additional experiments are required to confirm these data and exclude off-target effects of pharmacological agonists of PPARβ/δ.

5.2. PPARγ-Dependent Regulation of miRNAs Expression. In contrast to the other PPAR isoforms, PPARγ was reported to regulate several miRNAs in distinct pathophysiological processes (see Table 2).

Endothelial Functions. miR-98, which is reduced in endothelial cells of patients suffering from idiopathic pulmonary hypertension (IPAH) and of mouse models of this disease, directly targets endothelin-1 (ET1). PPARγ was shown to exert a beneficial role in pulmonary hypertension (PH) by attenuating, likely through activation of miR-98, ET1 expression. In support of this hypothesis, activation of PPARγ with specific agonists (e.g., rosiglitazone) restores miR-98 expression in hypoxic mouse and in primary human pulmonary artery endothelial cells (PAECs); however whether PPARγ is a direct regulator of miR-98 was not assessed [103].

Adipocytes Differentiation and Function. PPARγ agonists (rosiglitazone and pioglitazone) modulated the expression of 27 different miRNAs in human subcutaneous and visceral adipocytes. Among those, miR-329, miR-145, and miR-339-5p are involved, based on predictive bioinformatics analyses,

TABLE 2: PPARα- and PPARγ-dependent miRNAs induction in specific tissues and pathophysiological processes.

(a) PPARα

miRNA	Biological process	Organism	Cell/tissue	Reference
Let-7	Proliferation	Mouse	Liver tissue, HCC cell line	Shah et al., 2007 [71]
miR-200c	Migration	Human	HCC cell line	Zhang et al., 2011 [132]

(b) PPARγ

miRNA	Biological process	Organism	Cell/tissue	Reference
miR-98	Endothelial dysfunction Pulmonary hypertension	Mouse Human	Primary pulmonary artery endothelial cells	Kang et al., 2016 [103]
miR-125b	Proliferation Apoptosis	Human	Ovarian cancer tissue, Ovarian cancer cell lines	Luo et al., 2015 [130]
miR-145	Inflammation Oxidative stress	Rat	Cerebral cortex, Pheochromocytoma cell line	Dharap et al., 2015 [17]
	Collagen synthesis	Human	Hypertrophic scar fibroblasts	Zhu et al., 2015 [131]
	Cell cycle Invasion Differentiation	Human	Colorectal cancer tissue and colorectal cancer cell lines	Panza et al., 2014 [96]
miR-223	Inflammation	Mouse	Bone marrow derived macrophages Adipocyte-derived stromal cells Primary adipocytes	Ying et al., 2015 [133]
miR-329	Inflammation Oxidative stress	Rat	Cerebral cortex, Pheochromocytoma cell line	Dharap et al., 2015 [17]
miR-339-5p	Adipocyte differentiation	Human	White adipose tissue Isolated preadipocytes	Yu et al. 2014 [134]
miR-378	Adipocyte differentiation	Human	White adipose tissue Primary adipose derived stromal cells	Yu et al., 2014 [134]

in metabolic (e.g., insulin signaling) and proliferative (e.g., Wnt/β-catenin signaling) pathways [17, 134]. Interestingly, miR-329 and miR-145 contain a PPRE in their promoters and both miRNAs also bind to PPARγ 3′UTR, thus suggesting the existence of positive feedback loop mechanisms regulating expressions of these miRNAs and PPARγ [17]. In human subcutaneous adipocytes and bovine preadipocytes, PPARγ also induces the expression of miR-378, which is located in the first intron of PPARγ coactivator-1β (PGC1β) [98, 134, 137]. Finally, a list of potential miRNAs, directly regulated by PPARγ and involved in 3T3-L1 adipose differentiation, was identified by crossing datasets of miRNAs containing putative PPARγ binding site with datasets of miRNAs altered during 3T3-L1 differentiation. Authors of this study identified miR-103-1, miR-182/miR-96/miR-183, miR-205, and miR-378 as potential PPARγ-regulated miRNAs, whose expression was further induced in 3T3-L1 cells treated by rosiglitazone. Chip analyses also revealed that these miRNAs are directly regulated by PPARγ through PPRE present in their host genes (PanK3 and PGC1β) [138].

Inflammation. Exposure of bone marrow derived macrophages (BMDMs) to Th2 stimuli (i.e., IL-4) triggers the expression of miR-223 through a direct binding of PPARγ in PPREs within the promoter of pre-miR-223. This effect was

further enhanced by a PPARγ agonist (i.e., pioglitazone) and inhibited by a PPARγ antagonist (i.e., GW9662). Since PPARγ-dependent M2 activation is inhibited in BMDMs from miR-223 knockout mice, these data suggest that miR-223 and its target genes (e.g., *Rasal* and *genuine*) are key effectors of macrophages polarization [133].

Fibrosis. Whether PPARγ may control fibrotic processes through miRNAs-dependent mechanisms is not well established, but one study supports this concept. Indeed, Dharap et al., reported that miR-145, which contains a PPAR response element in its promoter [17, 96], was increased in rosiglitazone-treated hypertrophic scar fibroblasts (HSFDs), thus leading to a direct decrease of SMAD3 expression and collagen synthesis [131].

Carcinogenesis. A direct effect of PPARγ on the expression of specific miRNAs through binding of PPRE in their promoters was demonstrated for three different types of cancer cell lines. In hepatoma HepG2 cells, miR-122 was strongly induced in cells treated with DNA methylation or histone deacetylase inhibitors *via* a direct binding of PPARγ/RXRα in the pre-miR-122 promoter [139]. In ovarian cancer cells (i.e., Ovcar3, CaOv3, and Skov3 cells), PPARγ also directly regulates the transcription of miR-125b and silencing of miR-125 impaired the growth inhibitory capacity of PPARγ agonists [130]. Finally, miR-145, which is downregulated in colorectal cancer cells (Caco2, Sw480, HCT116, and HT29) and colorectal tumor tissues, is induced by the PPARγ agonist (i.e., rosiglitazone) *via* direct binding of PPARγ to PPRE in the promoter encoding pre-miR-145 [96, 131].

6. miRNAs-Based Therapies to Target PPARs Expression/Activity

Targeting tissue-specific miRNAs with pharmacological compounds may represent novel and valuable alternative therapeutic approaches to PPAR agonists or antagonists [10–13]. Different methods have been developed to modulate miRNA expressions in vivo. Of particular interest are chemically modified synthetic oligonucleotides inhibiting or mimicking endogenous miRNAs that display increased affinity for their targets and great stability in the serum. Currently, these oligonucleotides bear modifications on the $2'$- or $3'$-position of the nucleic acid ribose backbone. For example, antagomiRs ($3'$-cholesterol-conjugated, $2'$-O-Me oligonucleotides with terminal phosphorothioate modifications), antisense modified oligonucleotides (AMO) ($2'$-O-methoxyethyl phosphorothioate modified antisense oligonucleotide or $2'$-fluoro-modified antisense oligonucleotides), or locked nucleic acids (LNA) represent potent inhibitors of miRNAs expression/activity. These synthetic nucleotides are usually administered by intravenous injection and hopefully soon orally with a good efficiency [140, 141]. When administered by intravenous injection they can broadly reach every tissue but tends to accumulate in particular organs, such as the liver or the kidneys [26]. Special formulations such as liposomes or polyethylenimine-formulated nanoparticles as miRNA nanocarriers have been developed to improve tissue-specific distribution, circulation time, and clearance of the miRNAs-like compounds [26, 142, 143]. Of particular interest, microvesicles (MVs) were shown to represent efficient and functional miRNA delivery tools as it was demonstrated in animals and in the case of miR-130b [144, 145]. Other alternative methods to target specific tissues have been also developed such as inclusion of oligonucleotides into liposomal or oleic-based nanoparticles, which target preferentially the liver [142]. Finally, viruses with specific tropisms, for example, adenoassociated viruses (AAV), have been used in animal models to robustly express or inhibit specific miRNAs in particular tissues and may represent an interesting alternative to chemically modified nucleotides [26]. Importantly, abnormal levels of circulating miRNAs stimulate toll-like receptors therefore promoting inflammation and favoring the development of chronic diseases such as metabolic and cardiovascular disorders as well as cancers. Interestingly, chemically modified synthetic oligonucleotides, in particular those modified in the $2'$ position of the ribose, have the ability to reduce, but not completely prevent, such unintended immune responses [26, 146].

Several miRNA inhibitors have been tested in preclinical studies with rodents or primates in the context of various pathologies (e.g., miR-155 in inflammatory diseases, miR-208 in cardiac remodeling) including metabolic diseases (e.g., miR-103/107 for type 2 diabetes and obesity) [26]. However, only few of them, for example, miR-122 inhibitors (Miravirsen) to treat HCV infection, are currently being tested in human clinical trials [26, 147–149]. Unfortunately, none of the miRNAs known to potentially target PPAR isoforms are under clinical trials in human. Only preclinical studies were performed for miR-33 and miR-21 [26], which targets directly PPARα (Figures 2-3). In African green monkeys, inhibition of mir-33a/b with specific antagomiRs increased the hepatic expression of ABCA1, thus leading to an increase of HDL (high density lipoprotein) and a decrease in VLDL (very low density lipoproteins) and triglycerides plasma levels [150]. Inhibition of miR-21 in mice with an anti-sense oligonucleotide prevented hepatic lipid accumulation in animals fed an obesogenic diet [151].

The (pre)clinical use of synthetic nucleotides mimicking endogenous miRNAs is less developed compared to miRNAs inhibitors and currently only miR-34 mimics nucleotides are tested to treat some cancers [26, 152]. MRX34, a liposome-formulated miR-34 mimic-based drug is currently in phase I study for melanoma patients. This miR-34 mimic achieved positive outcomes as a monotherapeutic agent in patients with renal cell carcinoma, acral melanoma, and HCC (http://www.mirnatherapeutics.com/pipeline/mirna-pipeline.html) [26]. However, other in vivo studies indicated that miR-34a/c could also activate hepatic stellate cells and promote fibrogenesis by targeting PPARγ and repressing RXRα and Sirt1 [52, 109]. Other miRNAs, such as miR-27 or miR-9, are also able to regulate the expression/activities of different PPARs isoforms in distinct tissues. Therefore, although miRNAs-based therapies are promising, the potential pleiotropic effects of systemic administration of pharmacological miRNAs inhibitors or mimics call also for cautiousness in their therapeutic use since they can likely lead, as in the case of PPARs agonists/antagonists, to conflicting and unwanted side effects.

7. Conclusion

The pivotal role of abnormal PPARs signaling in the development and the progression of various pathologies including metabolic diseases, inflammation, and cancer is now well established. However, the mechanisms and extent to which miRNAs contribute to alterations of PPARs expressions and/or activities in physiopathological conditions are currently still poorly understood and represent an important developing field of research. Conversely, the fact that PPARs can drive the expression of specific miRNAs, which may target in turn hundreds of different mRNAs, opens also a new dimension in our understanding of the physiological and pathological roles of PPARs isoforms. Given the tissue-specific and pleiotropic action of PPARs in various cellular processes described herein, it is likely that posttranscriptional regulation of PPARs and related cofactors by miRNAs is tissue- and process-specific. In addition, the simplistic view that only changes in the intracellular levels of miRNAs impact the expression of target genes is likely incorrect. Indeed increasing evidence indicates that the activity and bioavailability of miRNAs are also key factors to consider in these regulatory mechanisms. This concept is further supported by the emerging role of long noncoding RNAs [31] and RNA-binding proteins, which could interfere with the activity/expression of specific miRNAs [153, 154] and regulation of their target genes. Further studies are thus required to deepen our knowledge of miRNAs-based posttranscriptional regulatory mechanisms controlling PPARs expressions and activities.

Abbreviations

AP-1:	Activator protein-1
ApoA:	Apolipoprotein-A
BAT:	Brown adipose tissue
CD36:	Cluster of differentiation 36
FAT:	Fatty acid translocase
C/EBPα:	CCAAT/enhancer-binding protein α
C. elegans:	Caenorhabditis elegans
COX-2:	Cyclooxygenase-2
CRC:	Colorectal carcinoma
CREB:	cAMP response element-binding protein
CVD:	Cardiovascular disease
DEN:	Diethylnitrosamine
DGCR8:	DiGeorge syndrome chromosomal region 8
ECM:	Extracellular matrix
FABP:	Fatty acid binding protein
Glut4:	Glucose-transporter 4
HCC:	Hepatocellular carcinoma
HCV/HBV:	Hepatitis C/B virus
HFD:	High fat diet
HSC:	Hepatic stellate cells
IRS-1/2:	Insulin receptor substrates-1/2
lncRNA:	Long noncoding RNA
LPL:	Lipoprotein lipase
LPS:	Lipopolysaccharide
LRH-1:	Liver receptor homolog-1
MCP-1:	Monocyte chemoattractant protein-1
miRNA:	MicroRNA
MSC:	Mesenchymal stem cell
NAFLD:	Nonalcoholic fatty liver disease
NASH:	Nonalcoholic steatohepatitis
NCOR:	Nuclear receptor corepressor
ncRNA:	Noncoding RNA
NFκB:	Nuclear factor-κB
PGE2:	Prostaglandin E2
PGC1:	Peroxisome proliferator-activated receptor gamma coactivator-1
PPAR:	Peroxisome proliferator-activated receptor
PPRE:	Peroxisome proliferator response element
Prdm16:	PR domain-containing 16
RISC:	RNA-induced silencing complex
ROS:	Reactive oxygen species
RXR:	Retinoid-X-Receptor
siRNA:	Small interfering RNA
Sirt1:	Sirtuin 1
SMRT:	Silencing mediator for retinoid and thyroid hormone receptor
sncRNA:	Small noncoding RNA
STAT1:	Signal transducer and activator of transcription 1
T2DM:	Type 2 diabetes mellitus
TARP2:	T-cell receptor gamma-chain constant region
TNF-α:	Tumor necrosis factor-α
TZD:	Thiazolidinedione
UCP-1:	Uncoupling protein-1
UTR:	Untranslated region
VCAM:	Vascular cell adhesion protein
WAT:	White adipose tissue.

Competing Interests

The authors declare that they have no competing interests.

Authors' Contributions

Dorothea Portius and Cyril Sobolewski have equal contributions.

Acknowledgments

Work in the Foti laboratory is supported by the Swiss National Science Foundation (Grant nos. 310030-152618 and CRSII3-160717), the Swiss Cancer Research Foundation (Grant no. KFS-3246-08-2013), the Bo & Kerstin Hjelt Diabetes Foundation, the FLAGS Foundation, the Fondation Romande pour la Recherche sur le Diabetes, and the EFSD/Lilly European Diabetes Research Programme.

References

[1] I. Issemann and S. Green, "Activation of a member of the steroid hormone receptor superfamily by peroxisome proliferators," *Nature*, vol. 347, no. 6294, pp. 645–650, 1990.

[2] R. M. Evans, G. D. Barish, and Y.-X. Wang, "PPARs and the complex journey to obesity," *Nature Medicine*, vol. 10, no. 4, pp. 355–361, 2004.

[3] S. Polvani, "Peroxisome proliferator activated receptors at the crossroad of obesity, diabetes, and pancreatic cancer," *World Journal of Gastroenterology*, vol. 22, no. 8, pp. 2441–2459, 2016.

[4] G. M. G. Attianese and B. Desvergne, "Integrative and systemic approaches for evaluating PPARβ/δ (PPARD) function," *Nuclear Receptor Signaling*, 2015.

[5] M. Ahmadian, J. M. Suh, N. Hah et al., "PPARγ signaling and metabolism: the good, the bad and the future," *Nature Medicine*, vol. 19, no. 5, pp. 557–566, 2013.

[6] B. Grygiel-Górniak, "Peroxisome proliferator-activated receptors and their ligands: nutritional and clinical implications—a review," *Nutrition Journal*, vol. 13, no. 1, article no. 17, 2014.

[7] J. M. Peters, Y. M. Shah, and F. J. Gonzalez, "The role of peroxisome proliferator-activated receptors in carcinogenesis and chemoprevention," *Nature Reviews Cancer*, vol. 12, no. 3, pp. 181–195, 2012.

[8] A. S. Laganà, S. G. Vitale, A. Nigro et al., "Pleiotropic actions of Peroxisome Proliferator-Activated Receptors (PPARs) in dysregulated metabolic homeostasis, inflammation and cancer: current evidence and future perspectives," *International Journal of Molecular Sciences*, vol. 17, no. 7, article 999, 2016.

[9] E. Fuentes, L. Guzmán-Jofre, R. Moore-Carrasco, and I. Palomo, "Role of PPARs in inflammatory processes associated with metabolic syndrome (Review)," *Molecular Medicine Reports*, vol. 8, no. 6, pp. 1611–1616, 2013.

[10] C. J. Bailey, A. A. Tahrani, and A. H. Barnett, "Future glucose-lowering drugs for type 2 diabetes," *The Lancet Diabetes and Endocrinology*, vol. 4, no. 4, pp. 350–359, 2016.

[11] B. Gross and B. Staels, "PPAR agonists: multimodal drugs for the treatment of type-2 diabetes," *Best Practice and Research in Clinical Endocrinology and Metabolism*, vol. 21, no. 4, pp. 687–710, 2007.

[12] S. Sugii and R. M. Evans, "Epigenetic codes of PPARγ in metabolic disease," *FEBS Letters*, vol. 585, no. 13, pp. 2121–2128, 2011.

[13] C. V. Rizos, A. Kei, and M. S. Elisaf, "The current role of thiazolidinediones in diabetes management," *Archives of Toxicology*, vol. 90, no. 8, pp. 1861–1881, 2016.

[14] R. Barres and J. R. Zierath, "DNA methylation in metabolic disorders," *American Journal of Clinical Nutrition*, vol. 93, no. 4, pp. 897S–900S, 2011.

[15] K. Fujiki, F. Kano, K. Shiota, and M. Murata, "Expression of the peroxisome proliferator activated receptor γ gene is repressed by DNA methylation in visceral adipose tissue of mouse models of diabetes," *BMC Biology*, vol. 7, article no. 38, 2009.

[16] M. K. Ramlee, Q. Zhang, M. Idris et al., "Histone H3 K27 acetylation marks a potent enhancer element on the adipogenic master regulator gene Pparg2," *Cell Cycle*, vol. 13, no. 21, pp. 3414–3422, 2014.

[17] A. Dharap, C. Pokrzywa, S. Murali, B. Kaimal, and R. Vemuganti, "Mutual induction of transcription factor PPARγ and microRNAs miR-145 and miR-329," *Journal of Neurochemistry*, vol. 135, no. 1, pp. 139–146, 2015.

[18] W. Liu, P. Bi, T. Shan et al., "miR-133a regulates adipocyte browning in vivo," *PLOS Genetics*, vol. 9, no. 7, Article ID e1003626, 2013.

[19] V. Rottiers and A. M. Näär, "MicroRNAs in metabolism and metabolic disorders," *Nature Reviews Molecular Cell Biology*, vol. 13, no. 4, pp. 239–251, 2012.

[20] Z. Yang, T. Cappello, and L. Wang, "Emerging role of microRNAs in lipid metabolism," *Acta Pharmaceutica Sinica B*, vol. 5, no. 2, pp. 145–150, 2015.

[21] J. A. Deiuliis, "MicroRNAs as regulators of metabolic disease: pathophysiologic significance and emerging role as biomarkers and therapeutics," *International Journal of Obesity*, vol. 40, no. 1, pp. 88–101, 2016.

[22] C. L. Holley and V. K. Topkara, "An introduction to small non-coding RNAs: miRNA and snoRNA," *Cardiovascular Drugs and Therapy*, vol. 25, no. 2, pp. 151–159, 2011.

[23] S. L. Ameres and P. D. Zamore, "Diversifying microRNA sequence and function," *Nature Reviews Molecular Cell Biology*, vol. 14, no. 8, pp. 475–488, 2013.

[24] M. A. Goldgraben, R. Russell, O. M. Rueda, C. Caldas, and A. Git, "Double-stranded microRNA mimics can induce length- and passenger strand-dependent effects in a cell type-specific manner," *RNA*, vol. 22, no. 2, pp. 193–203, 2016.

[25] C. Fernandez-Hernando, C. M. Ramírez, L. Goedeke, and Y. Suárez, "MicroRNAs in metabolic disease," *Arteriosclerosis, Thrombosis, and Vascular Biology*, vol. 33, no. 2, pp. 178–185, 2013.

[26] E. van Rooij and S. Kauppinen, "Development of microRNA therapeutics is coming of age," *EMBO Molecular Medicine*, vol. 6, no. 7, pp. 851–864, 2014.

[27] A. Lujambio and S. W. Lowe, "The microcosmos of cancer," *Nature*, vol. 482, no. 7385, pp. 347–355, 2012.

[28] G. A. Calin and C. M. Croce, "MicroRNA signatures in human cancers," *Nature Reviews Cancer*, vol. 6, no. 11, pp. 857–866, 2006.

[29] C. Sobolewski, N. Calo, D. Portius, and M. Foti, "MicroRNAs in fatty liver disease," *Seminars in Liver Disease*, vol. 35, no. 1, pp. 12–25, 2015.

[30] A. Drakaki, M. Hatziapostolou, C. Polytarchou et al., "Functional microRNA high throughput screening reveals miR-9 as a central regulator of liver oncogenesis by affecting the PPARA-CDH1 pathway," *BMC Cancer*, vol. 15, no. 1, article no. 542, 2015.

[31] M. Cui, Z. Xiao, Y. Wang et al., "Long noncoding RNA HULC modulates abnormal lipid metabolism in hepatoma cells through an mir-9-mediated RXRA signaling pathway," *Cancer Research*, vol. 75, no. 5, pp. 846–857, 2015.

[32] L. Zheng, G.-C. Lv, J. Sheng, and Y.-D. Yang, "Effect of miRNA-10b in regulating cellular steatosis level by targeting PPAR-α expression, a novel mechanism for the pathogenesis of NAFLD," *Journal of Gastroenterology and Hepatology*, vol. 25, no. 1, pp. 156–163, 2010.

[33] J. Zhou, K.-C. Wang, W. Wu et al., "MicroRNA-21 targets peroxisome proliferators-activated receptor-α in an autoregulatory loop to modulate flow-induced endothelial inflammation," *Proceedings of the National Academy of Sciences of the United States of America*, vol. 108, no. 25, pp. 10355–10360, 2011.

[34] X. Loyer, V. Paradis, C. Hénique et al., "Liver microRNA-21 is overexpressed in non-alcoholic steatohepatitis and contributes to the disease in experimental models by inhibiting PPARa expression," *Gut*, vol. 65, no. 11, pp. 1882–1894, 2015.

[35] Z.-J. Li, P.-H. Ou-Yang, and X.-P. Han, "Profibrotic effect of miR-33a with Akt activation in hepatic stellate cells," *Cellular Signalling*, vol. 26, no. 1, pp. 141–148, 2014.

[36] W. Hu, X. Wang, X. Ding et al., "MicroRNA-141 represses HBV replication by targeting PPARA," *PLoS ONE*, vol. 7, no. 3, Article ID e34165, 2012.

[37] B. Li, Z. Zhang, H. Zhang et al., "Aberrant miR199a-5p/caveolin1/PPARα axis in hepatic steatosis," *Journal of Molecular Endocrinology*, vol. 53, no. 3, pp. 393–403, 2014.

[38] J. L. Tong, C. P. Zhang, F. Nie et al., "MicroRNA 506 regulates expression of PPAR alpha in hydroxycamptothecin-resistant human colon cancer cells," *FEBS Letters*, vol. 585, no. 22, pp. 3560–3568, 2011.

[39] R. Martinelli, C. Nardelli, V. Pilone et al., "MiR-519d overexpression is associated with human obesity," *Obesity*, vol. 18, no. 11, pp. 2170–2176, 2010.

[40] P. Gurha, T. Wang, A. H. Larimore et al., "microRNA-22 promotes heart failure through coordinate suppression of PPAR/ERR-nuclear hormone receptor transcription," *PLoS ONE*, vol. 8, no. 9, Article ID e75882, 2013.

[41] L. Sun and M. Trajkovski, "MiR-27 orchestrates the transcriptional regulation of brown adipogenesis," *Metabolism: Clinical and Experimental*, vol. 63, no. 2, pp. 272–282, 2014.

[42] D. Baek, J. Villén, C. Shin, F. D. Camargo, S. P. Gygi, and D. P. Bartel, "The impact of microRNAs on protein output," *Nature*, vol. 455, no. 7209, pp. 64–71, 2008.

[43] H. El Azzouzi, S. Leptidis, E. Dirkx et al., "The Hypoxia-Inducible MicroRNA Cluster miR-199a~214 targets myocardial PPARδ and impairs mitochondrial fatty acid oxidation," *Cell Metabolism*, vol. 18, no. 3, pp. 341–354, 2013.

[44] P. Thulin, T. Wei, O. Werngren et al., "MicroRNA-9 regulates the expression of peroxisome proliferator-activated receptor δ in human monocytes during the inflammatory response," *International Journal of Molecular Medicine*, vol. 31, no. 5, pp. 1003–1010, 2013.

[45] Y.-Y. Xiao, P.-J. Fan, S.-R. Lei, M. Qi, and X.-H. Yang, "MiR-138/peroxisome proliferator-activated receptor β signaling regulates human hypertrophic scar fibroblast proliferation and movement in vitro," *Journal of Dermatology*, vol. 42, no. 5, pp. 485–495, 2015.

[46] J.-F. Zhang, W.-M. Fu, M.-L. He et al., "MiRNA-20a promotes osteogenic differentiation of human mesenchymal stem cells by co-regulating BMP signaling," *RNA Biology*, vol. 8, no. 5, pp. 829–838, 2011.

[47] S. Li, J. Li, B.-Y. Fei et al., "MiR-27a promotes hepatocellular carcinoma cell proliferation through suppression of its target gene peroxisome proliferator-activated receptor γ," *Chinese Medical Journal*, vol. 128, no. 7, pp. 941–947, 2015.

[48] B.-Y. Kang, K. K. Park, D. E. Green et al., "Hypoxia mediates mutual repression between microRNA-27a and PPARγ in the pulmonary vasculature," *PLoS ONE*, vol. 8, no. 11, Article ID e79503, 2013.

[49] C. Jennewein, A. Von Knethen, T. Schmid, and B. Brüne, "MicroRNA-27b contributes to lipopolysaccharide-mediated peroxisome proliferator-activated receptor γ (PPARγ) mRNA destabilization," *Journal of Biological Chemistry*, vol. 285, no. 16, pp. 11846–11853, 2010.

[50] M. Karbiener, C. Fischer, S. Nowitsch et al., "microRNA miR-27b impairs human adipocyte differentiation and targets PPARgamma," *Biochemical and Biophysical Research Communications*, vol. 390, no. 2, pp. 247–251, 2009.

[51] J.-J. Lee, A. Drakaki, D. Iliopoulos, and K. Struhl, "MiR-27b targets PPARγ to inhibit growth, tumor progression and the inflammatory response in neuroblastoma cells," *Oncogene*, vol. 31, no. 33, pp. 3818–3825, 2012.

[52] X. Li, Y. Chen, S. Wu et al., "MicroRNA-34a and microRNA-34c promote the activation of human hepatic stellate cells by targeting peroxisome proliferator-activated receptor γ," *Molecular Medicine Reports*, vol. 11, no. 2, pp. 1017–1024, 2015.

[53] D. Povero, N. Panera, A. Eguchi et al., "Lipid-induced hepatocyte-derived extracellular vesicles regulate hepatic stellate cells via microRNA targeting Peroxisome Proliferator-Activated Receptor-γ," *CMGH Cellular and Molecular Gastroenterology and Hepatology*, vol. 1, no. 6, pp. 646.e4–663.e4, 2015.

[54] E. K. Lee, M. J. Lee, K. Abdelmohsen et al., "miR-130 suppresses adipogenesis by inhibiting peroxisome proliferator-activated receptor γ expression," *Molecular and Cellular Biology*, vol. 31, no. 4, pp. 626–638, 2011.

[55] K. Tu, X. Zheng, C. Dou et al., "MicroRNA-130b promotes cell aggressiveness by inhibiting peroxisome proliferator-activated receptor gamma in human hepatocellular carcinoma," *International Journal of Molecular Sciences*, vol. 15, no. 11, pp. 20486–20499, 2014.

[56] Y. Jiao, M. Zhu, X. Mao et al., "MicroRNA-130a expression is decreased in Xinjiang Uygur patients with type 2 diabetes mellitus," *American Journal of Translational Research*, vol. 7, no. 10, pp. 1984–1991, 2015.

[57] Z. Yang, C. Bian, H. Zhou et al., "MicroRNA hsa-miR-138 inhibits adipogenic differentiation of human adipose tissue-derived mesenchymal stem cells through adenovirus EID-1," *Stem Cells and Development*, vol. 20, no. 2, pp. 259–267, 2011.

[58] J. Sun, Y. Wang, Y. Li, and G. Zhao, "Downregulation of PPARγ by miR-548d-5p suppresses the adipogenic differentiation of human bone marrow mesenchymal stem cells and enhances their osteogenic potential," *Journal of Translational Medicine*, vol. 12, no. 1, article no. 168, 2014.

[59] S. Y. Kim, A. Y. Kim, H. W. Lee et al., "miR-27a is a negative regulator of adipocyte differentiation via suppressing PPARγ expression," *Biochemical and Biophysical Research Communications*, vol. 392, no. 3, pp. 323–328, 2010.

[60] X. Hou, J. Tian, J. Geng et al., "MicroRNA-27a promotes renal tubulointerstitial fibrosis via suppressing PPARγ pathway in diabetic nephropathy," *Oncotarget*, vol. 7, no. 30, pp. 47760–47776, 2016.

[61] J. Wang, Y. Song, Y. Zhang et al., "Cardiomyocyte overexpression of miR-27b induces cardiac hypertrophy and dysfunction in mice," *Cell Research*, vol. 22, no. 3, pp. 516–527, 2012.

[62] C. Kim, H. Lee, Y. M. Cho, O.-J. Kwon, W. Kim, and E. K. Lee, "TNFα-induced miR-130 resulted in adipocyte dysfunction during obesity-related inflammation," *FEBS Letters*, vol. 587, no. 23, pp. 3853–3858, 2013.

[63] L. Lu, J. Wang, H. Lu et al., "MicroRNA-130a and -130b enhance activation of hepatic stellate cells by suppressing PPARγ expression: a rat fibrosis model study," *Biochemical and Biophysical Research Communications*, vol. 465, no. 3, pp. 387–393, 2015.

[64] X.-D. Liu, F. Cai, L. Liu, Y. Zhang, and A.-L. Yang, "MicroRNA-210 is involved in the regulation of postmenopausal osteoporosis through promotion of VEGF expression and osteoblast differentiation," *Biological Chemistry*, vol. 396, no. 4, pp. 339–347, 2015.

[65] H. Li, M. Xue, J. Xu, and X. Qin, "MiR-301a is involved in adipocyte dysfunction during obesity-related inflammation via suppression of PPARγ," *Pharmazie*, vol. 71, no. 2, pp. 84–88, 2016.

[66] B.-C. Jeong, I.-H. Kang, and J.-T. Koh, "MicroRNA-302a inhibits adipogenesis by suppressing peroxisome proliferator-activated receptor γ expression," *FEBS Letters*, vol. 588, no. 18, pp. 3427–3434, 2014.

[67] L. Chen, Y. Chen, S. Zhang et al., "MiR-540 as a novel adipogenic inhibitor impairs adipogenesis via suppression of PPARγ," *Journal of Cellular Biochemistry*, vol. 116, no. 6, pp. 969–976, 2015.

[68] M. Pawlak, P. Lefebvre, and B. Staels, "Molecular mechanism of PPARα action and its impact on lipid metabolism, inflammation and fibrosis in non-alcoholic fatty liver disease," *Journal of Hepatology*, vol. 62, no. 3, pp. 720–733, 2015.

[69] P. Misra and J. K. Reddy, "Peroxisome proliferator-activated receptor-α activation and excess energy burning in hepatocarcinogenesis," *Biochimie*, vol. 98, no. 1, pp. 63–74, 2014.

[70] R. K. Lyn, R. Singaravelu, S. Kargman et al., "Stearoyl-CoA desaturase inhibition blocks formation of hepatitis C virus-induced specialized membranes," *Scientific Reports*, vol. 4, article 4549, 2014.

[71] Y. M. Shah, K. Morimura, Q. Yang, T. Tanabe, M. Takagi, and F. J. Gonzalez, "Peroxisome proliferator-activated receptor α regulates a microRNA-mediated signaling cascade responsible for hepatocellular proliferation," *Molecular and Cellular Biology*, vol. 27, no. 12, pp. 4238–4247, 2007.

[72] N. Calo, P. Ramadori, C. Sobolewski et al., "Stress-activated *miR-21/miR-21** in hepatocytes promotes lipid and glucose metabolic disorders associated with high-fat diet consumption," *Gut*, vol. 65, no. 11, pp. 1871–1881, 2016.

[73] J. Ji, J. Zhang, G. Huang, J. Qian, X. Wang, and S. Mei, "Over-expressed microRNA-27a and 27b influence fat accumulation and cell proliferation during rat hepatic stellate cell activation," *FEBS Letters*, vol. 583, no. 4, pp. 759–766, 2009.

[74] M. Karbiener and M. Scheideler, "MicroRNA functions in brite/brown fat—novel perspectives towards anti-obesity strategies," *Computational and Structural Biotechnology Journal*, vol. 11, no. 19, pp. 101–105, 2014.

[75] Y. Wu, J. Zuo, Y. Zhang et al., "Identification of miR-106b-93 as a negative regulator of brown adipocyte differentiation," *Biochemical and Biophysical Research Communications*, vol. 438, no. 4, pp. 575–580, 2013.

[76] D. Iliopoulos, K. N. Malizos, P. Oikonomou, and A. Tsezou, "Integrative MicroRNA and proteomic approaches identify novel osteoarthritis genes and their collaborative metabolic and inflammatory networks," *PLoS ONE*, vol. 3, no. 11, article e3740, 2008.

[77] W.-L. W. Wang, J. E. Welsh, and M. Tenniswood, "1,25-Dihydroxyvitamin D_3 modulates lipid metabolism in prostate cancer cells through miRNA mediated regulation of PPARA," *The Journal of Steroid Biochemistry and Molecular Biology*, vol. 136, no. 1, pp. 247–251, 2013.

[78] L. Salvadó, L. Serrano-Marco, E. Barroso, X. Palomer, and M. Vázquez-Carrera, "Targeting PPARβ/δ for the treatment of type 2 diabetes mellitus," *Expert Opinion on Therapeutic Targets*, vol. 16, no. 2, pp. 209–223, 2012.

[79] S. A. Ross and C. D. Davis, "MicroRNA, nutrition, and cancer prevention," *Advances in Nutrition*, vol. 2, no. 6, pp. 472–485, 2011.

[80] C. H. Lee, P. Olson, A. Hevener et al., "PPARdelta regulates glucose metabolism and insulin sensitivity," *Proceedings of the National Academy of Sciences of the United States of America*, vol. 103, no. 9, pp. 3444–3449, 2006.

[81] Y.-X. Wang, C.-H. Lee, S. Tiep et al., "Peroxisome-proliferator-activated receptor δ activates fat metabolism to prevent obesity," *Cell*, vol. 113, no. 2, pp. 159–170, 2003.

[82] E. Ehrenborg and A. Krook, "Regulation of skeletal muscle physiology and metabolism by peroxisome proliferator-activated receptor δ," *Pharmacological Reviews*, vol. 61, no. 3, pp. 373–393, 2009.

[83] B. Gross, M. Pawlak, P. Lefebvre, and B. Staels, "PPARs in obesity-induced T2DM, dyslipidaemia and NAFLD," *Nature Reviews Endocrinology*, vol. 13, no. 1, pp. 36–49, 2016.

[84] R. L. Stephen, M. C. U. Gustafsson, M. Jarvis et al., "Activation of peroxisome proliferator-activated receptor δ stimulates the proliferation of human breast and prostate cancer cell lines," *Cancer Research*, vol. 64, no. 9, pp. 3162–3170, 2004.

[85] J. M. Peters, F. J. Gonzalez, and R. Müller, "Establishing the Role of PPARβ/δ in Carcinogenesis," *Trends in Endocrinology & Metabolism*, vol. 26, no. 11, pp. 595–607, 2015.

[86] D. Gatfield, G. Le Martelot, C. E. Vejnar et al., "Integration of microRNA miR-122 in hepatic circadian gene expression," *Genes and Development*, vol. 23, no. 11, pp. 1313–1326, 2009.

[87] M. Aprile, M. R. Ambrosio, V. D'Esposito et al., "PPARG in human adipogenesis: differential contribution of canonical transcripts and dominant negative isoforms," *PPAR Research*, vol. 2014, Article ID 537865, 11 pages, 2014.

[88] M. Pancione, L. Sabatino, A. Fucci et al., "Epigenetic silencing of peroxisome proliferator-activated receptor γ is a biomarker for colorectal cancer progression and adverse patients' outcome," *PLoS ONE*, vol. 5, no. 12, Article ID e14229, 2010.

[89] M. Peyrou, P. Ramadori, L. Bourgoin, and M. Foti, "PPARs in liver diseases and cancer: epigenetic regulation by microRNAs," *PPAR Research*, vol. 2012, Article ID 757803, 16 pages, 2012.

[90] J. Mann, D. C. K. Chu, A. Maxwell et al., "MeCP2 controls an epigenetic pathway that promotes myofibroblast transdifferentiation and fibrosis," *Gastroenterology*, vol. 138, no. 2, pp. 705.e4–714.e4, 2010.

[91] T. Shirasaki, M. Honda, T. Shimakami et al., "MicroRNA-27a regulates lipid metabolism and inhibits hepatitis C virus replication in human hepatoma cells," *Journal of Virology*, vol. 87, no. 9, pp. 5270–5286, 2013.

[92] L. Q. Cao, X. L. Wang, Q. Wang et al., "Rosiglitazone sensitizes hepatocellular carcinoma cell lines to 5-fluorouracil antitumor activity through activation of the PPARgamma signaling pathway," *Acta Pharmacologica Sinica*, vol. 30, no. 9, pp. 1316–1322, 2009.

[93] J. Yu, B. Shen, E. S. H. Chu et al., "Inhibitory role of peroxisome proliferator-activated receptor gamma in hepatocarcinogenesis in mice and in vitro," *Hepatology*, vol. 51, no. 6, pp. 2008–2019, 2010.

[94] K. L. Schaefer, K. Wada, H. Takahashi et al., "Peroxisome proliferator-activated receptor γ inhibition prevents adhesion to the extracellular matrix and induces anoikis in hepatocellular carcinoma cells," *Cancer Research*, vol. 65, no. 6, pp. 2251–2259, 2005.

[95] K. Yoshizawa, D. P. Cioca, S. Kawa, E. Tanaka, and K. Kiyosawa, "Peroxisome proliferator-activated receptor γ ligand troglitazone induces cell cycle arrest and apoptosis of hepatocellular carcinoma cell lines," *Cancer*, vol. 95, no. 10, pp. 2243–2251, 2002.

[96] A. Panza, C. Votino, A. Gentile et al., "Peroxisome proliferator-activated receptor γ-mediated induction of microRNA-145 opposes tumor phenotype in colorectal cancer," *Biochimica et Biophysica Acta—Molecular Cell Research*, vol. 1843, no. 6, pp. 1225–1236, 2014.

[97] B.-C. Jeong, I.-H. Kang, and J.-T. Koh, "MicroRNA-302a inhibits adipogenesis by suppressing peroxisome proliferator-activated receptor γ expression," *FEBS Letters*, vol. 588, no. 18, pp. 3427–3434, 2014.

[98] Q. Lin, Z. Gao, R. M. Alarcon, J. Ye, and Z. Yun, "A role of miR-27 in the regulation of adipogenesis," *FEBS Journal*, vol. 276, no. 8, pp. 2348–2358, 2009.

[99] H. Li, T. Li, S. Wang et al., "MiR-17-5p and miR-106a are involved in the balance between osteogenic and adipogenic differentiation of adipose-derived mesenchymal stem cells," *Stem Cell Research*, vol. 10, no. 3, pp. 313–324, 2013.

[100] M. Sun, X. Zhou, L. Chen et al., "The regulatory roles of microRNAs in bone remodeling and perspectives as biomarkers in osteoporosis," *BioMed Research International*, vol. 2016, Article ID 1652417, 11 pages, 2016.

[101] C. S. Lutz and A. L. Cornett, "Regulation of genes in the arachidonic acid metabolic pathway by RNA processing and RNA-mediated mechanisms," *Wiley Interdisciplinary Reviews: RNA*, vol. 4, no. 5, pp. 593–605, 2013.

[102] A. Croasdell, P. F. Duffney, N. Kim, S. H. Lacy, P. J. Sime, and R. P. Phipps, "PPARγ and the innate immune system mediate the resolution of inflammation," *PPAR Research*, vol. 2015, Article ID 549691, 20 pages, 2015.

[103] B. Kang, K. K. Park, J. M. Kleinhenz et al., "Peroxisome proliferator–activated receptor γ and microRNA 98 in hypoxia-induced endothelin-1 signaling," *American Journal of Respiratory Cell and Molecular Biology*, vol. 54, no. 1, pp. 136–146, 2016.

[104] D. E. Green, R. L. Sutliff, and C. M. Hart, "Is peroxisome proliferator-activated receptor gamma (PPARγ) a therapeutic target for the treatment of pulmonary hypertension?" *Pulmonary Circulation*, vol. 1, no. 1, pp. 33–47, 2011.

[105] T. Liu, H. Tang, Y. Lang, M. Liu, and X. Li, "MicroRNA-27a functions as an oncogene in gastric adenocarcinoma by targeting prohibitin," *Cancer Letters*, vol. 273, no. 2, pp. 233–242, 2009.

[106] Y. Tsuchiya, M. Nakajima, S. Takagi, T. Taniya, and T. Yokoi, "MicroRNA regulates the expression of human cytochrome P450 1B1," *Cancer Research*, vol. 66, no. 18, pp. 9090–9098, 2006.

[107] R. Zhou, X. Li, G. Hu, A.-Y. Gong, K. M. Drescher, and X.-M. Chen, "MiR-16 targets transcriptional corepressor SMRT and modulates NF-kappaB-regulated transactivation of interleukin-8 gene," *PLoS ONE*, vol. 7, no. 1, Article ID e30772, 2012.

[108] L. Tombolan, M. Zampini, S. Casara et al., "MicroRNA-27a contributes to rhabdomyosarcoma cell proliferation by suppressing RARA and RXRA," *PLoS ONE*, vol. 10, no. 4, Article ID e0125171, 2015.

[109] Y. Oda, M. Nakajima, K. Tsuneyama et al., "Retinoid X receptor α in human liver is regulated by miR-34a," *Biochemical Pharmacology*, vol. 90, no. 2, pp. 179–187, 2014.

[110] M. J. Ochs, D. Steinhilber, and B. Suess, "MicroRNA involved in inflammation: control of eicosanoid pathway," *Frontiers in Pharmacology*, vol. 2, article no. 39, 2011.

[111] S.-E. Choi and J. K. Kemper, "Regulation of SIRT1 by microRNAs," *Molecules and Cells*, vol. 36, no. 5, pp. 385–392, 2013.

[112] B. M. Alrfaei, R. Vemuganti, and J. S. Kuo, "microRNA-100 targets SMRT/NCOR2, reduces proliferation, and improves survival in glioblastoma animal models," *PLoS ONE*, vol. 8, no. 11, Article ID e80865, 2013.

[113] D. Guérit, D. Philipot, P. Chuchana et al., "Sox9-regulated miRNA-574-3p inhibits chondrogenic differentiation of mesenchymal stem cells," *PLoS ONE*, vol. 8, no. 4, Article ID e62582, 2013.

[114] Y. K. Adlakha, S. Khanna, R. Singh, V. P. Singh, A. Agrawal, and N. Saini, "Pro-apoptotic miRNA-128-2 modulates ABCA1, ABCG1 and RXRα expression and cholesterol homeostasis," *Cell Death & Disease*, vol. 4, article e780, 2013.

[115] P. Seale, B. Bjork, W. Yang et al., "PRDM16 controls a brown fat/skeletal muscle switch," *Nature*, vol. 454, no. 7207, pp. 961–967, 2008.

[116] H. Yin, A. Pasut, V. D. Soleimani et al., "MicroRNA-133 controls brown adipose determination in skeletal muscle satellite cells by targeting Prdm16," *Cell Metabolism*, vol. 17, no. 2, pp. 210–224, 2013.

[117] M. Trajkovski, K. Ahmed, C. C. Esau, and M. Stoffel, "MyomiR-133 regulates brown fat differentiation through Prdm16," *Nature Cell Biology*, vol. 14, no. 12, pp. 1330–1335, 2012.

[118] R. B. Vega, J. M. Huss, and D. P. Kelly, "The coactivator PGC-1 cooperates with peroxisome proliferator-activated receptor α in transcriptional control of nuclear genes encoding mitochondrial fatty acid oxidation enzymes," *Molecular and Cellular Biology*, vol. 20, no. 5, pp. 1868–1876, 2000.

[119] Z. Fang, P. Li, W. Jia, T. Jiang, Z. Wang, and Y. Xiang, "miR-696 plays a role in hepatic gluconeogenesis in ob/ob mice by targeting PGC-1α," *International Journal of Molecular Medicine*, vol. 38, no. 3, pp. 845–852, 2016.

[120] J.-Y. Huang, S.-F. Chou, J.-W. Lee et al., "MicroRNA-130a can inhibit hepatitis B virus replication via targeting PGC1α and PPARγ," *RNA*, vol. 21, no. 3, pp. 385–400, 2015.

[121] C. Cantó and J. Auwerx, "Targeting sirtuin 1 to improve metabolism: all you need is NAD$^+$?" *Pharmacological Reviews*, vol. 64, no. 1, pp. 166–187, 2012.

[122] H. Yin, M. Hu, R. Zhang, Z. Shen, L. Flatow, and M. You, "MicroRNA-217 promotes ethanol-induced fat accumulation in hepatocytes by down-regulating SIRT1," *Journal of Biological Chemistry*, vol. 287, no. 13, pp. 9817–9826, 2012.

[123] B. Zhou, C. Li, W. Qi et al., "Downregulation of miR-181a upregulates sirtuin-1 (SIRT1) and improves hepatic insulin sensitivity," *Diabetologia*, vol. 55, no. 7, pp. 2032–2043, 2012.

[124] C. L. Kurtz, E. E. Fannin, C. L. Toth, D. S. Pearson, K. C. Vickers, and P. Sethupathy, "Inhibition of miR-29 has a significant lipid-lowering benefit through suppression of lipogenic programs in liver," *Scientific Reports*, vol. 5, Article ID 12911, 2015.

[125] X.-F. Tian, F.-J. Ji, H.-L. Zang, and H. Cao, "Activation of the miR-34a/SIRT1/p53 signaling pathway contributes to the progress of liver fibrosis via inducing apoptosis in hepatocytes but not in HSCs," *PLoS ONE*, vol. 11, no. 7, Article ID e0158657, 2016.

[126] F. Zhang, J. Cui, X. Liu et al., "Roles of microRNA-34a targeting SIRT1 in mesenchymal stem cells," *Stem Cell Research and Therapy*, vol. 6, no. 1, article 195, 2015.

[127] A. L. McCubbrey, J. D. Nelson, V. R. Stolberg et al., "MicroRNA-34a negatively regulates efferocytosis by tissue macrophages in part via SIRT1," *Journal of Immunology*, vol. 196, no. 3, pp. 1366–1375, 2016.

[128] K. Duan, Y.-C. Ge, X.-P. Zhang et al., "miR-34a inhibits cell proliferation in prostate cancer by downregulation of SIRT1 expression," *Oncology Letters*, vol. 10, no. 5, pp. 3223–3227, 2015.

[129] X. Liu, X. Chen, X. Yu et al., "Regulation of microRNAs by epigenetics and their interplay involved in cancer," *Journal of Experimental and Clinical Cancer Research*, vol. 32, no. 1, article 96, 2013.

[130] S. Luo, J. Wang, Y. Ma, Z. Yao, and H. Pan, "PPARγ inhibits ovarian cancer cells proliferation through upregulation of miR-125b," *Biochemical and Biophysical Research Communications*, vol. 462, no. 2, pp. 85–90, 2015.

[131] H.-Y. Zhu, C. Li, Z. Zheng et al., "Peroxisome proliferator-activated receptor-γ (PPAR-γ) agonist inhibits collagen synthesis in human hypertrophic scar fibroblasts by targeting Smad3 via miR-145," *Biochemical and Biophysical Research Communications*, vol. 459, no. 1, pp. 49–53, 2015.

[132] Y. Zhang, Z. Yang, R. Whitby, and L. Wang, "Regulation of miR-200c by nuclear receptors PPARα, LRH-1 and SHP," *Biochemical and Biophysical Research Communications*, vol. 416, no. 1-2, pp. 135–139, 2011.

[133] W. Ying, A. Tseng, R. C.-A. Chang et al., "MicroRNA-223 is a crucial mediator of PPARγ-regulated alternative macrophage activation," *Journal of Clinical Investigation*, vol. 125, no. 11, pp. 4149–4159, 2015.

[134] J. Yu, X. Kong, J. Liu et al., "Expression profiling of PPARγ-regulated MicroRNAs in human subcutaneous and visceral adipogenesis in both genders," *Endocrinology*, vol. 155, no. 6, pp. 2155–2165, 2014.

[135] C.-M. Wong, L. Wei, S. L.-K. Au et al., "MiR-200b/200c/429 subfamily negatively regulates Rho/ROCK signaling pathway to suppress hepatocellular carcinoma metastasis," *Oncotarget*, vol. 6, no. 15, pp. 13658–13670, 2015.

[136] X. Fang, L. Fang, A. Liu, X. Wang, B. Zhao, and N. Wang, "Activation of PPAR-δ induces microRNA-100 and decreases the uptake of very low-density lipoprotein in endothelial cells,"

British Journal of Pharmacology, vol. 172, no. 15, pp. 3728–3736, 2015.

[137] S.-Y. Liu, Y.-Y. Zhang, Y. Gao et al., "MiR-378 plays an important role in the differentiation of bovine preadipocytes," *Cellular Physiology and Biochemistry*, vol. 36, no. 4, pp. 1552–1562, 2015.

[138] E. John, A. Wienecke-Baldacchino, M. Liivrand, M. Heinäniemi, C. Carlberg, and L. Sinkkonen, "Dataset integration identifies transcriptional regulation of microRNA genes by PPARγ in differentiating mouse 3T3-L1 adipocytes," *Nucleic Acids Research*, vol. 40, no. 10, pp. 4446–4460, 2012.

[139] K. Song, C. Han, J. Zhang et al., "Epigenetic regulation of microRNA-122 by peroxisome proliferator activated receptor-gamma and hepatitis b virus X protein in hepatocellular carcinoma cells," *Hepatology*, vol. 58, no. 5, pp. 1681–1692, 2013.

[140] L. G. Tillman, R. S. Geary, and G. E. Hardee, "Oral delivery of antisense oligonucleotides in man," *Journal of Pharmaceutical Sciences*, vol. 97, no. 1, pp. 225–236, 2008.

[141] S. Mitragotri, P. A. Burke, and R. Langer, "Overcoming the challenges in administering biopharmaceuticals: formulation and delivery strategies," *Nature Reviews Drug Discovery*, vol. 13, no. 9, pp. 655–672, 2014.

[142] X. Wang, B. Yu, W. Ren et al., "Enhanced hepatic delivery of siRNA and microRNA using oleic acid based lipid nanoparticle formulations," *Journal of Controlled Release*, vol. 172, no. 3, pp. 690–698, 2013.

[143] C. J. Cheng, W. M. Saltzman, and J. F. Slack, "Canonical and non-canonical barriers facing antimiR cancer therapeutics," *Current Medicinal Chemistry*, vol. 20, no. 29, pp. 3582–3593, 2013.

[144] S. Pan, X. Yang, Y. Jia, R. Li, and R. Zhao, "Microvesicle-shuttled miR-130b reduces fat deposition in recipient primary cultured porcine adipocytes by inhibiting PPAR-γ expression," *Journal of Cellular Physiology*, vol. 229, no. 5, pp. 631–639, 2014.

[145] S. Pan, X. Yang, Y. Jia et al., "Intravenous injection of microvesicle-delivery miR-130b alleviates high-fat diet-induced obesity in C57BL/6 mice through translational repression of PPAR-γ," *Journal of Biomedical Science*, vol. 22, article 86, 2015.

[146] F. Olivieri, M. R. Rippo, F. Prattichizzo et al., "Toll like receptor signaling in "inflammaging": microRNA as new players," *Immunity and Ageing*, vol. 10, article no. 11, 2013.

[147] R. E. Lanford, E. S. Hildebrandt-Eriksen, A. Petri et al., "Therapeutic silencing of microRNA-122 in primates with chronic hepatitis C virus infection," *Science*, vol. 327, no. 5962, pp. 198–201, 2010.

[148] S. Ottosen, T. B. Parsley, L. Yang et al., "*In vitro* antiviral activity and preclinical and clinical resistance profile of miravirsen, a novel anti-hepatitis C virus therapeutic targeting the human factor miR-122," *Antimicrobial Agents and Chemotherapy*, vol. 59, no. 1, pp. 599–608, 2015.

[149] J. Stenvang, A. Petri, M. Lindow, S. Obad, and S. Kauppinen, "Inhibition of microRNA function by antimiR oligonucleotides," *Silence*, vol. 3, no. 1, article 1, 2012.

[150] K. J. Rayner, C. C. Esau, F. N. Hussain et al., "Inhibition of miR-33a/b in non-human primates raises plasma HDL and lowers VLDL triglycerides," *Nature*, vol. 178, no. 7369, pp. 404–407, 2011.

[151] H. Wu, R. Ng, X. Chen, C. J. Steer, and G. Song, "MicroRNA-21 is a potential link between non-alcoholic fatty liver disease and hepatocellular carcinoma via modulation of the HBP1-p53-Srebp1c pathway," *Gut*, vol. 65, no. 11, pp. 1850–1860, 2015.

[152] M. Agostini and R. A. Knight, "miR-34: from bench to bedside," *Oncotarget*, vol. 5, no. 4, pp. 872–881, 2014.

[153] L. E. Young, A. E. Moore, L. Sokol, N. Meisner-Kober, and D. A. Dixon, "The mRNA stability factor HuR inhibits MicroRNA-16 targeting of COX-2," *Molecular Cancer Research*, vol. 10, no. 1, pp. 167–180, 2012.

[154] S. Geisler and J. Coller, "RNA in unexpected places: long non-coding RNA functions in diverse cellular contexts," *Nature Reviews Molecular Cell Biology*, vol. 14, no. 11, pp. 699–712, 2013.

16

Chiglitazar Preferentially Regulates Gene Expression via Configuration-Restricted Binding and Phosphorylation Inhibition of PPARγ

De-Si Pan,[1] **Wei Wang,**[2] **Nan-Song Liu,**[1] **Qian-Jiao Yang,**[1] **Kun Zhang,**[1] **Jing-Zhong Zhu,**[1] **Song Shan,**[1] **Zhi-Bin Li,**[1] **Zhi-Qiang Ning,**[1] **Laiqiang Huang,**[2] **and Xian-Ping Lu**[1]

[1]*Shenzhen Chipscreen Biosciences Ltd., Shenzhen, Guangdong 518057, China*
[2]*Shenzhen Key Lab of Gene & Antibody Therapy, Division of Life & Health Sciences, Graduate School at Shenzhen, Tsinghua University, Shenzhen, Guangdong 518057, China*

Correspondence should be addressed to Xian-Ping Lu; xplu@chipscreen.com

Academic Editor: Xinran Ma

Type 2 diabetes mellitus is often treated with insulin-sensitizing drugs called thiazolidinediones (TZD), which improve insulin resistance and glycemic control. Despite their effectiveness in treating diabetes, these drugs provide little protection from eminent cardiovascular disease associated with diabetes. Here we demonstrate how chiglitazar, a configuration-restricted non-TZD peroxisome proliferator-activated receptor (PPAR) pan agonist with moderate transcription activity, preferentially regulates *ANGPTL4* and *PDK4*, which are involved in glucose and lipid metabolism. CDK5-mediated phosphorylation at serine 273 (S273) is a unique regulatory mechanism reserved for PPARγ, and this event is linked to insulin resistance in type 2 diabetes mellitus. Our data demonstrates that chiglitazar modulates gene expression differently from two TZDs, rosiglitazone and pioglitazone, via its configuration-restricted binding and phosphorylation inhibition of PPARγ. Chiglitazar induced significantly greater expression of *ANGPTL4* and *PDK4* than rosiglitazone and pioglitazone in different cell models. These increased expressions were dependent on the phosphorylation status of PPARγ at S273. Furthermore, ChIP and AlphaScreen assays showed that phosphorylation at S273 inhibited promoter binding and cofactor recruitment by PPARγ. Based on these results, activities from pan agonist chiglitazar can be an effective part of a long-term therapeutic strategy for treating type 2 diabetes in a more balanced action among its targeted organs.

1. Introduction

Metabolic syndromes, including type 2 diabetes mellitus (T2DM) and its associated complications (e.g., obesity, cardiovascular symptoms, and dyslipidemia), have significant worldwide impact. Current antidiabetic treatments, especially the insulin-sensitizing class of drugs called thiazolidinediones (TZD) (i.e., rosiglitazone (Ros) and pioglitazone (Pio)), improve insulin resistance and glycemic control with benefit of improvement in rental complication. However, they offer ambiguous protection from eminent cardiovascular risks associated with the diseases. Moreover, the related side effects, such as water retention and body weight gain, rather impair their extended uses in long-term management of diabetic patients. Nevertheless, the TZD class of peroxisome proliferator-activated receptor γ (PPARγ) agonists is one major and important therapeutic that directly targets insulin resistance by protecting pancreatic β-islet cells, dysregulated transcription program on glucolipid modulation, and imparting anti-inflammatory protection. These drugs also exhibit a more preventive effect and provide more durable HbA1c control than other diabetes treatments [1, 2]. In China, less than one-third of T2D patients received a durable control of HbA1c and only 5.6% of T2D patients with dysregulated metabolic function achieved a comprehensive control of glucose, lipid, and blood pressure [3]. Therefore, development of new type of insulin sensitizers for treating type 2 diabetes and associated complications remains of great interest and potential.

PPARγ, a primary target of TZDs along with PPARα and PPARδ, is a ligand-activated member of the nuclear hormone receptor superfamily which is expressed in various tissues with overlapping or distinct biological activity in controlling glucose, lipid, and energy homeostasis. In brief, PPARγ is predominantly present in adipose tissue and macrophages and functions to repartition fatty acids (FAs) to adipose tissue from muscle, liver, and circulation, thus improving insulin resistance [4]. PPARα is mainly expressed in liver, heart, muscle, and kidney, where it stimulates FA oxidation and improves lipoprotein metabolism [5]. Although PPARδ is expressed ubiquitously, its function is less defined and PPARδ is mainly considered as an important regulator of FA metabolism and thermogenesis [6]. All three subtypes also exert pleiotropic anti-inflammatory effects via distinct mechanisms in modulating proliferation or cholesterol turnover in vascular endothelial cells and macrophages [7]. Controversially, PPARα and PPARδ promote osteoblast activity in bone, while PPARγ promotes osteoclast activity [8]. Considering their mutually compensatory and sometimes antagonistic effects, a less potent and well-balanced agonist that targets all three PPAR subtypes may provide more comprehensive protection from metabolic dysfunction and accompanied cardiovascular disease, as well as offset of undesired side effect such as weight gain and bone fracture associated with highly active PPARγ agonists in T2DM patients [9, 10]. Thus far, no clinically proven drugs have been developed by such strategies, most likely due to difficulty in discriminating one effect from another for the same target or in bringing well-balanced activities from different subtypes.

Recently, several studies reported that specific inhibition of PPARγ phosphorylation, induced by "pathological stimuli" such as a high-fat diet, obesity, and inflammation, at serine 273 (S273) by TZD and synthetic ligands, resulted in alterations in gene expression profile which led to insulin resistance in animals and humans. Therefore, this event may play a unique role in discriminating insulin-sensitizing from other adverse effects, such as weight gain and edema, used to be linked to PPARγ activation by TZDs [11–14].

Chiglitazar (Chi) is a configuration-restricted non-TZD PPAR pan agonist, with AC50 of 1.2, 0.08, and 1.7 μM in CV-1 cells for PPARα, PPARγ, and PPARδ, respectively, which is currently in phase III clinical development in China. This compound is a moderate transcriptional activator of all three PPAR subtypes and induces different patterns of gene regulation compared to the TZD class of drugs in vitro and in vivo [15, 16]. In animal studies, compared with Ros, Chi demonstrated comparable antidiabetic effects but with fewer adverse effects on body weight and fat pad weight increases in KKAy and db/db diabetic mouse models [16]. This compound also produced a much improved lipid profile in monosodium L-glutamate- (MSG-) induced obese rats [15].

In this article, we report that Chi preferentially induced two important PPAR target genes, ANGPTL4 (angiopoietin-like 4) and PDK4 (pyruvate dehydrogenase kinase, isozyme 4), which are involved in lipid metabolism and insulin sensitization, relative to Ros and Pio. These genes are regulated mainly by PPARδ and to a lesser extent by other PPAR subtypes [17, 18]. The differential induction by Chi did not seem to be entirely due to its pan agonist activity. Instead, our results demonstrated that both genes were directly regulated by CDK5- (cell division protein kinase 5-) mediated phosphorylation of PPARγ at S273, which affects cofactor recruitment by the receptor and binding of a PPARγ-containing transcription complex to PDK4 and ANGPTL4 promoters. The unique structure of Chi allows its distinct binding and interactions with the receptor, which results in significantly stronger inhibition of site-specific phosphorylation leading to higher induction of ANGPTL4 and PDK4 expression. Since the phosphorylation status of PPARγ is directly linked to "pathological stimuli" such as a high-fat diet, obesity, and inflammation commonly seen in T2DM patients, the prominent activity of Chi in this regard in addition to its pan agonist activity can thus act cooperatively to rebalance glucose, FA uptake, and substrate utilization in energy production upon insulin resistance and obesity, which may improve the clinical prognosis of T2DM patients over time.

2. Materials and Methods

2.1. Chemicals. Chiglitazar was discovered and synthesized by Chipscreen Biosciences Ltd. [14]. Rosiglitazone and pioglitazone were provided by Jiangsu Depei Chemical Co. Ltd. (Jintan, China). Roscovitine, Sutent, U0126, SR1664, and VX680 were purchased from Selleck Chemicals (Houston, TX, USA). All chemicals were supplied with purity qualified.

2.2. Cell Lines. Human preadipocyte-visceral (HPA-v) cells were purchased from ScienCell (Carlsbad, CA, USA) and cultured in preadipocyte medium (PAM, ScienCell) containing 10% fetal bovine serum. The human normal liver cell line L-02 was purchased from the Shanghai cell bank of the Chinese Academy of Sciences (Shanghai, China) and cultured in RPMI-1640 medium containing 10% fetal bovine serum, 50 μg/ml streptomycin, and 50 units/ml penicillin at 37°C in a humidified incubator with 5% CO_2.

2.3. Molecular Docking Simulation (MDS). The published crystal structures of PPARγ binding to its ligands were downloaded from the Protein Data Bank (PDB code: 2PRG, 2XKW) [19]. Images of structures were generated using UCSF Chimera [20]. MDS was performed using the Molegro Virtual Docker (MVD) [21]. The conformation with the lowest docked energy produced by Chiglitazar against either 2PRG or 2XKW was chosen as the proposed mode. The MDS modes for rosiglitazone and pioglitazone were referenced from published sources [18, 19]. The output structure figures were prepared with PyMOL (DeLano Scientific LLC) [22].

2.4. Gene Expression Analysis by Real-Time RT-PCR and Immunoblot. HPA-v cells were cultured overnight in 6-well plates with the appropriate medium before use. After a 24-hour incubation with the tested compounds at varying concentrations or vehicle control (0.1% vol/vol dimethyl sulfoxide (DMSO)), cells were collected and total RNA was extracted using TRIzol reagent (Invitrogen, Life Technologies, Carlsbad, CA, USA) followed by purification using the RNeasy Mini Kit (Qiagen, Venlo, Germany, USA). The concentration of RNA was assessed using the UV spectrometer DU520 (Beckman Coulter, Brea, CA, USA). First-strand cDNA was synthesized by SuperScript II reverse transcriptase (Invitrogen) according to the manufacturer's instructions. Real-time PCR was performed with StepOnePlus™ (Applied Biosystems, Life Technologies, Carlsbad, CA, USA) using the FastStart High Fidelity PCR kit (Roche, Molecular Biochemicals, Indianapolis, IN, USA). Primer sequences used were as follows: *CD36*, F: 5′ CATCGCTGGGGCTGTCATT 3′, R: 5′ GCGTCCTGGGTTACATTTTCC 3′; *ANGPTL4*, F: 5′ GCAGCCATTCCAACCTCAA 3′, R: 5′ CAAGAGTCACCGTCTTTCGTG 3′; *PDK4*, F: 5′ ATGTCATTGGCAAGAGGAAGAA 3′, R: 5′ ATTACCAGAAGCACCACAACACT 3′; *LIPE* (lipase, hormone-sensitive), F: 5′ CCCTGCTCCTCCGAGACTT 3′, R: 5′ GGACTTGCGCCCACTTAACT 3′; *β*-actin, F: 5′ AGTTGCGTTACACCCTTTC 3′, R: 5′ TGTCACCTTCACCGTTCC 3′. The relative gene expression level was normalized against *β*-actin. The fold change of expression induced by the various treatments was calculated as the relative expression level in treated samples divided by the vehicle sample or treatment control.

HPA-v cells were cultured in 60 mm plates overnight and then incubated with the indicated compounds at varying concentrations or vehicle control (0.1% *(vol/vol)* DMSO) for 48 hours. Proteins were extracted using the NE-PER Nuclear and Cytoplasmic Extraction Kit and quantitated with Pierce Micro BCA Protein Assay kit according to the manufacturer's instructions (Thermo Fisher Scientific, Waltham, MA, USA). The appropriate quantity of protein was loaded and separated by sodium dodecyl sulfate-polyacrylamide gel electrophoresis (SDS-PAGE) and then transferred to polyvinylidene difluoride membrane (Amersham Biosciences, GE Healthcare Life Sciences, Piscataway, NJ, USA). Blots were blocked for 1 hour at room temperature in TBST buffer (Tris-buffered saline-Tween 20) with 5% nonfat dry milk and subsequently incubated with individual primary antibodies. Primary antibodies for PPAR*γ* (Cell Signaling Technologies (CST), Danvers, MA; 81B8), phospho-(Ser) CDKs substrates (CST; 2324), *β*-Actin (Santa Cruz Biotechnology, San Jose, CA; 69879), LIPE (Abcam, Cambridge, UK; ab45422), CD36 (Abcam; ab17044), PDK4 (Abcam; ab71240), and ANGPTL4 (Abcam; ab95194) were used according to the manufacturer's recommendation. After three washes with TBST buffer, membranes were incubated at room temperature for 1 hour with the respective secondary antibodies according to the manufacturer's recommendation. The bands were visualized with Super ECL Plus Detection Reagent (Applygen, China) and exposed to Kodak X-OMAT film. The film was scanned and transformed to gray-scale graphs with the Bio-Print gel scanner and accessory software (Vilber Lourmat, France).

2.5. Cell Transfection for Reporter Gene Assay and Gene Expression Analysis. Cell transfection was performed as described previously using the same constructs for the luciferase reporter assay [12, 13]. Briefly, L-02 cells were seeded into 96-well plates the day before transfection to obtain 50–80% confluence at the time of transfection. For the reporter assay, plasmids expressing hRXR (10 ng), pGFP (10 ng), the relevant PPAR isoform (10 ng), and the corresponding reporter plasmid (30 ng) were cotransfected using FuGENE 6 transfection reagent (Roche) according to the manufacturer's instructions. At 48 hours after transfection, cells were treated with the indicated compounds at various concentrations or vehicle control (0.1% *(vol/vol)* DMSO) for 24 hours. Luciferase activity was measured using a luciferase assay kit from Promega (Madison, WI, USA). GFP fluorescence and luciferase activity were sequentially detected using the Fluoroskan Ascent FL reader (Thermo Labsystems, Helsinki, Finland). Reporter gene expression as represented by luciferase activity was normalized against GFP fluorescence in the same well. Reporter induction by the tested compounds was compared with the vehicle control (i.e., DMSO).

To detect changes in gene expression, L-02 cells were seeded into 6-well plates and cotransfected with plasmids expressing hRXR and different PPAR subtypes. At 48 hours after transfection, cells were incubated with the tested compounds at the indicated concentrations or vehicle control (0.1% *(vol/vol)* DMSO) for 24 hours. Total RNA was extracted and then real-time RT-PCR was performed as described above.

2.6. Immunoprecipitation (IP) and Immunoblot of PPARγ. HPA-v cells were cultured in 60 mm plates overnight and then incubated with the indicated compounds or DMSO. Cell lysates were dissolved in Pierce IP Lysis Buffer (Thermo Fisher Scientific) and then incubated with anti-PPAR*γ* primary antibody (CST, 81B8) at 4°C overnight prior to mixing with protein G-Sepharose beads (Thermo Fisher Scientific) for 2 hours. The beads were washed three times with lysis buffer, and the immunoprecipitates were recovered and dissolved in SDS loading buffer. Equal amounts of immunoprecipitates were loaded and separated by SDS-PAGE prior to immunoblot analysis using primary antibodies against PPAR*γ* (CST; 81B8) and phospho-(Ser) CDKs substrates (CST; 2324).

2.7. Site-Directed Mutagenesis. Site-directed mutagenesis of amino acid sites in human PPAR*γ*2 (serine 289, glutamine 343, and tyrosine 473) [23] was conducted by inserting full-length human *PPARγ2* into the pcDNA3.1 vector using the QuikChange site-directed mutagenesis kit (Stratagene, La Jolla, CA, USA) as recommended by the manufacturer. The following primer pairs were used for site-directed mutagenesis: PPAR*γ* S289A, F: 5′ GCTGCCAGTTTCGC**G**CCGTGGAGGCTGT 3′, R: 5′ ACAGCCTCCACGGCGC-GAAACTGGCAGC 3′, where TCC (serine) was substituted with GCC (Alanine); Y473D, F: 5′ CTCCTGCAGGAGATC**G**ACAAGGACTTGTACTAG 3′, R: 5′ CTAGTACAAGTCCTTGTCGATCTCCTGCAGGAG 3′, where TAC (tyrosine) was substituted with GAC (aspartic acid); E343A, F: 5′ GGGTTCTCATATCCG**C**GGGCCAAGGCTTCA 3′, R: 5′ TGAAGCCTTGGCCCGCGGATATGAGAACCC 3′, where GAG (glutamate acid) was substituted with GCG (alanine). The primer pair and its endonuclease site for subcloning were as follows: NheI F: 5′ CTGGCTAGCGT-TATGGGTGAAACTCTGG 3′, XhoI R: 5′ GGCCTCGAGC-TAGTACAAGTCCTTGTA 3′. All constructs were confirmed by full-length sequencing.

2.8. Chromatin Immunoprecipitation (ChIP).

2.8. Chromatin Immunoprecipitation (ChIP). The Chromatin Immunoprecipitation (ChIP) assay kit (Upstate/Millipore, Temecula, CA, USA) was used according to the manufacturer's instructions. Briefly, after incubation with the indicated treatments, HPA-v cells were fixed with 1% formaldehyde at 37°C for 15 minutes and then sonicated using the XO-900D Ultrasonic cell disruption apparatus (Nanjing, China). After removing debris with protein A-agarose beads, an aliquot of supernatant was taken as the input control. The same sample volume was subjected to immunoprecipitation with anti-PPARγ antibody (CST; 81B8) as described above. The DNA fragments were subsequently recovered using a QIAquick column (Qiagen). Real-time PCR was performed as described above using the following sequence-specific primer pairs against target gene promoters: *ANGPTL4*, F: 5′ TGAGCT-CTTCTCCGTTCATCTCGAACCAC 3′, R: 5′ GAGTCTAGA-CATCTCAGAGGCTCTGCCTG 3′; *PDK4*, F: 5′ GGATTT-CAACAGCCAGTGCT 3′, R: 5′ ATAGTGCTGCCCAGTGT-GTG 3′; *CD36*, F: 5′ ATTTGTGGTTGGTTGCCAAG 3′, R: 5′ AGGTGATGGGTCTTCACCAG 3′; *LIPE*, F: 5′ CAA-GTGATTGGGATGAAGCA 3′, R: 5′ CTAGCCAGCCCA-GTCTTCAG 3′; insulin, F: 5′ CTTCAGCCCAGTTGAC-CAAT 3′, R: 5′ AGGGAGGAGGAAAGCAGAAC 3′. Real-time PCR of the *insulin* promoter was used as a negative control. The respective input samples were taken as internal (loading) controls. Real-time PCR was performed as described above. Promoter binding was evaluated by normalizing the Ct (threshold cycle of PCR) value of samples immunoprecipitated with anti-PPARγ antibody against the Ct of respective Input controls.

2.9. In Vitro Phosphorylation and the Cofactor Recruitment Assay.

2.9. In Vitro Phosphorylation and the Cofactor Recruitment Assay. Active heterodimer of CDK5/p25 was purchased from Millipore (cat. number 14-516). Recombinant human His-PPARγ-LBD fragment was expressed and purified as described previously [24]. *In vitro* phosphorylation of PPARγ-LBD (ligand binding domain) was performed in a 50 μl reaction volume consisting of the individual tested agonists or vehicle control (DMSO) at the indicated concentration, 1 μg of His-PPARγ-LBD, 30–50 ng of active CDK5/p25, and 100 mM ATP in 1x kinase buffer. The reaction was incubated at 30°C for 30 minutes and then subjected to immunoblot analysis or the AlphaScreen assay of cofactor binding.

The representative LXXLL peptide motifs of different cofactors were synthesized according to published literature. The binding of various peptide motifs to PPARγ-LBD was determined using the AlphaScreen assay (AlphaScreen® Histidine (Nickel Chelate) Detection Kit, Perkin-Elmer, Waltham, MA, USA) as described previously [24]. The conventional assay was conducted with approximately 40 nM His-tagged PPARγ-LBD and 40 nM of the respective biotinylated peptides in the presence of 5 μg/ml donor and acceptor beads in a buffer containing 50 nM MOPS, 50 mM

NaF, 50 mM CHAPS, and 0.1 mg/ml bovine serum albumin, pH 7.4. For the cofactor binding assay with phosphorylated PPARγ-LBD, *in vitro* phosphorylation was first performed as described above followed by the conventional AlphaScreen procedure. The phosphorylation status of PPARγ-LBD was varied depending on the presence of CDK5/p25, ATP, or tested agonists or their order of addition into the *in vitro* phosphorylation reaction. For example, "LBD + CDK5 − ATP + agonist" represents no ATP in the phosphorylation reaction; "LBD + CDK5 + ATP + agonist" represents that all components were present in the phosphorylation reaction. Furthermore, "(LBD + CDK5 + ATP) + agonist" denotes that *in vitro* phosphorylation was completed before agonist was added. The representative biotinylated peptide motifs used were as follows: NCOR2 (nuclear receptor corepressor 2): Biotin-GHSFADPASNLGLEDIIRKALMGSF; PGC1a (peroxisome proliferator-activated receptor gamma, coactivator 1 alpha): Biotin-QEAEEPSLLKKLLLAPANTQ; SRC1-2 (nuclear receptor coactivator 1): Biotin-SPSSHSSLTERHKILHRLLQEGSP; SRC2-3 (nuclear receptor coactivator 2): Biotin-SPKKKENALLRYLLDKDDT; SRC3-3 (nuclear receptor coactivator 3): Biotin-SPKKKENALL-RYLLDRDD; TRAP1b (mediator complex subunit 1, MED1): Biotin-FSKVSQNPILTSLLQITGN.

The fold change of baseline cofactor recruitment induction is represented as the ratio of the relative luciferase unit (RLU) value from the ligand-free binding reaction with cofactor divided by the value with no peptide in presence. The fold change of cofactor recruitment induction by the tested agonists was calculated as the ratio of the RLU value from the binding reaction with agonist divided by vehicle control (DMSO).

2.10. Statistical Analysis. Student's *t*-test was performed to determine statistical significance as needed. Statistical significance between the different comparisons was defined as $p < 0.01$.

3. Results

3.1. Differential Induction of ANGPTL4 and PDK4 Expression by Chiglitazar and TZD Class Compounds. During the process of investigating the differential effects of Chi and the TZD compounds on the expression of genes involved in lipid metabolism and insulin sensitization, we identified two genes among multiple known PPARγ targets (Supplementary Figure 1 in Supplementary Material available online at https://doi.org/10.1155/2017/4313561), *ANGPTL4* and *PDK4*, which were preferentially induced by Chi. As shown in Figure 1, in human preadipocyte HPA-v cells, mRNA and protein from *ANGPTL4* and *PDK4* were significantly induced by Chi compared to Ros or Pio. Consistent with previous findings [16], the expressions of *CD36* and *LIPE*, two well-established PPARγ target genes, were similar following the treatments with each compound (Figure 1(c)).

ANGPTL4 and *PDK4* are regulated by PPARδ and to a lesser extent by other PPAR subtypes [17, 18]. Is the PPARδ activity from pan agonist Chi the only factor that contributes to the observed significantly higher induction of these two

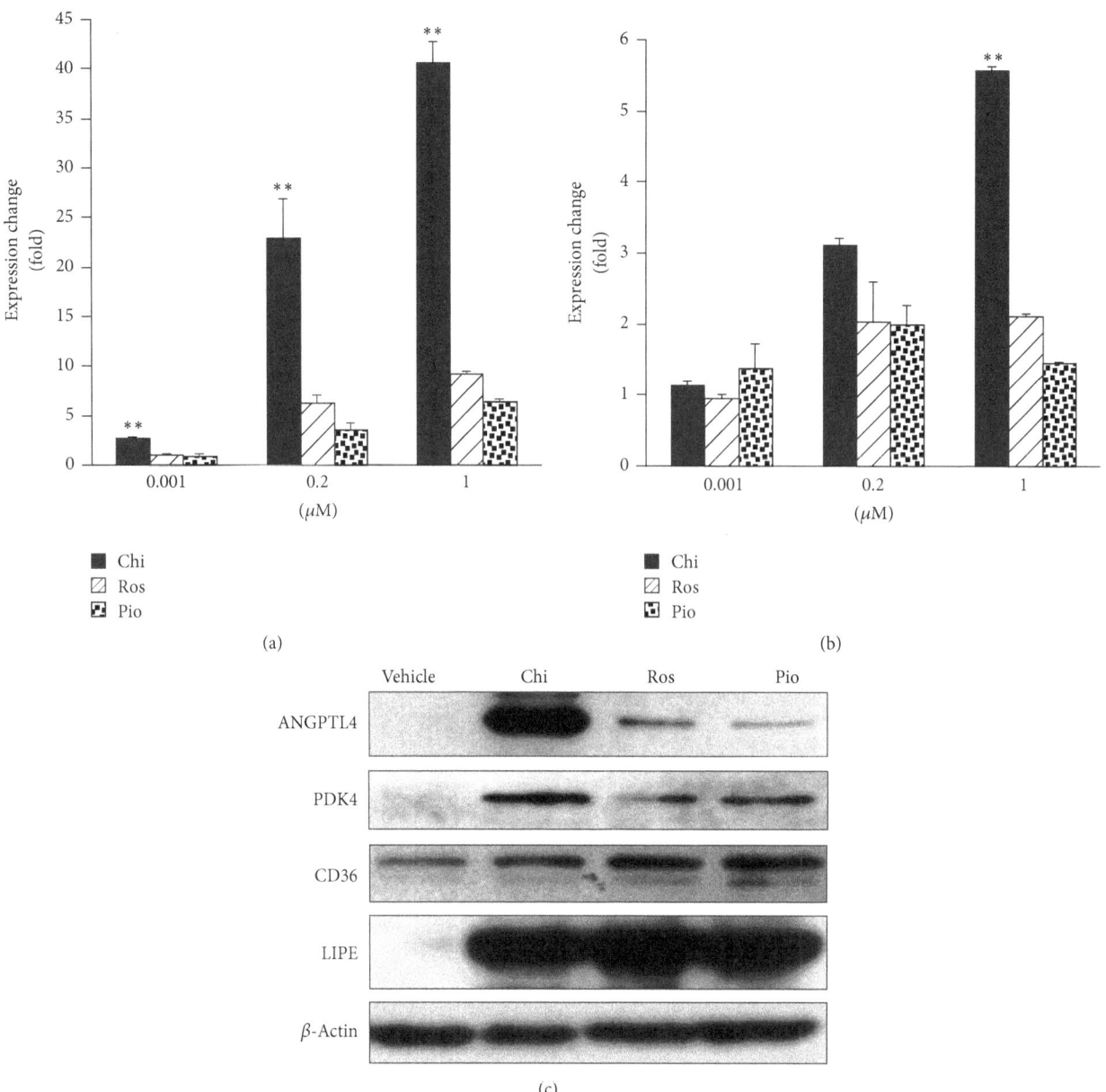

FIGURE 1: Preferential induction of *ANGPTL4* and *PDK4* mRNA and protein by chiglitazar. (a) and (b) Human preadipocyte HPA-v cells were incubated with different concentrations of the three agonists for 24 hours before total RNA was collected and purified. Real-time RT-PCR was performed as described in *Materials and Methods*. The dose-dependent changes in *ANGPTL4* (a) and *PDK4* (b) expression induced by the different agonists were normalized against the sample treated with vehicle (0.01% *(vol/vol)* DMSO) only. (c) HPA-v cells were incubated with 1 μM of each agonist for 48 hours. Protein levels were assessed by immunoblot analysis using the respective primary antibodies (β-Actin, 1:1000; LIPE, 1:1000; CD36, 1:1000; PDK4, 1:500; ANGPTL4, 1:500) as described in *Materials and Methods*. Chi: chiglitazar; Ros: rosiglitazone; Pio: pioglitazone; LIPE: lipase, hormone-sensitive (HSL). Data represent the average and standard deviation of three independent experiments. $**$ represents statistically significant differences in expression induction by Chi relative to Ros and Pio ($p < 0.01$).

genes? We treated a human hepatocyte cell line, L-02, which expresses little endogenous PPARs and their target genes, including *ANGPTL4* and *PDK4*, when treating the cells with Chi, Ros, and Pio (Supplementary Figure 2). As shown in Figure 2, while Chi induced *ANGPTL4* and *PDK4* significantly in PPARδ-transfected cells, this PPAR pan agonist also upregulated both genes even more significantly in PPARγ- but not PPARα-transfected cells compared to Ros and Pio

in this cell model. These results suggest that *ANGPTL4* and *PDK4* expressions are upregulated not only in response to PPARδ activation but also by PPARγ. However, this induction of gene expression following agonist treatments does not appear to be correlated with PPARγ transactivity, since Chi consistently produces less potent PPARγ transactivation relative to Ros in different cell model systems [16]. Consistent with this, reporter assays demonstrate that treatment of L-02

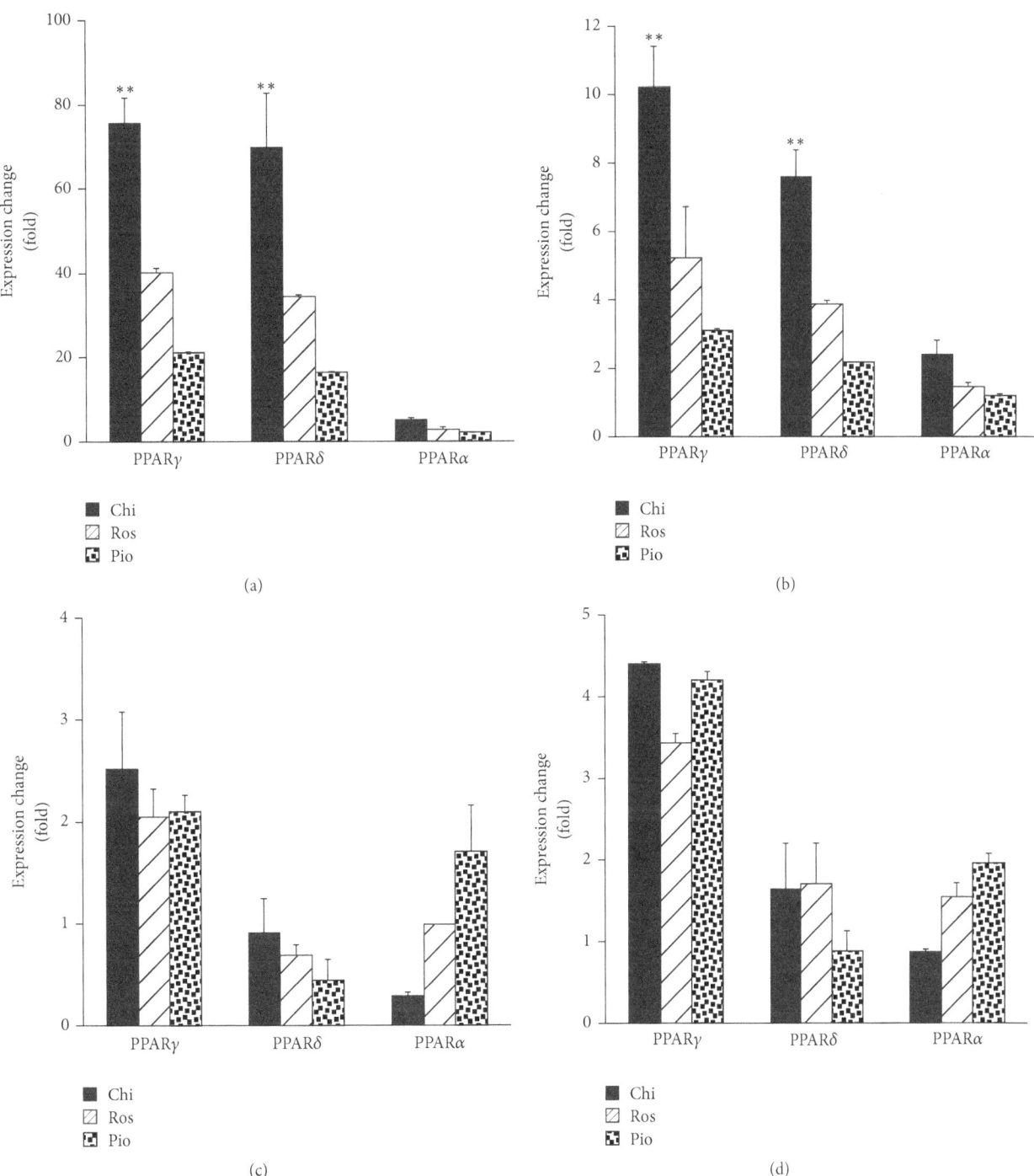

FIGURE 2: Chiglitazar preferentially induced *ANGPTL4* and *PDK4* expression via both PPARγ and PPARδ. Human hepatic L-02 cells were cotransfected with plasmids expressing the three PPAR subtypes or an empty vector and hRXR. At 48 hours after transfection, cells were incubated with 1 μM of each agonist or the vehicle control (0.1% *(vol/vol)* DMSO) for 24 hours. The mRNA level of each target gene was determined by real-time RT-PCR as described in *Materials and Methods*. Induced expression changes of ANGPTL4 (a), PDK4 (b), CD36 (c), and LIPE (d) were evaluated by comparison against the vehicle control. Data represent the average and standard deviation of three independent experiments. ** represents statistically significant differences in expression induction by Chi relative to Ros and Pio ($p < 0.01$).

cells with Chi, Ros, and Pio yielded AC_{50} for PPARγ transitivity of 0.120 ± 0.047, 0.035 ± 0.037, and 0.288 ± 0.514 μM, respectively (mean ± SD, Supplementary Figure 3).

3.2. Chiglitazar and TZD Class Compounds Differentially Bind to PPARγ and Inhibit CDK5-Mediated Phosphorylation. Chi possesses a non-TZD structure with a relatively restricted configuration. Simulated molecular docking with the published PPARγ crystal structure [19] revealed that both Ros (Figure 3(a)) and Pio (Figure 3(b)) form hydrogen bonds with PPARγ via Tyr-473 of helix 12 and His-323 of helix 5, which is consistent with a typical full agonist binding model [25, 26]. However, Chi (Figure 3(c)) did not exhibit any hydrogen bond donor or acceptors in proximity to helices 12 and 5; this compound most likely does not form hydrogen bonds with these two sites. Instead, Chi forms hydrogen bonds with Ser-289 and Arg-288 of helix 3 and Glu-343 of the β-sheet. To verify the different binding modes between them, we performed serial site-directed mutations of the referred residues on the receptor including Tyr-473Asp (Y473D), Ser-289Ala (S289A), and Glu-343Ala (E343A), respectively. Unexpectedly, the Y473D mutation significantly diminished the transactivity of Chi as well as Ros and Pio in reporter gene assay (Figures 3(d)–3(f)), despite no hydrogen bond between Chi and PPARγ at this region, which is different from SR1664, a known partial PPARγ agonist, showing no interaction with Y473 (Supplementary Figure 4) [11]. Among other interaction residues, only S289A mutation attenuates the transactivity of Chi which is different from Ros and Pio (Figures 3(d)–3(f)). It seems that Chi might act like a full agonist fashion in terms of ligand-receptor interaction with helices 12 and 5 but differently affect the receptor activity via its configuration-restricted binding mode with particular residues in other regions. Recent studies have shown that PPARγ activity can be modulated by CDK5-mediated phosphorylation at S273 [12], and Glu-343 is adjacent to the reported phosphorylation pocket. Based on this unique receptor-ligand binding model, we hypothesized that, compared with TZDs, Chi might interact with PPARγ by preferentially inhibiting the receptor phosphorylation and, thus, producing a differential pattern of the PPARγ-targeted gene regulation.

To test this hypothesis, the preadipocyte HPA-v cells were incubated with the ligands in the presence or absence of TNFα, an inducer of CDK5-mediated PPARγ phosphorylation [12]. The cell extracts were immunoprecipitated using antibody against PPARγ and then the immunoprecipitates were visualized by immunoblotting using anti-phospho-(Ser) CDKs substrate antibody. While Chi and the two TZDs all exhibited dose-dependent inhibition in TNFα-enhanced phosphorylation of PPARγ in HPA-v cells, Chi produced a stronger inhibitory effect even at 0.05 and 0.2 μM (Figure 4(a)). To confirm this result, we performed an *in vitro* phosphorylation reaction with purified recombinant human His-PPARγ ligand binding domain (LBD) [24] and the active heterodimer of CDK5/p25. Our results show that 0.2 and 2 μM Chi inhibits CDK5-mediated phosphorylation of the PPARγ-LBD significantly greater than the two TZDs tested (Figure 4(b)). These experiments demonstrated that Chi exhibited a stronger inhibitory effect on CDK5-mediated

PPARγ phosphorylation compared with that of the two TZD compounds.

To investigate the role of CDK5-mediated PPARγ phosphorylation in regulating target gene expression, we examined PPAR target gene expression in TNFα-treated HPA-v cells incubated with a panel of kinase inhibitors (Sutent for VEGFRs and PDGFRs, VX680 for AURK A/B/C, U0126 for MEK1/2, and roscovitine for CDK5). Expressions of *ANGPTL4* and *PDK4* were only induced by roscovitine treatment, indicating that this event is CDK5 kinase-dependent. Meanwhile, induction of the classic PPARγ target genes, *CD36* and *LIPE*, was not changed in HPA-v cells by the treatment with above-mentioned kinase inhibitors (Figure 5), suggesting, at least, that the induction of these two target genes is unlikely due to the phosphorylation status of PPARγ. These results suggest a direct link between CDK5-mediated PPARγ phosphorylation and *ANGPTL4* and *PDK4* expression. Taken together, this differential inhibitory effect of Chi on CDK5-mediated PPARγ phosphorylation perhaps explains why this compound induces *ANGPTL4* and *PDK4* expressions greater than TZDs.

3.3. Chiglitazar Differentially Affects Promoter Binding of PPARγ-Containing Transcription Complex and Cofactor Recruitment upon CDK5-Mediated Phosphorylation. PPARs heterodimerize with the retinoid X receptor (RXR) to recruit cofactors (e.g., coactivators or corepressors) upon specific ligand binding or to induce protein-protein interactions (e.g., with chromatin-binding proteins) that result in formation of a transcriptome that regulates downstream target genes [27, 28]. Studies have reported that the unique β-sheet region of the PPARγ-LBD, in which S273 is located, interacts with the RXRα DNA binding domain (DBD) [29, 30]. Thus, it is highly possible that phosphorylation of PPARγ at S273 may affect its interaction with RXR and subsequent promoter binding. We performed ChIP assays to test the promoter binding of PPARγ-containing transcription complex induced by Chi, Ros, and Pio in the presence and absence of S273 phosphorylation. In absence of TNFα, it is clear that Chi induced greater recruitment of PPARγ-containing complexes to the *ANGPTL4* and *PDK4* promoters than *CD36* and *LIPE* (Figure 6). Most strikingly, TNFα stimulation repressed the binding of PPARγ-containing complexes to all four target gene promoters examined in HPA-v cells treated with the agonists, while Chi seems to keep stronger recruitment of PPARγ-containing complexes to the *ANGPTL4* and *PDK4* promoters compared with the *CD36* and *LIPE* promoters (Figure 6). These results suggest a general, rather than gene-specific, repression of promoter binding by PPARγ in response to TNFα via S273 phosphorylation and possibly ERK signaling [31].

Next, we performed an AlphaScreen assay using purified recombinant PPARγ-LBD to see whether specific cofactor recruitment is affected by S273 phosphorylation during target gene regulation. Our data show, for the first time, that *in vitro* phosphorylation of PPARγ by CDK5 inhibited cofactor recruitment (Figure 7). Among the six cofactors examined, recruitments of coactivator PGC1a and corepressor NCOR2, which displayed significant baseline binding activity to the

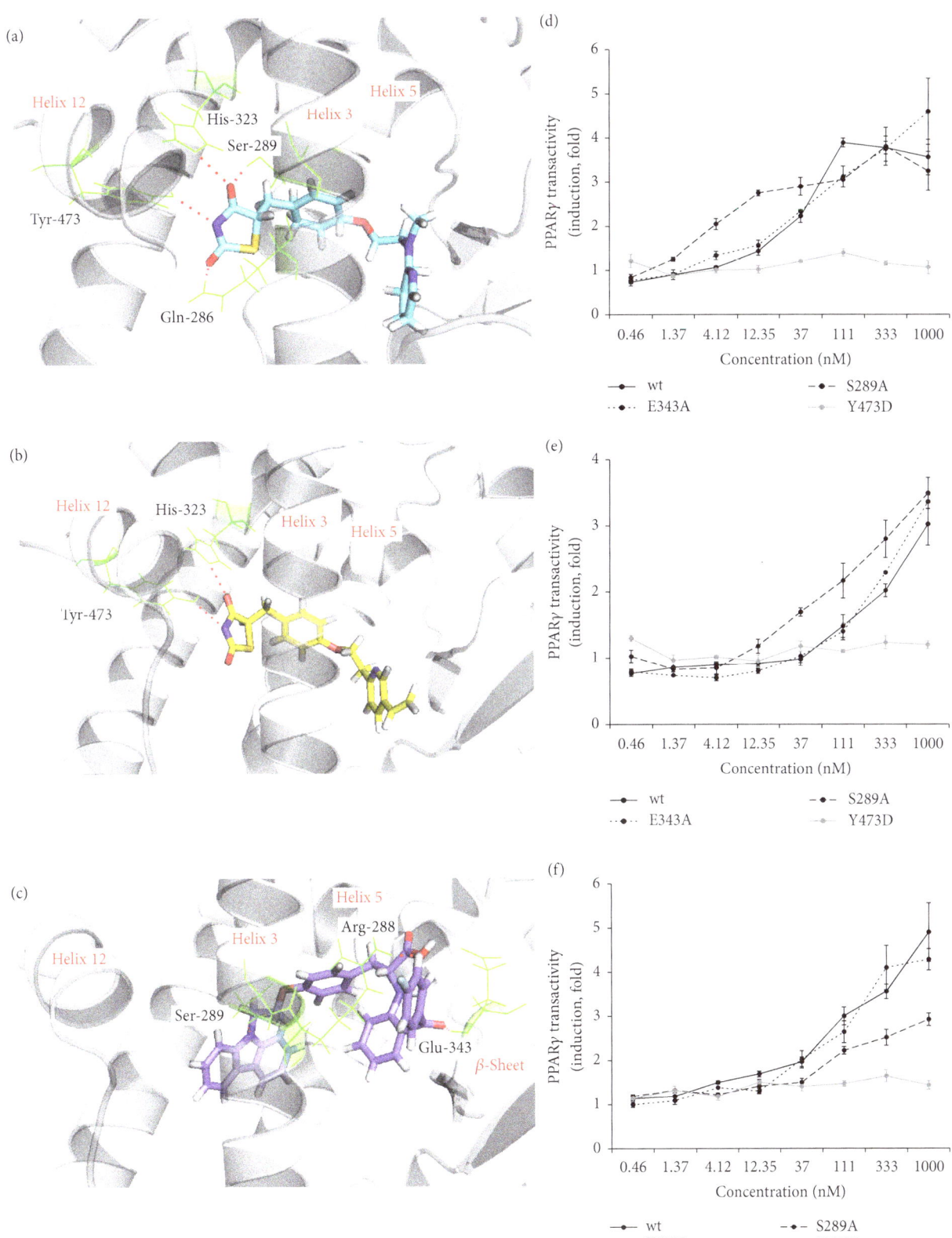

FIGURE 3: Chiglitazar binds PPARγ differently from rosiglitazone and pioglitazone. (a)–(c) Simulated molecular docking of each agonist to the crystal structure of PPARγ (PDB code: 2PRG, 2XKW as shown in gray) was performed using Molegro Virtual Docker software. Ros ((a), in cyan, docking to 2PRG) and Pio ((b), in yellow, docking to 2XKW) have typical modes of interaction with the receptor via hydrogen bonding to helix 12 (Tyr-473) and helix 5 (His-323) (residues in green, hydrogen bonds shown in dotted red lines). In this conformation, helix 12, along with helices 3–5, forms the coactivator-binding site (AF-2) responsible for full agonist activity. Chi ((c), in blue, docking to 2XKW) does not form typical hydrogen bonding to helices 12 and 5 but rather forms alternative hydrogen bonds to helix 3 and the receptor β-sheet (residues in green). This conformation is highly similar to the partial agonist MRL-24. (d)–(g) Site-directed mutation of PPARγ differently affects transactivity of different agonists (Ros (d), Pio (e), and Chi (f)) compared with wild-type receptor by reporter gene assay. PPARγ with site-directed mutation at Y473D, E343A, or S289A, respectively, was constructed and applied in reporter gene assay as described in *Materials and Methods*.

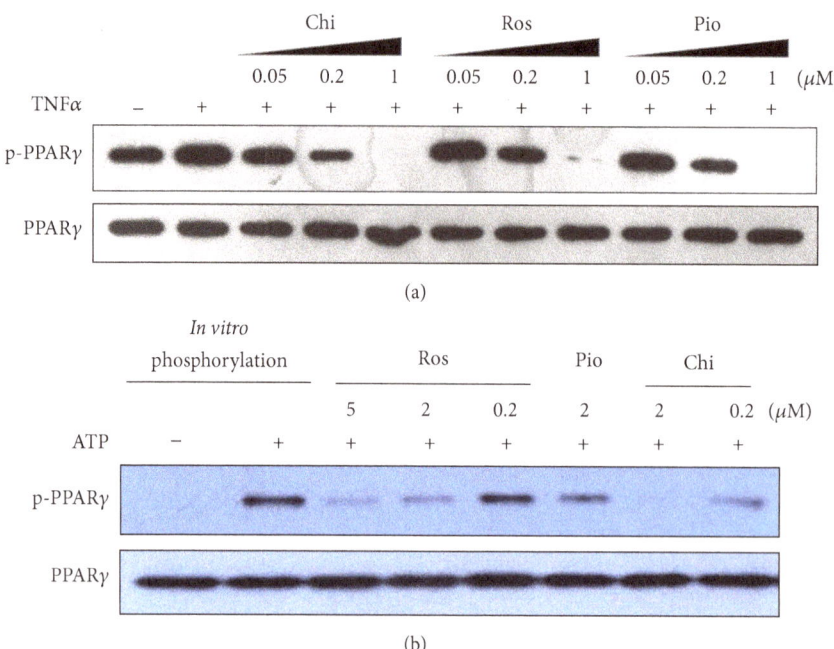

(a)

(b)

FIGURE 4: Chiglitazar inhibited TNFα-induced and CDK5-mediated phosphorylation of PPARγ. (a) HPA-v cells were cultured in 10 cm plates and incubated with each agonist at the indicated concentration in the presence or absence of TNFα (5 ng/ml). Cells were lysed and then subjected to immunoprecipitation (IP) with primary anti-PPARγ antibody followed by SDS-PAGE and immunoblot analysis as described in *Materials and Methods*. (b) *In vitro* phosphorylation was performed using purified active CDK5/p25 (5 ng/mL) and purified recombinant human PPARγ-LBD. Chi, Ros, and Pio were added to the reaction, respectively, at the indicated concentrations in presence of TNFα (5 ng/ml) and then incubated for 30 minutes at 30°C. Immunoblot analysis was performed to determine the levels of the specified proteins.

LBD independent of ligand binding (Supplementary Figure 5), were not significantly affected by the phosphorylation status of PPARγ at S273. Nevertheless, recruitments of other coactivators, namely, SRC1, SRC2, SRC3, and TRAP1b (MED1), were significantly inhibited by CDK5-mediated phosphorylation of the receptor. The inhibition was partially and differentially restored upon additions of the three ligands, consistent with their inhibition potency on *in vitro* phosphorylation at S273 (Figure 4(b)). NCOR2 served as major corepressor to recruit HDAC (histone deacetylase) to form a complex and further repress transcription activity of PPARγ. Noticeably, there are significantly more chi-bound PPARγ-LBD dissociated from NCOR2 complex than the two TZDs-bound PPARγ-LBD; this differential phenomenon cannot be observed in reporter gene assay.

4. Discussion

Although TZD-like drugs such as Ros and Pio are promising therapeutics for the treatment of T2DM patients [1, 2], the potential safety risks linked to cardiovascular diseases and other undesired effects greatly limit their application [32, 33]. New generation of PPAR ligands designated as subtype-selective PPAR modulator, transcriptional-inactive PPARγ synthetic ligand, or pan agonist is currently under preclinical or clinical development [9, 15, 34–38]. The different PPAR subtypes possess overlapping and sometimes antagonistic effects on different aspects of glucose-lipid metabolism, inflammatory regulation, and other biological pathways. The

limitations of current knowledge regarding exact mechanism of each subtype and partial inability to further differentiate each other generally halt the development progress [39]. Recent studies have revealed that specific phosphorylation of S273 on PPARγ by obesity-linked or high-fat-diet-induced activation of CDK5, which leads to insulin resistance in animals and humans, can be ameliorated by treatment with TZDs or ligands without transactivation of PPARγ via inhibition of CDK5-mediated S273 phosphorylation [11, 14]. Considering that S273 phosphorylation by CDK5 is unique to PPARγ, this event is important for dictating binding to the promoter of potential target genes related to glucose and lipid regulation, since PPARγ heterodimerizes with DBD region of RXRα via the β-sheet domain in which S273 resides. Thus, it is essential to understand how the effects of this phosphorylation functionally differentiate PPARγ from other subtypes and the subsequent role of configuration-restricted non-TZD ligands in generating a more balanced or beneficial effect during modulation of glucose/lipid/energy metabolism.

Chi moderately but significantly activates all three PPAR subtypes and the AC_{50} values of them are clinically achievable concentrations. Results from our docking study with the crystal structure of PPARγ demonstrated that Chi does not form a typical binding model as that of TZD-type PPARγ full agonist (e.g., Ros) (Figure 3). Instead, Chi forms hydrogen bonds with Arg-288 of helix H3 and Glu-343 of the β-sheet adjacent to the CDK5 phosphorylation pocket. This binding model is very similar to that of MRL-24, a partial agonist of PPARγ

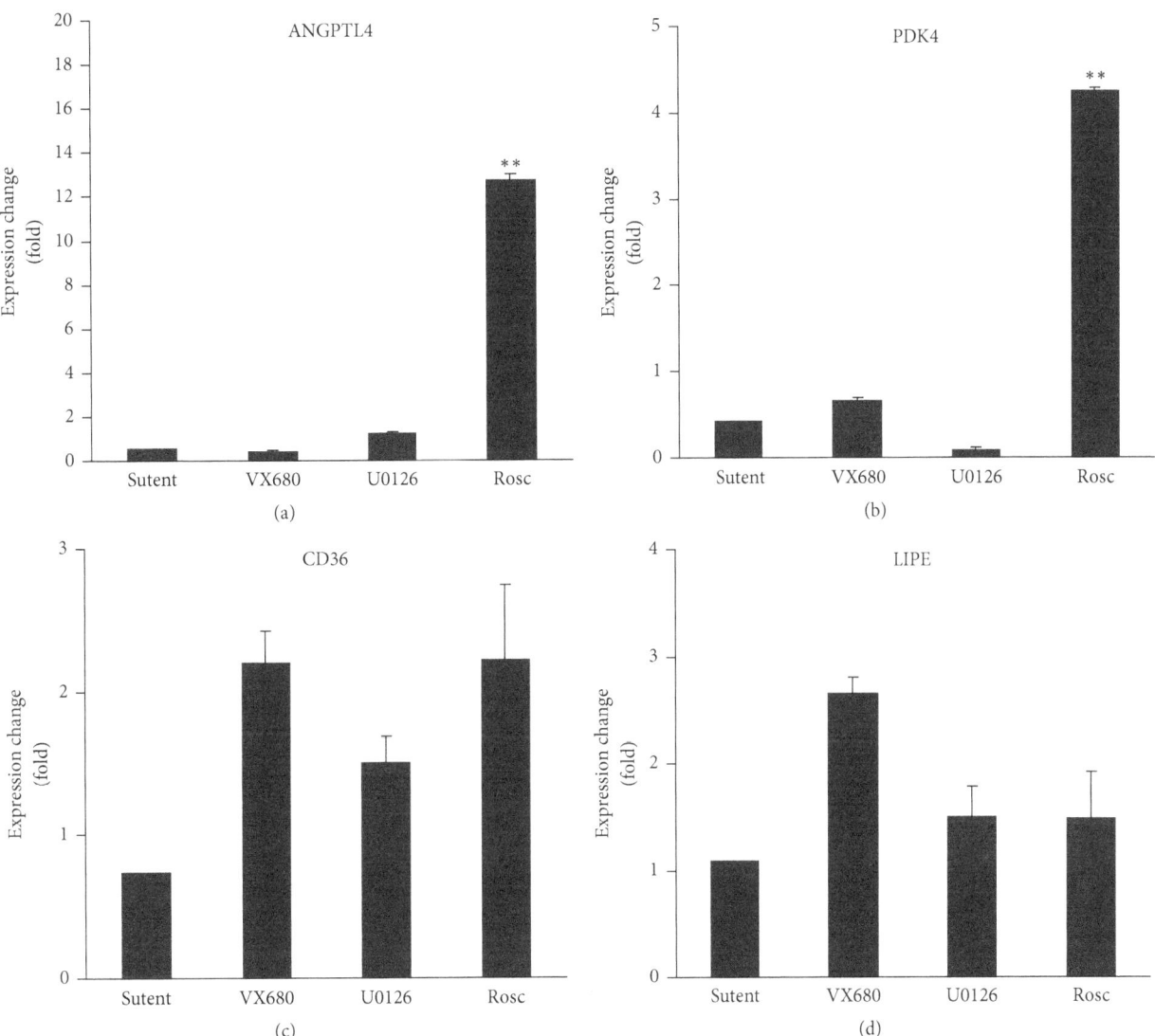

FIGURE 5: Increased *ANGPTL4* and *PDK4* expressions are associated with inhibition of TNFα-induced and CDK5-mediated phosphorylation of PPARγ. HPA-v cells were incubated with different protein kinases (i.e., VEGFR and PDGFR inhibitor Sutent (1 μM), AURK A/B/C inhibitor VX680 (0.1 μM), MEK1/2 inhibitor U0126 (1 μM), and CDK5 inhibitor roscovitine (Rosc, 10 μM) or vehicle control (0.1% *(vol/vol)* DMSO) in the presence of TNFα (5 ng/ml) for 24 hours. Total RNA was extracted and subjected to real-time RT-PCR as described in *Materials and Methods*. Data represent the average and standard deviation of three independent experiments. ∗∗ represents statistically significant differences in expression induction by roscovitine compared to all other inhibitors ($p < 0.01$).

[26]. Different agonists binding to the receptor could induce unique conformational changes, as revealed in a recent study utilizing nuclear magnetic resonance, hydrogen/deuterium exchange, and docking [40–42]. Ros has been shown to stabilize the AF2 domain and the β-sheet upon binding to the receptor, while MRL-24 mainly stabilizes the β-sheet. Despite the lack of cocrystal data for Chi, our docking study and reporter gene activation result with serial site-directed mutations are consistent with published literature showing that stabilization of the β-sheet is important in phosphorylation inhibition. As expected, Chi exhibited much stronger inhibition of CDK5-mediated phosphorylation of PPARγ at S273 in HPA-v cells (Figure 4(a)) and *in vitro* phosphorylation assays (Figure 4(b)) than the other two TZDs tested.

The increase in S273 phosphorylation has been linked to insulin resistance in obesity or T2DM patients, probably due to altered expression of genes involved in glucose, lipid, and energy homeostasis [11, 12]. Here, we demonstrated that S273 phosphorylation was directly related to the transcriptional regulation of two insulin resistance-related genes, *ANGPTL4* and *PDK4*. In the human preadipocyte HPA-v cell line, Chi differentially regulated a different set of target genes compared to Ros and Pio. Among them, expression of *ANGPTL4* and *PDK4* was dramatically higher following Chi treatment (Figure 1). This induction was specifically related to TNFα stimulation and CDK5-mediated S273 phosphorylation of PPARγ, since the CDK5 kinase inhibitor roscovitine mimicked the effect of Chi (Figure 5). Most strikingly, the expression of *ANGPTL4* and *PDK4* at the gene and protein

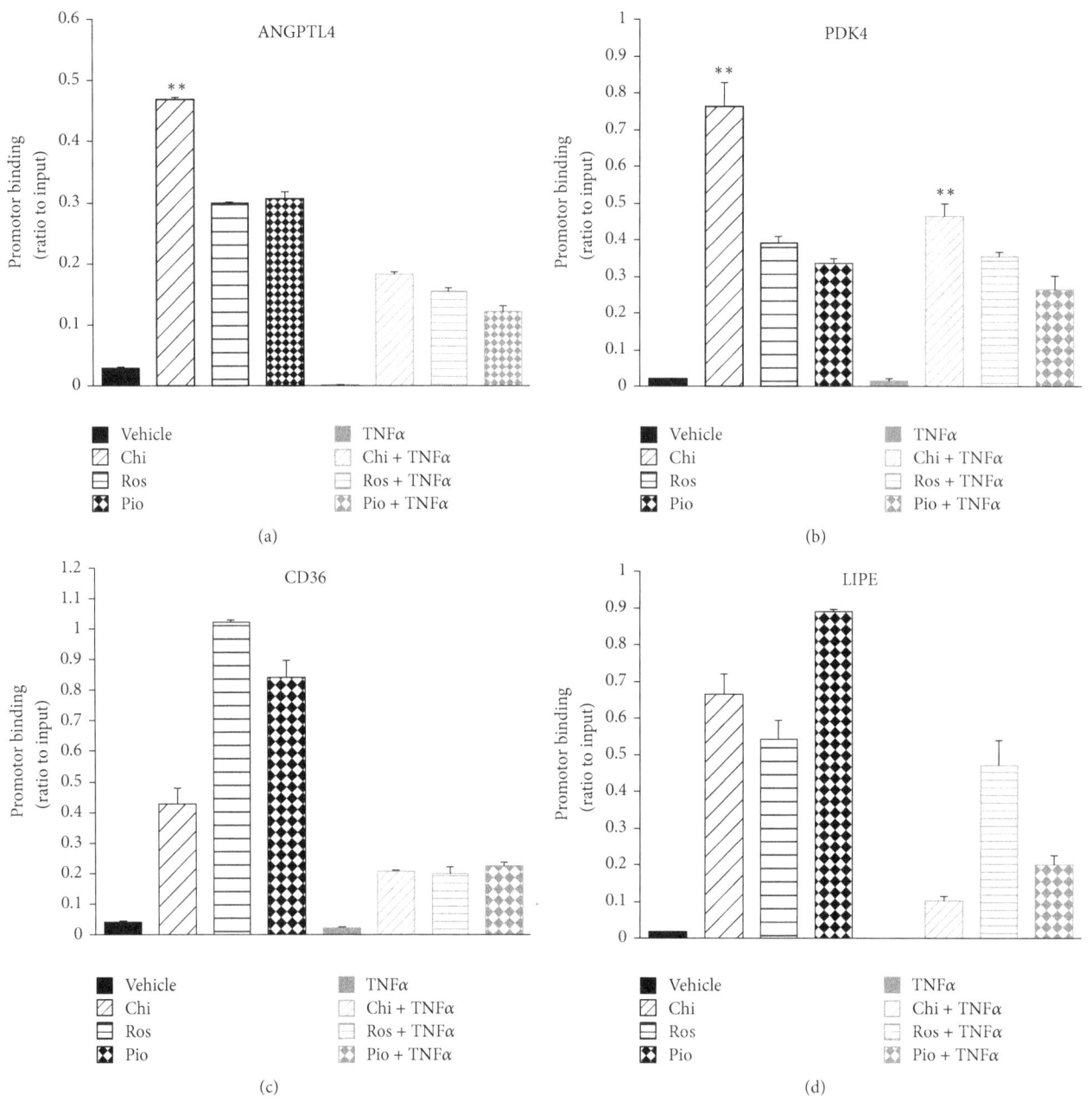

FIGURE 6: Chiglitazar differentially affects promoter binding of PPARγ-containing transcription complexes. HPA-v cells were incubated with Chi (1 μM), Ros (1 μM), Pio (1 μM), and vehicle control (0.1% (vol/vol) DMSO) in the presence or absence of TNFα (5 ng/ml) for 24 hours. ChIP assays using anti-PPARγ antibody were then performed as described in *Materials and Methods*. The relative abundance of promoters bound to PPARγ was normalized against the input control sample. The diagrammed results represent the average of two independent experiments. ∗∗ represents statistically significant differences in promoter binding induced by chiglitazar compared to the other two TZDs ($p < 0.01$).

levels appeared to be preferentially induced by Chi. However, other insulin sensitization-related genes such as *CD36* and *LIPE*, which are apparently not regulated by TNFα or CDK5-mediated S273 phosphorylation on PPARγ (Figure 5), displayed comparable expression with all three agonists (Figures 1 and 2). These results suggest a clear distinction between TZD and non-TZD type compounds such as Chi in regulation of insulin resistance, consistent with other reports demonstrating that CDK5-mediated S273 phosphorylation

on PPARγ independently regulates a specific set of insulin-sensitizing related genes [11, 12].

Our ChIP and AlphaScreen assays revealed that TNFα stimulation and CDK5-mediated phosphorylation indeed inhibit the promoter binding of PPARγ-containing transcription complexes on target genes, as well as cofactor recruitment. Chi could partially restore the recruitment activity of some cofactors (i.e., SRC1, SRC2, SRC3, and TRAP1b) but not others (i.e., NCOR2 and PGC1α) inhibited

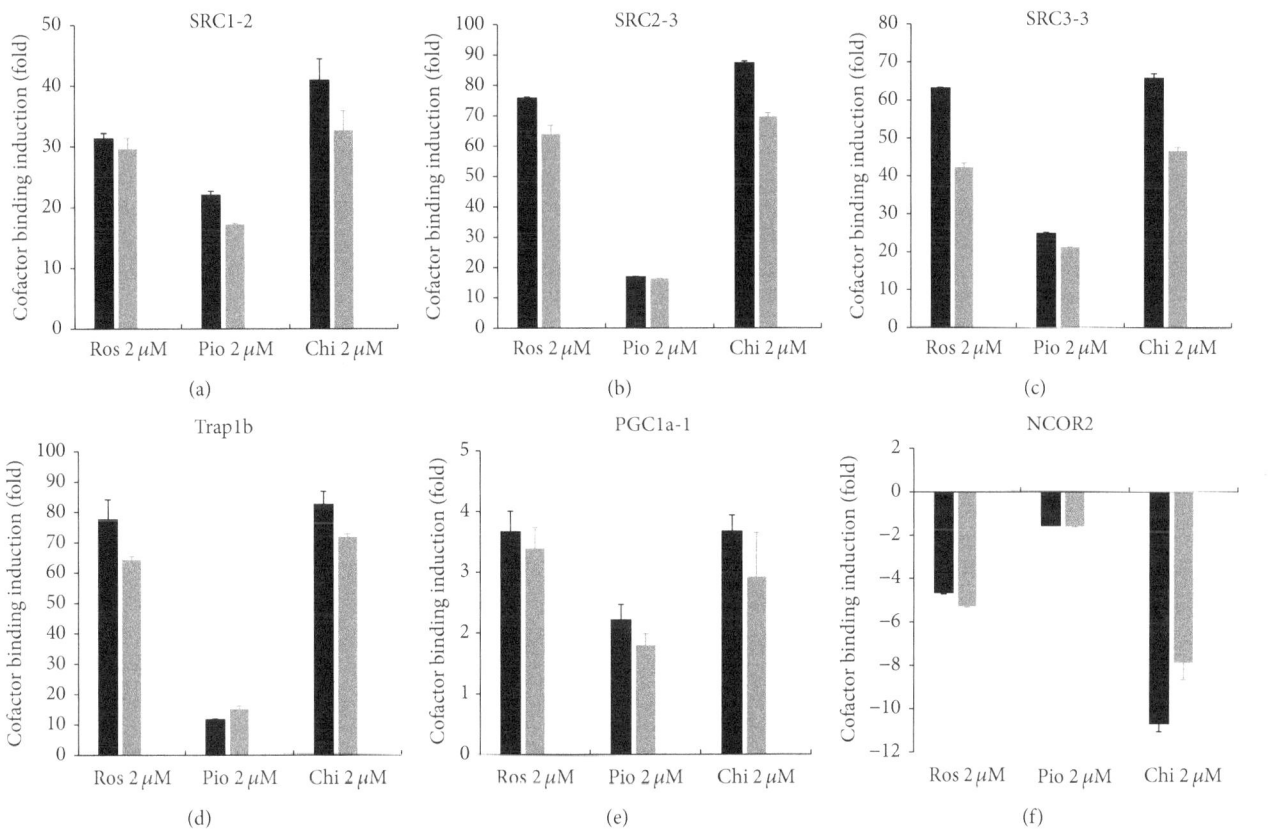

FIGURE 7: Chiglitazar differentially affects cofactor recruitment upon CDK5-mediated phosphorylation. AlphaScreen assay was performed to evaluate the recruitment of six representative LXXLL peptides to PPARγ-LBD following treatment with $2\,\mu M$ of Chi, Ros, and Pio as described in *Materials and Methods*. The S273 phosphorylation status of PPARγ-LBD was varied by adding different components to the *in vitro* phosphorylation reaction as indicated. For instance, "LBD + CDK5 − ATP + agonist" denotes no phosphorylation completed by active CDK5/p25 without ATP in the reaction (indicated as black bar). "LBD + CDK5 + ATP + agonist" indicates that the phosphorylation was partially repressed in the presence of agonist (indicated as grey bar). Finally, "(LBD + CDK5 + ATP) + agonist" signifies that the phosphorylation was completed before the addition of agonist to the reaction (indicated as light grey bar). All reactions were then directly applied to the AlphaScreen assay following a conventional procedure as described in *Materials and Methods*. The baseline for cofactor recruitment, independent of ligand binding, was calculated using RLUs from reactions performed in the presence of cofactor peptides divided by control reactions lacking peptide (background signal). Induction of cofactor recruitment by agonist is represented in fold change using RLUs from the cofactor binding reaction with agonist divided by the vehicle control sample (0.1% *(vol/vol)* DMSO).

by CDK5-mediated S273 phosphorylation (Figure 7). These data are supported by a previous structural study suggesting that SRC3 interacts with a PPARγ region located far from helix 12 yet near the β-sheet containing the CDK5 binding site [11]. Although a previous study indicated that the PPARγ A/B-domain (N-terminal ligand-independent activation function 1, AF-1) was specifically involved in the recruitment or stabilization of cAMP response element-binding protein and p300-containing cofactor complexes to a subset of target genes [43], our understanding of how a particular target gene is regulated by an individual cofactor recruited by PPAR remains poor. We have not identified the differences in recruitment among the six cofactors tested, which may contribute to the increased *ANGPTL4* and *PDK4* expressions promoted by Chi compared with the other two TZDs. In contrast, we found that Chi more significantly dissociates corepressor NCOR2 from PPARγ-LBD than Ros in AlphaScreen assay; knockout NCOR in adipocyte was

recently reported to repress PPARγ S273 phosphorylation and increase insulin sensitivity in mouse model [13]; the more potency on dissociation of NCOR2 from PPARγ by Chi partially contributes to its phosphorylation inhibition. In contrast, another report demonstrated that short chain FA butyrate could induce a unique set of PPAR target genes, including *ANGPTL4*, even though no significant activity in cofactor recruitment (except for induced binding of two corepressors NCOR1 and NCOR2 binding) was observed by PamChip® arrays [44]. Butyrate is a HDAC inhibitor, which may be recruited by NCOR2 into PPARγ transcriptome; it is possible to induce *ANGPTL4* expression via interfering in the interaction of HDAC and NCOR2. Considering the pathophysiological and therapeutic relevance of PPARγ S273 phosphorylation in T2DM and its associated complications, the impact of this biological process on specific target gene regulation and cofactor recruitment is worthy of further investigation.

Insulin resistance, T2DM, and its cardiovascular complications reflect a very complex outcome due to dysfunction in the mutually compensatory interactions among glucose, lipid, and energy utilization in relevant tissues. One consequence, namely, lipid overload in adipose tissue, liver, muscle, and heart tissue due to a metabolic syndrome often seen in T2D patients, is a critical factor leading to body weight gain, heart failure, and other cardiovascular conditions. Therefore, treatments that restore glucose, lipid, and energy homeostasis would potentially provide the most clinical benefit. Among the three subtypes, PPARα and PPARδ could contribute additional effects to lipid metabolism over PPARγ. In fact, Pio brings cardiovascular benefits to patients most likely due to weaker PPARγ and PPARα activation compared with Ros [45, 46]. Such a complex mechanism of action for insulin sensitization by PPARγ and other PPAR subtypes may not only explain the drastic differences in clinical outcomes, such as CV events, resulting from the same chemical class of TZDs (e.g., Pio versus Ros) but also potentially enable the development of configuration-restricted non-TZD molecules with fewer side effects associated with PPARγ activation.

Beyond its moderate pan agonist activity, Chi greatly induces two target genes, ANGPTL4 and PDK4, involved in glucose and lipid metabolism via inhibition of PPARγ phosphorylation. Dietary saturated fatty acids (SFAs) can be presented to cells in the form of circulating free fatty acids (FFAs) or FAs hydrolyzed by lipoprotein lipase (LDL) from chylomicrons or VLDL in the lymph nodes and blood. SFAs are strong proinflammatory nutrients that can trigger activation of intracellular inflammatory pathways in innate immune cells such as macrophages, as well as the main insulin target cells, adipocytes, myocytes, and hepatocytes, leading to insulin resistance, obesity, and cardiovascular disease [47, 48]. ANGPTL4 is an endogenous inhibitor of LDL activity and plays a crucial role in preventing fat-induced inflammation elicited by SFAs, diet-induced obesity, and myocardial infarction through preservation of vascular integrity [49–51]. ANGPTL4 decreases circulating FFAs derived from triglyceride- (TG-) rich lipoproteins to enhance insulin sensitivity of target organs. The positive relationship of ANGPTL4 activity with increased plasma level of TG-rich VLDL lipoproteins is seen in human with less-of-function variance ANGPTL4 E40K as well as ANGPTL4-deficient or liver-specific overexpression transgenic mice [52–54]; however, transgenic overexpression of ANGPTL4 suppresses foam cell formation to reduce atherosclerosis development in atherosclerosis-prone E3L mice [55]. Similar to lipotoxic cardiomyopathy caused by cardiac-specific overexpression of LPL, heart function is also impaired in transgenic mice with cardiac-specific overexpression of ANGPTL4 [56], highlighting the importance of balanced FFA demand and availability for normal cardiac function. Thus, ANGPTL4 may potentially contribute to increased lipid accumulation (i.e., lipid overload) in the liver, muscle, and heart [57], which is a "side effect" that can be overcome by increased β-oxidation in these tissues through the additional activation of PPARα and PPARδ activity [58]. Indeed, plasma TG level was increased by Ros but was reduced by Pio in clinical application. It could be partially due to stronger induction of ANGPTL4 by Ros

and a weak PPARα transactivity of Pio [44, 59]. In preclinical studies of various animal models, Chi exhibited different gene expression profiles, including the preferential induction of UCP-1 in fat and skeletal tissues [15]. Furthermore, no body weight gain in leptin-positive KKAy mice and less fat pad weight increase in leptin-negative db/db mice were noted after treatment by Chi [16]. Much less effect on increase in heart weight in long-term toxicity rat study and no increase of heart weight in dog upon Chi treatments were also observed [16].

Increased insulin sensitivity occurs following enhanced FA reesterification in adipose tissue, reduced FA efflux, and limited ectopic lipid deposition. PDK4 inactivates the pyruvate dehydrogenase complex, which leads to reliance on β-oxidization of FFA as a primary energy source rather than glucose. The glycerol-3-phosphate catalyzed from glucose thus serves to immobilize circulating FFA in adipose tissue, which further enhances the insulin sensitivity of other glucose-utilizing organs. PDK4 is upregulated in skeletal muscle in insulin-resistant states and proposed to be involved in the etiology of insulin resistance [60]. However, systemic PDK4 knockout in mice has no obvious phenotype change and no effect on blood glucose levels and insulin sensitivity in the fed state and only leads to hypoglycemia after the prolonged starvation [61], which is consistent with the essential role of PDK4 for glucose homoeostasis. Although cardiac-specific overexpression of PDK4 exacerbates hypertrophic cardiomyopathy caused by calcineurin stress-activated pathway in PDK4/CnA double transgenic mice [62], it exerts a protective effect against cardiac ischemia-reperfusion injury via chronic metabolic adaptation in similar cardiac-specific PDK4 transgenic mice [63]. Myocardiocytes in T2DM patients exert less substrate flexibility for energy production and manifest diabetic cardiomyopathy or later stage of heart failure in absence of other macrovascular complications. In addition to PDK4, distinct metabolic modulation profile of PPARδ from two other PPAR subtypes and cardiac protection in ischemia/reperfusion mice as previously reported [64] may endow PPAR pan agonist such as Chi benefit in the prevention of diabetic cardiac dysfunction.

5. Conclusions

In summary, we demonstrate that regulation of the expression of ANGPTL4 and PDK4, which are important regulators of glucose and lipid metabolism and insulin resistance, is directly linked to S273 phosphorylation of PPARγ in response to common T2DM factors such as a high-fat diet, obesity, and inflammation. Chi preferentially induced ANGPTL4 and PDK4 expressions by inhibiting these cascades most likely via its unique configuration-restricted binding to the receptor, which influenced cofactor recruitment and promoter binding of the PPARγ-containing transcription complex. Further investigation is required to elucidate the detailed mechanism for gene-specific regulation by the phosphorylated receptor. Nevertheless, the effect of Chi on the regulation of insulin resistance-related gene expression by PPARγ, together with its moderate activity on PPARα and δ, could rebalance glucose and FA uptake and substrate utilization in adipose tissue, muscle, liver, and heart upon insulin resistance and obesity, which may provide comprehensive clinical benefits to T2DM patients in the future.

Conflicts of Interest

All authors have no conflicts of interest to declare.

Authors' Contributions

De-Si Pan and Wei Wang contributed equally to this work.

Acknowledgments

The authors thank Dr. Li Yong and Ms. Jin Lihua from the School of Life Sciences, Xiamen University, for providing technical assistance in the AlphaScreen assay. This study was supported by grants from the Chinese National "863" Project (no. 2002AA2Z3146), National "New Drug Initiative" (2008ZX09101-002), China NSFC (81641051), and the Significant Project in Biotech Field from Guangdong Province (no. 2002A1090214) and Shenzhen City (nos. 2003-L1-013, ZDSYS20140509172959975, JCYJ20140418112611757, and GJHZ20140416153844269).

References

[1] S. E. Kahn, J. M. Lachin, B. Zinman et al., "Effects of rosiglitazone, glyburide, and metformin on β-cell function and insulin sensitivity in ADOPT," *Diabetes*, vol. 60, no. 5, pp. 1552–1560, 2011.

[2] W. L. Bennett, N. M. Maruthur, S. Singh et al., "Comparative effectiveness and safety of medications for type 2 diabetes: an update including new drugs and 2-drug combinations," *Annals of Internal Medicine*, vol. 154, no. 9, pp. 602–618, 2011.

[3] L. Ji, D. Hu, C. Pan et al., "Primacy of the 3B approach to control risk factors for cardiovascular disease in type 2 diabetes patients," *American Journal of Medicine*, vol. 126, no. 10, pp. 925–e22, 2013.

[4] R. K. Semple, V. K. K. Chatterjee, and S. O'Rahilly, "PPARγ and human metabolic disease," *The Journal of Clinical Investigation*, vol. 116, no. 3, pp. 581–589, 2006.

[5] P. Lefebvre, G. Chinetti, J. C. Fruchart, and B. Staels, "Sorting out the roles of PPARα in energy metabolism and vascular homeostasis," *The Journal of Clinical Investigation*, vol. 116, no. 3, pp. 571–580, 2006.

[6] G. D. Barish, V. A. Narkar, and R. M. Evans, "PPARδ: a dagger in the heart of the metabolic syndrome," *Journal of Clinical Investigation*, vol. 116, no. 3, pp. 590–597, 2006.

[7] W. Wahli and L. Michalik, "PPARs at the crossroads of lipid signaling and inflammation," *Trends in Endocrinology and Metabolism*, vol. 23, no. 7, pp. 351–363, 2012.

[8] J. M. Peters, Y. M. Shah, and F. J. Gonzalez, "The role of peroxisome proliferator-activated receptors in carcinogenesis and chemoprevention," *Nature Reviews Cancer*, vol. 12, no. 3, pp. 181–195, 2012.

[9] B. Pourcet, J.-C. Fruchart, B. Staels, and C. Glineur, "Selective PPAR modulators, dual and pan PPAR agonists: Multimodal drugs for the treatment of Type 2 diabetes and atherosclerosis," *Expert Opinion on Emerging Drugs*, vol. 11, no. 3, pp. 379–401, 2006.

[10] B. Gross, M. Pawlak, P. Lefebvre, and B. Staels, "PPARs in obesity-induced T2DM, dyslipidaemia and NAFLD," *Nature Reviews Endocrinology*, vol. 13, no. 1, pp. 36–49, 2016.

[11] J. H. Choi, A. S. Banks, J. L. Estall et al., "Anti-diabetic drugs inhibit obesity-linked phosphorylation of PPARγ 3 by Cdk5," *Nature*, vol. 466, no. 7305, pp. 451–456, 2010.

[12] J. H. Choi, A. S. Banks, T. M. Kamenecka et al., "Antidiabetic actions of a non-agonist PPARγ ligand blocking Cdk5-mediated phosphorylation," *Nature*, vol. 477, no. 7365, pp. 477–481, 2011.

[13] P. Li, W. Fan, J. Xu et al., "Adipocyte NCoR knockout decreases PPARγ phosphorylation and enhances PPARγ activity and insulin sensitivity," *Cell*, vol. 147, no. 4, pp. 815–826, 2011.

[14] C. Weidner, J. C. de Groot, A. Prasad et al., "Amorfrutins are potent antidiabetic dietary natural products," *Proceedings of the National Academy of Sciences of the United States of America*, vol. 109, no. 19, pp. 7257–7262, 2012.

[15] P.-P. Li, S. Shan, Y.-T. Chen et al., "The PPARα/γ dual agonist chiglitazar improves insulin resistance and dyslipidemia in MSG obese rats," *British Journal of Pharmacology*, vol. 148, no. 5, pp. 610–618, 2006.

[16] B. K. He, Z. Q. Ning, Z. B. Li et al., "In vitro and in vivo characterizations of chiglitazar, a newly identified PPAR pan-agonist," *PPAR Research*, Article ID 546548, 2012.

[17] P. Zhu, Y. Y. Goh, H. F. A. Chin, S. Kersten, and N. S. Tan, "Angiopoietin-like 4: a decade of research," *Bioscience Reports*, vol. 32, no. 3, pp. 211–219, 2012.

[18] M. C. Sugden, M. G. Zariwala, and M. J. Holness, "PPARs and the orchestration of metabolic fuel selection," *Pharmacological Research*, vol. 60, no. 3, pp. 141–150, 2009.

[19] H. M. Berman, J. Westbrook, Z. Feng et al., "The protein data bank," *Nucleic Acids Research*, vol. 28, no. 1, pp. 235–242, 2000.

[20] E. F. Pettersen, T. D. Goddard, C. C. Huang et al., "UCSF Chimera—a visualization system for exploratory research and analysis," *Journal of Computational Chemistry*, vol. 25, no. 13, pp. 1605–1612, 2004.

[21] R. Thomsen and M. H. Christensen, "MolDock: a new technique for high-accuracy molecular docking," *Journal of Medicinal Chemistry*, vol. 49, no. 11, pp. 3315–3321, 2006.

[22] W. L. DeLano, *The PyMol Users Manual*, DeLano Scientific, CA, San Carlos, 2002.

[23] K. A. Burns and J. P. Vanden Heuvel, "Modulation of PPAR activity via phosphorylation," *Biochimica et Biophysica Acta*, vol. 1771, no. 8, pp. 952–960, 2007.

[24] Y. Li, M. Choi, K. Suino et al., "Structural and biochemical basis for selective repression of the orphan nuclear receptor liver receptor homolog 1 by small heterodimer partner," *Proceedings of the National Academy of Sciences of the United States of America*, vol. 102, no. 27, pp. 9505–9510, 2005.

[25] K. W. Nettles, "Insights into PPARgamma from structures with endogenous and covalently bound ligands," *Nature Structural and Molecular Biology*, vol. 15, no. 9, pp. 893–895, 2008.

[26] J. B. Bruning, M. J. Chalmers, S. Prasad et al., "Partial agonists activate PPARγ using a helix 12 independent mechanism," *Structure*, vol. 15, no. 10, pp. 1258–1271, 2007.

[27] A. Koppen and E. Kalkhoven, "Brown vs white adipocytes: The PPARγ coregulator story," *FEBS Letters*, vol. 584, no. 15, pp. 3250–3259, 2010.

[28] N. Viswakarma, Y. Jia, L. Bai et al., "Coactivators in PPAR-regulated gene expression," *PPAR Research*, vol. 2010, Article ID 250126, 21 pages, 2010.

[29] V. Chandra, P. Huang, Y. Hamuro et al., "Structure of the intact PPAR-γ-RXR-α nuclear receptor complex on DNA," *Nature*, vol. 456, no. 7220, pp. 350–356, 2008.

[30] D. Moras, "Structure of Full-Length PPARγ-RXRα: A Snapshot of a Functional Complex?" *Cell Metabolism*, vol. 9, no. 1, pp. 8–10, 2009.

[31] A. Lombardi, G. Cantini, E. Piscitelli et al., "A new mechanism involving ERK contributes to rosiglitazone inhibition of tumor necrosis factor-alpha and interferon-gamma inflammatory effects in human endothelial cells," *Arteriosclerosis Thrombosis and Vascular Biology*, vol. 28, no. 4, pp. 718–724, 2008.

[32] S. E. Nissen and K. Wolski, "Rosiglitazone revisited: an updated meta-analysis of risk for myocardial infarction and cardiovascular mortality," *Archives of Internal Medicine*, vol. 170, no. 14, pp. 1191–1201, 2010.

[33] D. Hillaire-Buys, J.-L. Faillie, and J.-L. Montastruc, "Pioglitazone and bladder cancer," *The Lancet*, vol. 378, no. 9802, pp. 1543-1544, 2011.

[34] F. M. Gregoire, F. Zhang, H. J. Clarke et al., "MBX-102/JNJ39659100, a novel peroxisome proliferator-activated receptor-ligand with weak transactivation activity retains antidiabetic properties in the absence of weight gain and edema," *Molecular Endocrinology*, vol. 23, no. 7, pp. 975–988, 2009.

[35] L. S. Higgins and C. S. Mantzoros, "The development of INT131 as a selective PPARgamma modulator: approach to a safer insulin sensitizer," *PPAR Research*, vol. 2008, Article ID 936906, 9 pages, 2008.

[36] Y. Li, Z. Wang, N. Furukawa et al., "T2384, a novel antidiabetic agent with unique peroxisome proliferator-activated receptor γ binding properties," *The Journal of Biological Chemistry*, vol. 283, no. 14, pp. 9168–9176, 2008.

[37] R. R. Henry, A. M. Lincoff, S. Mudaliar, M. Rabbia, C. Chognot, and M. Herz, "Effect of the dual peroxisome proliferator-activated receptor-α/γ agonist aleglitazar on risk of cardiovascular disease in patients with type 2 diabetes (SYNCHRONY): a phase II, randomised, dose-ranging study," *The Lancet*, vol. 374, no. 9684, pp. 126–135, 2009.

[38] A. A. Amato, S. Rajagopalan, and J. Z. Lin, "GQ-16, a novel peroxisome proliferator-activated receptor γ (PPARγ) ligand, promotes insulin sensitization without weight gain," *The Journal of Biological Chemistry*, vol. 287, no. 33, pp. 28169–28179, 2012.

[39] D. Jones, "Potential remains for PPAR-targeted drugs," *Nature Reviews Drug Discovery*, vol. 9, no. 9, pp. 668-669, 2010.

[40] T. S. Hughes, M. J. Chalmers, S. Novick et al., "Ligand and receptor dynamics contribute to the mechanism of graded PPARγ agonism," *Structure*, vol. 20, no. 1, pp. 139–150, 2012.

[41] S. Yu and H. E. Xu, "Couple dynamics: PPARγ and its ligand partners," *Structure*, vol. 20, no. 1, pp. 2–4, 2012.

[42] R. R. V. Malapaka, S. Khoo, J. Zhang et al., "Identification and mechanism of 10-carbon fatty acid as modulating ligand of peroxisome proliferator-activated receptors," *The Journal of Biological Chemistry*, vol. 287, no. 1, pp. 183–195, 2012.

[43] A. Bugge, L. Grøntved, M. M. Aagaard, R. Borup, and S. Mandrup, "The PPARγ2 A/B-domain plays a gene-specific role in transactivation and cofactor recruitment," *Molecular Endocrinology*, vol. 23, no. 6, pp. 794–808, 2009.

[44] S. Alex, K. Lange, and T. Amolo, "Short chain fatty acids stimulate Angiopoietin-like 4 synthesis in human colon adenocarcinoma cells by activating, A-?" *Molecular Cellular Biology*, vol. 33, no. 7, p. pp, 2013.

[45] R. B. Goldberg, D. M. Kendall, M. A. Deeg et al., "A comparison of lipid and glycemic effects of pioglitazone and rosiglitazone in patients with type 2 diabetes and dyslipidemia," *Diabetes Care*, vol. 28, no. 7, pp. 1547–1554, 2005.

[46] G. Orasanu, O. Ziouzenkova, P. R. Devchand et al., "The peroxisome proliferator-activated receptor-γ agonist pioglitazone represses inflammation in a peroxisome proliferator-activated receptor-α-dependent manner in vitro and in vivo in mice," *Journal of the American College of Cardiology*, vol. 52, no. 10, pp. 869–881, 2008.

[47] A. Guilherme, J. V. Virbasius, V. Puri, and M. P. Czech, "Adipocyte dysfunctions linking obesity to insulin resistance and type 2 diabetes," *Nature Reviews Molecular Cell Biology*, vol. 9, no. 5, pp. 367–377, 2008.

[48] F. Karpe, J. R. Dickmann, and K. N. Frayn, "Fatty acids, obesity, and insulin resistance: time for a reevaluation," *Diabetes*, vol. 60, no. 10, pp. 2441–2449, 2011.

[49] A. Georgiadi, L. Lichtenstein, T. Degenhardt et al., "Induction of cardiac angptl4 by dietary fatty acids is mediated by peroxisome proliferator-activated receptor β/δ and protects against fatty acid-induced oxidative stress," *Circulation Research*, vol. 106, no. 11, pp. 1712–1721, 2010.

[50] O. Osborn, D. D. Sears, and J. M. Olefsky, "Fat-induced inflammation unchecked," *Cell Metabolism*, vol. 12, no. 6, pp. 553-554, 2010.

[51] L. Bird, "Macrophages: Preventing lipid overload," *Nature Reviews Immunology*, vol. 11, no. 2, p. 73, 2011.

[52] S. Romeo, L. A. Pennacchio, Y. Fu et al., "Population-based resequencing of ANGPTL4 uncovers variations that reduce triglycerides and increase HDL," *Nature Genetics*, vol. 39, no. 4, pp. 513–516, 2007.

[53] A. Xu, M. C. Lam, K. W. Chan et al., "Angiopoietin-like protein 4 decreases blood glucose and improves glucose tolerance but induces hyperlipidemia and hepatic steatosis in mice," *Proceedings of the National Academy of Sciences of the United States of America*, vol. 102, no. 17, pp. 6086–6091, 2005.

[54] A. Köster, Y. B. Chao, M. Mosior et al., "Transgenic angiopoietin-like (Angptl)4 overexpression and targeted disruption of Angptl4 and Angptl3: Regulation of triglyceride metabolism," *Endocrinology*, vol. 146, no. 11, pp. 4943–4950, 2005.

[55] A. Georgiadi, Y. Wang, and R. Stienstra, "Overexpression of angiopoietin-like protein 4 protects against atherosclerosis development," *Arteriosclerosis Thrombosis Vascular Biology*, vol. 33, no. 7, pp. 1529–1537, 2013.

[56] X. Yu, S. C. Burgess, H. Ge et al., "Inhibition of cardiac lipoprotein utilization by transgenic overexpression of Angptl4 in the heart," *Proceedings of the National Academy of Sciences of the United States of America*, vol. 102, no. 5, pp. 1767–1772, 2005.

[57] L. Lichtenstein, J. F. P. Berbée, S. J. van Dijk et al., "Angptl4 upregulates cholesterol synthesis in liver via inhibition of LPL- and HL-dependent hepatic cholesterol uptake," *Arteriosclerosis, Thrombosis, and Vascular Biology*, vol. 27, no. 11, pp. 2420–2427, 2007.

[58] G. D. Lopaschuk, J. R. Ussher, C. D. L. Folmes, J. S. Jaswal, and W. C. Stanley, "Myocardial fatty acid metabolism in health and disease," *Physiological Reviews*, vol. 90, no. 1, pp. 207–258, 2010.

[59] M. A. Deeg, J. B. Buse, R. B. Goldberg et al., "Pioglitazone and rosiglitazone have different effects on serum lipoprotein particle concentrations and sizes in patients with type 2 diabetes and dyslipidemia," *Diabetes Care*, vol. 30, no. 10, pp. 2458–2464, 2007.

[60] K. Chokkalingam, K. Jewell, L. Norton et al., "High-fat/low-carbohydrate diet reduces insulin-stimulated carbohydrate oxidation but stimulates nonoxidative glucose disposal in humans: An important role for skeletal muscle pyruvate dehydrogenase kinase 4," *Journal of Clinical Endocrinology and Metabolism*, vol. 92, no. 1, pp. 284–292, 2007.

[61] N. H. Jeoung, P. Wu, M. A. Joshi et al., "Role of pyruvate dehydrogenase kinase isoenzyme 4 (PDHK4) in glucose homoeostasis during starvation," *Biochemical Journal*, vol. 397, no. 3, pp. 417–425, 2006.

[62] G. Zhao, H. J. Nam, S. C. Burgess et al., "Overexpression of pyruvate dehydrogenase kinase 4 in heart perturbs metabolism and exacerbates calcineurin-induced cardiomyopathy," *American Journal of Physiology - Heart and Circulatory Physiology*, vol. 294, no. 2, pp. H936–H943, 2008.

[63] K. T. Chambers, T. C. Leone, N. Sambandam et al., "Chronic inhibition of pyruvate dehydrogenase in heart triggers an adaptive metabolic response," *Journal of Biological Chemistry*, vol. 286, no. 13, pp. 11155–11162, 2011.

[64] E. M. Burkart, N. Sambandam, X. Han et al., "Nuclear receptors PPARβ/δ and PPARα direct distinct metabolic regulatory programs in the mouse heart," *The Journal of Clinical Investigation*, vol. 117, no. 12, pp. 3930–3939, 2007.

Permissions

The contributors of this book come from diverse backgrounds, making this book a truly international effort. This book will bring forth new frontiers with its revolutionizing research information and detailed analysis of the nascent developments around the world.

We would like to thank all the contributing authors for lending their expertise to make the book truly unique. They have played a crucial role in the development of this book. Without their invaluable contributions this book wouldn't have been possible. They have made vital efforts to compile up to date information on the varied aspects of this subject to make this book a valuable addition to the collection of many professionals and students.

This book was conceptualized with the vision of imparting up-to-date information and advanced data in this field. To ensure the same, a matchless editorial board was set up. Every individual on the board went through rigorous rounds of assessment to prove their worth. After which they invested a large part of their time researching and compiling the most relevant data for our readers.

The editorial board has been involved in producing this book since its inception. They have spent rigorous hours researching and exploring the diverse topics which have resulted in the successful publishing of this book. They have passed on their knowledge of decades through this book. To expedite this challenging task, the publisher supported the team at every step. A small team of assistant editors was also appointed to further simplify the editing procedure and attain best results for the readers.

Apart from the editorial board, the designing team has also invested a significant amount of their time in understanding the subject and creating the most relevant covers. They scrutinized every image to scout for the most suitable representation of the subject and create an appropriate cover for the book.

The publishing team has been an ardent support to the editorial, designing and production team. Their endless efforts to recruit the best for this project, has resulted in the accomplishment of this book. They are a veteran in the field of academics and their pool of knowledge is as vast as their experience in printing. Their expertise and guidance has proved useful at every step. Their uncompromising quality standards have made this book an exceptional effort. Their encouragement from time to time has been an inspiration for everyone.

The publisher and the editorial board hope that this book will prove to be a valuable piece of knowledge for researchers, students, practitioners and scholars across the globe.

List of Contributors

Izabela Wojtkowska and Janina Stępińska Institute of Cardiology, Intensive Cardiac Therapy Clinic, Alpejska St. 42, 04-628Warsaw, Poland

Tomasz A. Bonda and Maria M. Winnicka
Department of General and Experimental Pathology, Medical University of Bialystok, Mickiewicza St. 2c, 15-222 Bialystok, Poland

Jadwiga Wolszakiewicz, Jerzy Osak and Ryszard Piotrowicz
Institute of Cardiology, Department of Cardiac Rehabilitation and Noninvasive Electrocardiology, Alpejska St. 42,04-628 Warsaw, Poland

Andrzej Tysarowski, Katarzyna Seliga and Janusz A. Siedlecki
Institute of Oncology, Department of Molecular and Translational Oncology, Wawelska St. 15B, 02-034 Warsaw, Poland

Si-Yu Zeng and Hui-Qin Lu
Department of Drug Clinical Trials, Guangdong Second Provincial General Hospital, Guangzhou 510317, China

Qiu-Jiang Yan
Department of Cardiac & Thoracic Surgery, The Third Affiliated Hospital of Guangzhou Medical University, Guangzhou 510000, China

Jian Zou
Department of Pharmacy, The People's Hospital of Pengzhou, Chengdu 611900, China

Soonkyu Chung
Department of Nutrition and Health Sciences, University of Nebraska-Lincoln, Lincoln, NE, USA

Young Jun Kim
Department of Food & Biotechnology, KoreaUniversity, Sejong, Republic of Korea

Soo Jin Yang
Department of Food and Nutrition, Seoul Women's University, Seoul, Republic of Korea

Yunkyoung Lee
Department of Food Science and Nutrition, Jeju National University, Jeju, Republic of Korea

Myoungsook Lee
Department of Food and Nutrition and Research Institute of Obesity Science, SungshinWomen's University, Seoul, Republic of Korea

Hui Luo, Nan Wang, Jingjing Li, Kan Chen, Jiao Feng, Liwei Wu, Sainan Li, Tong Liu, Xiya Lu, Yujing Xia, Yanhong Shi, Yingqun Zhou and Jie Lu
Department of Gastroenterology, Shanghai Tenth People's Hospital, Tongji University School of Medicine, Shanghai 200072, China

Rui Kong
Department of Gastroenterology, Shanghai Tenth People's Hospital, Tongji University School of Medicine, Shanghai 200072, China
The School of Medicine, Soochow University, Suzhou 215006, China

Shizan Xu
Department of Gastroenterology, Shanghai Tenth People's Hospital, Tongji University School of Medicine, Shanghai 200072, China
Department of Gastroenterology, Shanghai Tenth Hospital, School of Clinical Medicine, Nanjing Medical University, Shanghai 200072, China

Weigang He and Yuejuan Zheng
Department of Immunology and Microbiology, Shanghai University of Traditional Chinese Medicine, Shanghai 201203, China

Qi Dai
The Eye Hospital, Wenzhou Medical University, Wenzhou City, Zhejiang 325027, China

Yajing Huo, Xuqing Wu, Jing Ding, Yang Geng, Anyan Ge, Cen Guo, Jianing Lv, Haifeng Bao and Wei Fan
Department of Neurology, Zhongshan Hospital, Fudan University, Shanghai 200032, China

Weiwei Qiao
Department of Laboratory Animal Science, Fudan University, Shanghai 200032, China

Prasad P. Devarshi, Aarin D. Jones, Erin M. Taylor, Barbara Stefanska and Tara M. Henagan
Department of Nutrition Science, Purdue University, West Lafayette, IN, USA

Aravind T. Reddy, Sowmya P. Lakshmi and Raju C. Reddy
Department of Medicine, Division of Pulmonary, Allergy and Critical Care Medicine, University of Pittsburgh School of Medicine, Pittsburgh, PA 15213, USA
Veterans Affairs Pittsburgh Healthcare System, Pittsburgh, PA 15240, USA

Salvatore Giovanni Vitale, Antonio Simone Laganà, Francesco Corrado and Rosario D'Anna
Unit of Gynecology and Obstetrics, Department of Human Pathology in Adulthood and Childhood "G. Barresi", University of Messina, Messina, Italy

Angela Nigro, Paola Rossetti and Massimo Buscema
Unit of Diabetology and Endocrino-Metabolic Diseases, Hospital for Emergency Cannizzaro, Catania, Italy

Valentina Lucia La Rosa
Unit of Psychodiagnostics and Clinical Psychology, University of Catania, Catania, Italy

Agnese Maria Chiara Rapisarda
Department of General Surgery and Medical Surgical Specialties, University of Catania, Catania, Italy

Sandro La Vignera and Rosita Angela Condorelli
Department of Clinical and Experimental Medicine-CRAMD (Research Centre of Motor Activity and Metabolic Rehabilitation in Diabetes), University of Catania, Catania, Italy

Jinghua Xu, Mingyue Pan, Xiaoli Wang, Lishi Xu, Lanfang Li and Cheng Xu
Department of Physiology, School of Life Science and Biopharmaceutics, Shenyang Pharmaceutical University, 103 Wenhua Road, Shenyang 110016, China

Rehana Parvin, Erika Noro, Akiko Saito-Hakoda, Hiroki Shimada, Susumu Suzuki, Kyoko Shimizu, Atsushi Yokoyama and Akira Sugawara
Department of Molecular Endocrinology, Tohoku University Graduate School of Medicine, Sendai, Miyagi, Japan

Hiroyuki Miyachi
Drug Discovery Initiative,The University of Tokyo, 7-3-1 Hongo, Bunkyo-ku, Tokyo, Japan

Aneta A. Koronowicz, Paula Banks, Dominik Domagała, Ewelina Piasna-Słupecka, Mariola Drozdowska and Elhbieta Sikora
Department of Human Nutrition, Faculty of Food Technology, University of Agriculture in Krakow, Balicka 122,30-149 Krakow, Poland

Adam Master
Department of Biochemistry and Molecular Biology, Medical Centre for Postgraduate Education, Marymoncka 99,01-813 Warsaw, Poland

Piotr Laidler
Department of Medical Biochemistry, Jagiellonian University Medical College, Kopernika 7, 31-034 Krakow, Poland

Hengbo Shi
College of Life Science, Zhejiang Sci-Tech University, Hangzhou, Zhejiang 310018, China
Zhejiang Provincial Key Laboratory of Silkworm Bioreactor and Biomedicine, Hangzhou, Zhejiang 310018, China

Changhui Zhang and Jun Luo
Shaanxi Key Laboratory ofMolecular Biology for Agriculture, College of Animal Science and Technology, Northwest A&F University, Yangling, Shaanxi 712100, China

Wangsheng Zhao
Shaanxi Key Laboratory ofMolecular Biology for Agriculture, College of Animal Science and Technology, Northwest A&F University, Yangling, Shaanxi 712100, China
School of Life Science and Engineering, Southwest University of Science and Technology, Mianyang 621010, China

Khuram Shahzad and Juan J. Loor
Mammalian NutriPhysioGenomics, Department of Animal Sciences and Division of Nutritional Sciences, University of Illinois, Urbana, IL 61801, USA

Yves Lecarpentier
Centre de Recherche Clinique, Hôpital de Meaux, Meaux, France

Victor Claes
Department of Pharmaceutical Sciences, University of Antwerp, Wilrijk, Belgium

Alexandre Vallée
CHU Amiens Picardie, Universit´e Picardie Jules Verne, Amiens, France
Experimental and Clinical Neurosciences Laboratory, INSERMU1084, University of Poitiers, France

Jean-Louis Hébert
Institut de Cardiologie, Hôpital de la Pitié-Salpêtrière, Assistance Publique-Hôpitaux de Paris, Paris, France

Fernanda Aparecida Heleno Batista, Artur Torres Cordeiro and Ana Carolina Migliorini Figueira
Brazilian Biosciences National Laboratory (LNBio), Brazilian Center for Research in Energy and Materials (CNPEM),13083-970 Campinas, SP, Brazil

Natália Bernardi Videira
Brazilian Biosciences National Laboratory (LNBio), Brazilian Center for Research in Energy and Materials (CNPEM),13083-970 Campinas, SP, Brazil
Graduate Programin Biosciences and Technology of Bioactive Products, Institute of Biology, State University of Campinas (Unicamp),Campinas, SP, Brazil

Dorothea Portius, Cyril Sobolewski and Michelangelo Foti
Department of Cell Physiology and Metabolism and Diabetes Center, Faculty of Medicine, University of Geneva, Geneva, Switzerland

De-Si Pan, Nan-Song Liu, Qian-Jiao Yang, Kun Zhang, Jing-Zhong Zhu, Song Shan, Zhi-Bin Li, Zhi-Qiang Ning and Xian-Ping Lu
Shenzhen Chipscreen Biosciences Ltd., Shenzhen, Guangdong 518057, China

Wei Wang and Laiqiang Huang
Shenzhen Key Lab of Gene & AntibodyTherapy, Division of Life & Health Sciences, Graduate School at Shenzhen,Tsinghua University, Shenzhen, Guangdong 518057, China

Index

CPSIA information can be obtained
at www.ICGtesting.com
Printed in the USA
BVHW011520250820
587256BV00003B/5